AEROMEDICAL TRANSPOR

Aeromedical Transportation
A Clinical Guide
2nd Edition

T. MARTIN
Royal Hampshire County Hospital, Winchester, UK

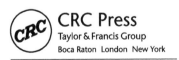

CRC Press
Taylor & Francis Group
Boca Raton London New York

CRC Press is an imprint of the
Taylor & Francis Group, an **informa** business

CRC Press
Taylor & Francis Group
6000 Broken Sound Parkway NW, Suite 300
Boca Raton, FL 33487-2742

© 2006 by T. Martin
CRC Press is an imprint of Taylor & Francis Group, an Informa business

No claim to original U.S. Government works

Printed on acid-free paper
Version Date: 20160226

International Standard Book Number-13: 978-0-7546-4148-3 (Paperback)

Visit the Taylor & Francis Web site at
http://www.taylorandfrancis.com

and the CRC Press Web site at
http://www.crcpress.com

Contents

PART IV   CLINICAL CONSIDERATIONS

PART V   ORGANIZATION AND ADMINISTRATION

List of Figures

List of Tables

Preface to the Second Edition

When the first edition of *Aeromedical Transportation* was published in 1996, I could not have predicted the acceleration in interest and enthusiasm that was to take place over the following decade. These years saw continued growth in aeromedical activities and an upsurge in publications which are starting to bring our specialty in from the cold. Many of these papers are still of the anecdotal and case study type design (level 5 evidence), but there has been enough original and well structured research to light the path for an optimistic future. For an author, the next best thing to seeing a new book published is acquisition of new facts and information from all the research and essential reading needed to update and enlarge a previous edition. As such, this work has been both a challenge and a pleasure to compile. In doing so, I have acknowledged many new friends and colleagues who have contributed in one way or another. To this list I must add the students who, under the guise of being taught by me, have often reversed the roles and encouraged me to look at aeromedical problems in a new light, to discover new ways of explaining complex information, or in helping me develop new skills and techniques of teaching. To paraphrase the words of Hippocrates 'Every doctor must be a teacher' (*to teach them this art, should they desire to learn [it]*), and my students have taught me well.

This book will continue to be the text for several aeromedical courses in English speaking nations around the world, and it is encouraging to hear that it is already being translated into Swedish and Spanish for wider use around Europe. However, like the first edition, I have included pet phrases from the medical and aviation communities on both sides of the Atlantic, and the language is still placed firmly somewhere halfway across the ocean. To ease the transition for those who still have difficulty, the glossary of terms has been enlarged to match the increase in material found in each chapter.

As well as more meat to each chapter, there are more references in the bibliographies, and two new chapters have been added. The first, chapter 16, looks more closely at the issues of critical care transfers – a rapidly growing subset of aeromedical transports due to the regionalization of expensive health care facilities and subspecialties. This new chapter takes a combined organizational and clinical approach to critical care retrievals and transfers, highlighting areas where room for improvement has been shown to exist, and offering tips to avoid the many potential pitfalls that are there to trap the unwary.

One of my profoundest discoveries in the last decade of teaching was that flight physicians often escort patients alone and yet have little concept of nursing care. Chapter 17 addresses this gap in knowledge by discussing the important issues that bring flight nursing skills out of the woodwork! Doctors are encouraged to utilize their time with flight nurse colleagues to develop a holistic approach to patient care.

Aeromedical transportation has come a long way since the first edition was published and is not so much a new kid on the specialty block anymore. However, the new age has brought new challenges. Increasing fuel costs, international terrorism, larger aircraft, advances in medical technology, critical 'expensive' care, demands for training, improvement and documentation of standards of care, and ever increasing legislation – these are just some of the challenges that are being met in hospitals, in helicopters, and high in the skies around the world on a daily basis.

Novel air medical courses offered by the Otago University in New Zealand are helping to take this new specialty forward, and the next decade will see postgraduates with masters and doctorates in patient transportation. This will be an exciting time for the academic development of the subject and for the establishment of new research programs and interests. As stated in the first edition, I look forward to chronicling these developments in future editions and my goals remain the same – not just to provide you, the reader, with an introduction to the world of aeromedical transport, but also to intrigue and entice you to learn more. As such, the book is intended as a basic primer for those who seek to work in transfer and retrieval medicine.

It wouldn't be surprising if you view the transfer of a patient as a move from one place of safety to another with a stressful and dangerous period of uncertainty between the two. This is a view often shared by our terrestrial medical and nursing colleagues! With this book as your flight companion, I hope you will acquire knowledge to plan well, skill to assess all dangers and potential problems, yet humility to withdraw when safety and wellbeing risk compromise.

Preface to the First Edition

Aeromedical transportation is the world of airborne cavalry coming to the rescue; of saving one's fellows by flying into the battle, borne on the wind, to snatch life from the jaws of death.

At least that's what the papers say! In truth, aeromedical practice usually comprises hours of tedium waiting for an assignment, interspersed with periods of sheer exhilaration and, just occasionally, moments of absolute terror. It is a fascinating mix of physics and physiology, of aeronautics, clinical care, and the thrill of flight, that combine to form one of the most unique and exciting fields of medicine. In the age of international travel, with the globe shrinking a little each day, aeromedical transport has become a routine facet of everyday life. No matter if you are just an occasional flyer, or if the thrill of the emergency helicopter is the stuff of your dreams, a career in aeromedical transportation may be your passport, and this book can serve as your visa – sufficient to allow entry, but you'll need a lifetime to really get to know it.

The reader will notice an imbalance in this book between the established science of aviation physiology and scientifically proven data and reports about clinical care while aloft. It must be remembered that aeromedical transportation is a new kid on the specialty block and, as such, does not yet possess the benefits and background of a fully developed research and literature base. It is hoped that, as aeromedical services continue to grow and document their efforts, this literature base will flourish. We look forward to chronicling these developments in future editions of this text. For now, the reader will find a relevant bibliography at the end of each chapter and a general reading list in chapter 2.

A note about language is in order. The authors of this book share the belief of George Bernard Shaw that Great Britain and America are two great English speaking nations separated only by a common language. As a result, we have each had to compromise on some pet phrases from the medical and aviation communities on both sides of the ocean. The reader will kindly accept our placement of language somewhere over the mid-Atlantic. To ease the transition for those who still have difficulty, a glossary of interchangeable terms has been included. Units of measurement throughout the book, are those most often used in either the aviation or the medical fraternity, not necessarily their *Système International* equivalents. Drug names are given as generics with alternative names following in parentheses. Lastly, to avoid the cumbersome use of multiple pronouns and adjectives, we have adopted the use of the male gender ('he', 'him', 'his') when, clearly, we mean to refer to either gender. Similarly the term 'man' should be taken to mean human of either sex.

Our goal is not just to provide you, the reader, with an introduction to the world of aeromedical transport, but also to intrigue and entice you to learn more. The book is intended as a basic reference for those who seek to work in transportation medicine, primarily doctors, but it will prove of great relevance and interest to flight nurses, paramedics and those who administer air ambulance organizations and other air medical flight programs. The book is now the standard text for the new *Clinical Considerations in Aeromedical Transportation* training course in the UK and, hopefully, will soon be adopted in other countries. The authorship reflects this international approach which, we trust, is emulated throughout the text. It is difficult, though, to fairly represent the vast variety of aeromedical systems that operate across the globe and we do not claim to have written the definitive text. Nevertheless, we have started the ball rolling, and we hope to have conveyed at least the flavor of this exciting field. One does not need to understand the minutiae of cavalry tactics to know that both Colonel Custer and the Light Brigade were deep in the mire. We hope that this book will allow you the knowledge and comfort to advance in confidence, and yet to retreat, quickly, when required.

Acknowledgements

We wish to thank all those who have taught and encouraged us over the years, on both sides of the Atlantic, on distant airfields, and in skies around the world. Special mention must be made of the Royal Air Force, the United States Air Force, Europ Assistance, the Royal London Hospital Helicopter Emergency Medical Service, ShandsCair Flight Program at Shands Hospital at the University of Florida, and Medical Rescue International in Johannesburg, South Africa.

In particular, we wish to thank those who have taken the time and trouble to read and give advice on this text. To the following, we are indebted: Lt Col John Crowley (US Army Medical Corps); Maj Philip Johnson (Royal Army Medical Corps); Dr Alexander Campbell (Medical and Dental Defence Union of Scotland); Ms Bridget Collier (Europ Assistance); Michael Spencer, Mrs Barbara Stone, Prof David Denison, Dr Rollin Stott, and Sgt René Metcalfe (Aeromedicine Department of the DERA Centre for Human Sciences). Thanks, also, to Sgt Andy Whittle, the Cornwall and Isles of Scilly Ambulance Service, and Bridget Collier, for kindly providing the photographs in Figures 1.2, 1.3 and 9.3 (respectively).

T.E. Martin and H.D. Rodenberg
July 1996

The text has been extensively reviewed in the second edition. I should like to thank the major contributors, Dr Michael Glanfield and Mr Ian MacLennan for their input to the new material. Some additional literature searches were undertaken by Dr Carmen de Andres and much of the proofreading was completed by Ms Melanie Robertson and Ms Hannah Shepherd. In thanking the above, I also take full responsibility for any errors, either factual or typographical, that remain in the text.

Finally, I welcome comments and correspondence, especially where disagreement exists, or where omissions and oversights have occurred.

T.E. Martin
2006

List of Abbreviations

AA	Automobile Association
AAMS	Association of Air Medical Services
ACLS	Advanced cardiac life support
ADM	Aeronautic decision making
AGL	Above ground level
AHA	American Heart Association
AIDS	Acquired immune deficiency syndrome
ALS	Advanced life support
AMI	Acute myocardial infarction
AMPA	Air Medical Physician's Association
AMS	Aerial Medical Service
APACHE	Acute physiology and chronic health evaluation
ARDS	Acute respiratory distress syndrome
ATLS	Advanced trauma life support
BAMPA	British Association of Aeromedical Practitioners
BASICS	British Association of Immediate Care (Schemes)
BLS	Basic life support
BMJ	British Medical Journal
BPAP	Bitlevel peak airway pressure
BSA	Body surface area
BVM	Bag-valve-mask system
CAA	Civil Aviation Authority
CAAMS	Commission on Accreditation of Aeromedical Services
casevac	Casualty evacuation
CCAT	Clinical Considerations in Aeromedical Transport (course)
CCU	Coronary care unit
CHF	Congestive heart failure
CPAP	Continuous positive airway pressure
CPR	Cardiopulmonary resuscitation
CQI	Continuous quality improvement
CRM	Cockpit resource management
CSD	Cabin service director
CSF	Cerebrospinal fluid
CT	Computerized tomography
CVA	Cerebrovascular accident
CVP	Central venous pressure

DCS	Decompression sickness
DEA	Drugs Enforcement Agency
EMS	Emergency medical services
EMT-P	Emergency medical technician – paramedic
ERC	European Resuscitation Council
ET	Endotracheal
ETCO2	End-tidal carbon dioxide
EURAMI	European Aero Medical Institute
FAA	Federal Aviation Administration
FiO$_2$	Inspired oxygen concentration
fpm	Feet per minute
GCS	Glasgow coma score (or scale)
GI	Gastrointestinal
GMT	Greenwich mean time
HAZMAT	Hazardous material
Hb	Hemoglobin
HbF	Fetal hemoglobin
HEMS	Helicopter emergency medical service
HIV	Human immunodeficiency virus
IABP	Intra-aortic balloon pump
ICAO	International Civil Aviation Organization
ICP	Intracranial pressure
ICU	Intensive care unit
IDL	International date line
IFR	Instrument flight rules
ILS	Instrument landing system
ISA	International standard atmosphere
ISAS	International Society of Aeromedical Services
ISS	Injury severity score
ITU	Intensive therapy unit
IV	Intravenous
kPa	Kilopascals
kt	Knot (one nautical mile per hour)
LOX	Liquid oxygen
m	Meters
mmHg	Millimeters of mercury
MAST	Military assistance to safety and traffic
MAST	Medical (or military) antishock trousers
MEDIF	Medical information form
MI	Myocardial infarction
mph	Miles per hour
mpm	Meters per minute
MV	Minute volume
MVA	Motor vehicle accident

NAAS	National Association of Air Ambulance Services (UK)
NHS	National Health Service
NICU	Neonatal intensive care unit
nm	Nautical miles
NTSB	National Transportation Safety Board
$PACO_2$	Alveolar partial pressure of carbon dioxide
$PaCO_2$	Arterial partial pressure of carbon dioxide
PAIP	Post-accident incident plan
PaO_2	Arterial partial pressure of oxygen
PASG	Pneumatic antishock garment
PEEP	Positive end expiratory pressure
PIH	Pregnancy induced hypertension
PO_2	Partial pressure of oxygen
PROM	Premature rupture of membranes
psi	Pounds per square inch
PTL	Preterm labor
QA	Quality assurance
QANTAS	Queensland and Northern Territories Air Service
RAF	Royal Air Force
RAPS	Rapid acute physiology score
REM	Rapid eye movement
SAMU	Service d'Aide Médicale Urgente
SAR	Search and Rescue
SAS	Scandinavian Air Services
SBP	Systolic blood pressure
SCBU	Special care baby unit
SCN	Suprachiasmatic nucleus
SIMV	Synchronized intermittent mandatory ventilation
SL	Sea level
SPO_2	Venous oxygen saturation
STOL	Short take-off and landing
SUMMA	Servicio de Urgencias Médicas de Madrid
SV	Stroke volume
TS	Trauma score
UH	Utility helicopter
UK	United Kingdom
US	United States (of America)
USA	United States of America
USAF	United States Air Force
UTC	Universal coordinated time
VFR	Visual flight rules
WC	Water closet (lavatory)

Glossary

The following words and phrases are used throughout the text. Where meaning may be ambiguous, an alternative word or description is given.

aeromedical	air medical
aeromedical escort	air medical attendant, medical flight crew
aeromedical team	doctor, nurse and/or paramedic flight crew
anesthesiologist	anaesthetist (UK)
antennas	aerials
chart	medical document, hospital or transport notes
desk doctor	doctor working in the office of a medical assistance organization
diapering	changing a nappy
dysrhythmia	arrhythmia
electrocardiogram	ECG, EKG
emergency room	accident and emergency unit
escort, attendant	member of aeromedical team
family practitioner	general practitioner, family doctor
fixed base operator	supplier of fuel, maintenance and other aviation services, based at an airport
flight crew	aircrew, pilot and copilot
flight following	a radar and/or radio means of keeping track of the whereabouts of an aircraft
flight physician	aeromedical doctor, flight doctor, flight surgeon
litter	stretcher
matériel	stores and supplies
medical flight crew	team of aeromedical personnel
off-line	supervision from a distance, e.g. by telemetry
on-line	supervision on board
physician	doctor (USA), doctor practising internal medicine (UK)
rotary wing	rotorwing, helicopter
scene flight	a primary response mission, that is, flight direct to the scene of an incident
scoop and run	to collect the patient from the scene of injury with little or no time or effort spent on stabilization before evacuation
stay and play	to spend time on scene in an effort to resuscitate or stabilize a patient prior to evacuation

stopover	overnight interruption during journey
stretcher	litter
veteran	retired military personnel, ex-serviceman

PART I
Introduction

Chapter 1

History of Aeromedical Transportation

Beginnings

Since earliest times, men have sought the gift of flight. As creatures grounded by nature, man's imagination took the form of gods drawn across the sky by chariots of fire or heroes borne to battle or their Valhalla on winged stallions. Mortals seldom experienced the power of flight. The Chinese Emperor Shun was said to have escaped his captors by 'donning the work clothes of a bird'. The Greek architect Daedalus (designer of the Maze of the Minotaur) and his son Icarus fled the isle of Crete by soaring to freedom on wings made of feathers and wax. Icarus was also the first aviation fatality. Enraptured by the joys of flight, he neglected the warnings of his father and flew too close to the sun, melting the fabric of his wings and plummeting down into the sea.

Myth became reality in 1783 when the first terrestrial creatures took to the air in a Montgolfier balloon. These pioneer aeronauts ascended to a height of 1700 feet. Upon landing, one of the aeronauts (Montauciel, a sheep) was noted to be calmly munching grass, while one colleague (a duck) was cowering in a corner and the other (a rooster) suffered a broken wing from being kicked by Montauciel prior to lift-off. As faith in the ability of living creatures to tolerate air travel had been vindicated, the first manned ascent was crewed by the French physician Pilatre de Rozier and the Marquis d'Arlandes in November of the same year.

One of the first balloon ascents was witnessed by Benjamin Franklin, American envoy to France. When a sceptic in the crowd noted that the balloon was, 'interesting, but what use is it?', Franklin remarked, 'What use is a newborn baby?' It was a portent of things to come, for in 1903 the owners of the Wright Cycle Factory in Dayton, Ohio, piloted the first successful heavier-than-air craft across the sand dunes at Kitty Hawk.

Less than a century later, aircraft and air travel have become part of our daily world. The phenomenon of flight has shrunk the globe and pushed back the frontiers of space. It is hardly surprising that aeromedical services form an integral part of the modern emergency care system.

Origins of aeromedical transportation

For many years it was popularly believed that the very first aeromedical flights evacuated patients from the besieged city of Paris during the Franco-Prussian War in 1870. However, contemporary records of the 67 balloons known to have left Paris during the siege make no mention of the carriage of any sick or wounded. The origin of this popular myth is unclear, but may have resulted from an error in the translation of the original French reports. Many of the balloons were under contract to the French postal service and carried letters, government dispatches, homing pigeons, and passengers on governmental or war related business. Like many other myths, perhaps the fabled medical evacuation flights should have happened, but there is verifiable documentary evidence that they did not. Some 20 years later a Dutch military doctor by the name of DeMooy proposed that casualties might be evacuated by horse-drawn tethered balloons but, again, there is no evidence that such flights actually took place.

The history of aeromedical transportation is therefore not quite as long as the history of flight itself, but certainly does not lag far behind it. Despite the statement reported in a French medical journal (*Le Caducée*) in 1912, that 'the use of the aeroplane for (medical) evacuation is, for the moment, in the realm of fiction', the first aeromedical flights were not long in coming. In fact, the earliest recorded evacuation of wounded casualties by aeroplane took place during the first world war, when Serbian patients were carried in an unmodified French fighter plane. In 1916, Dr Chassaing persuaded the French government to build an aircraft capable of carrying two stretchers. A year later it was being used successfully to evacuate the wounded from the battlefield at Amiens. As aviation technology progressed, the potential value of aircraft as airborne ambulances became obvious.

The first recorded British air ambulance flight took place in 1917 when a soldier in the Camel Corps in Turkey who had been shot in the ankle was flown to hospital in 45 minutes, thus avoiding a three-day journey on the ground. In the same year, the Reverend John Flynn, a Presbyterian minister with the Australian Inland Mission, conceived the idea of combining 'wireless', aviation, and medicine to produce a 'mantle of safety' across the outback. Over the next ten years, with the assistance of inventors, radio technicians, doctors, philanthropists and fellow missionaries, Flynn saw his dream literally take off. Although sporadic medical flights had been occurring for at least a year, the Inland Mission's Aerial Medical Service was the first organized program. The first official flight was from Cloncurry in Queensland on 17 May 1928; the aircraft was a de Havilland DH50 biplane, on secondment from the infant Queensland and Northern Territory Airline Service (now QANTAS, Australia's national carrier). The first communications network started out of Cloncurry at the same time, utilizing pedal powered radios developed by Alfred Traeger. Without radio, the Aerial Medical Service (AMS) would have been rendered worthless for want of a means of dispatch; it was to take the advent of microwave transmissions to make telephones widely available within the outback. Although it was initially a one-year experiment, flying continued for twelve years at Cloncurry and, until 1934, it was the sole AMS base.

Another vital component of Flynn's 'mantle of safety' was a network of Inland Mission hostels and hospitals staffed by nurses throughout the outback. The first hostel opened in 1912 at Oodnadatta. Within 14 years, ten hostels/hospitals had been established, all staffed by registered nurses. With few doctors in the outback, the concept of flying nurses was also developed. In 1939 a young nurse, Meg McKay flew from Cloncurry to Bulia to assist with immunisations and surgery, and the concept of a flying nurse was firmly established. The name of the organization was changed to the Flying Doctor Service (FDS) in 1942 and, by the end of the second world war, the military flight nurse concept was well proven. In 1945, the Victorian, South Australian, and New South Wales sections of the Flying Doctor Service jointly funded an experiment of a flying nurse based at Broken Hill. The FDS was probably the first aeromedical organization to train and employ flight nurses. By the time of Flynn's death in 1951, his concept had grown to a federation of six sections and a dozen bases. Its value to the people of the outback was recognized in 1955 with the granting of the 'Royal' prefix and it remains a vital part of outback Australian life to this day.

Between the wars, both the British and French employed aircraft for the transportation of casualties resulting from colonial conflicts. The Royal Air Force (RAF) first used aircraft in the casevac role in Somaliland, in 1919, when three patients were moved 175 miles on stretchers strapped to the fuselage of a de Havilland DH9 aircraft. A few years later, the French evacuated several thousand injured soldiers in confrontations with the Berber and Riffian tribesmen in Morocco.

Meanwhile, throughout the 1920s, military aeroplanes were used for disaster relief missions in the USA and, during the same period, the RAF operated an air ambulance service within a 100 mile radius of an airfield near to London. In 1933 the first UK civilian air ambulance service was instigated. Serving the Scottish Isles, the descendant of this service still operates today, carrying the sick and injured from the remote islands of Scotland to the mainland. Long distance, high altitude, aeromedical evacuation, however, was pioneered by the Luftwaffe. During the Spanish civil war (1936-41) they used trimotor Junkers JU 52 aircraft in missions lasting up to ten hours and flown at an altitude of 18 000 ft.

It was the Second World War, though, which heralded rapid advancement and created much work for the newly formed military casualty evacuation (casevac) organizations. Initially, the aeroplane supplemented ground and ship-borne evacuation of casualties but, in the latter years of the conflict, more than 90 per cent of allied casualties were evacuated by air. As more spacious aircraft became available, there was sufficient room for patient care to be continued in flight. In 1942 the US military began training flight transport personnel for the specific purpose of medical escort duties, and the first dedicated aeromedical unit (the 38th Medical Air Ambulance Squadron) was formed. Using transport aircraft such as the Douglas C-47 Skytrain and the C-54 Skymaster, over a million sick and wounded soldiers were airlifted to the United States during the last three years of the war.

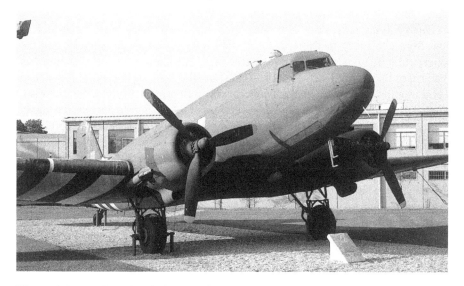

Figure 1.1   A Douglas C-47 used for casualty evacuation in World War II

The military continued to dominate the growth and development of aeromedical transportation in the immediate post-war period, a steady stream of conflicts and minor wars ensuring their interest. During this same period, other notable advances had a marked effect. The development of rotary wing aircraft was of particular significance because of their ability to operate in confined spaces. In fact, a helicopter was first used in the search and rescue (SAR) and casualty evacuation (casevac) role in Burma during the latter stages of the second world war. Lt Carter Harman, of the US Army Air Force, transported several wounded airmen near Mawlu in Burma on 23 April 1944. Details of this flight are not clear, but this WWII combat zone mission is believed to be the first time a helicopter was actually used to rescue and transport a trauma patient. However, the origin of the first helicopter SAR unit in January 1945 is well documented.

In an historic episode, a Sikorsky YR-4 helicopter (Figure 1.2) was dismantled at Wright Field, Dayton, Ohio in the USA, and flown half way around the world to Myitkyina, Burma where it was reassembled and flown over jungles and 5000 ft (1500 m) mountain peaks to accomplish its first mission. Although the original mission was to rescue downed aircrew, in the few days taken to airlift the helicopter and crew to Burma, these aircrew had already been rescued by ground forces.

However, soon after their arrival in Burma, news came in of a soldier who had accidentally shot himself through the hand with a .30 caliber machine gun while on duty at a weather station located on a mountain in the Naga hills, 160 miles northwest of Myitkyina. The soldier's hand was rapidly becoming infected and no experienced medical personnel were available to treat it. It would have taken approximately ten days for the man to walk from the station to a location where he could have medical care. The possibility of parachuting a medical officer on to the mountain had been considered but the nature of the terrain would have made it virtually impossible to get him down alive.

So it was on 26 January 1945 that the first mission took place. The helicopter had no radio and, since the American pilots, Capt Peterson and Lt Steiner, were unfamiliar with the country, it was decided that they would be escorted by two light fixed wing aircraft (L-5) of the Air Jungle Rescue Unit. The mission necessitated refuelling stops en route and personnel of the Royal Air Force provided support at a remote jungle clearing. The helicopter flew at tree top level with an average air speed of about 60 knots while that of the L-5s was 30 to 40 knots faster. Consequently, the L-5 pilots were forced to circle continuously to keep the helicopter in sight.

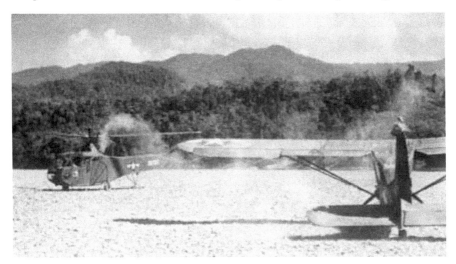

**Figure 1.2   Sikorsky YR-4 en route to the first helicopter casevac in
         Burma, 1945**
Source: US AAF, from the National Air and Space Museum archives, Washington DC.

The patient was a 21 year old soldier, Private Howard Ross, of North Tonawanda, New York. Although he had received a radio message that help was on the way, he had absolutely no idea in what form it would take. Little was he to know of his notable role in the history of helicopter rescue. Contemporaneous reports state that 'His hand was considerably swollen, but he was highly excited at his rescue. His recovery was uneventful.' (Holmes, 2005).

After this proving mission, Capt Peterson and Lt Steiner returned to Myitkyina and began to instruct the Air Jungle Rescue Unit personnel in the operation and maintenance of the helicopter, thus forming the first ever dedicated helicopter SAR and casevac unit.

The British later used helicopters in the casevac role in Malaya, immediately after the cessation of WWII hostilities, but the first real large scale evacuation of wounded soldiers by helicopter occurred during the Korean war. The Bell-47 and Sikorsky

S-51 were used to ferry patients from battalion aid stations to waiting hospital units. Patients were strapped to litters outside the aircraft, and covered with a canopy to prevent injury from wind or rotor wash. Over 20 000 wounded servicemen were transported in this fashion.

However, the Vietnam War was the definitive showcase for demonstrating the efficacy of helicopter medical transport in improving care for the injured. Under the codename 'Operation Dustoff', and using dedicated squadrons of Bell UH-1 Iroquois ('Huey') aircraft (Figure 1.3), over 400 000 patients were airlifted to hospital during the conflict. For the first time, casevac helicopters were used for the rapid removal of injured troops from close to the point of wounding. Casualties were then transported rapidly to nearby expert and specialist medical care for definitive treatment. This concept was called 'scoop and run', and may have accounted, at least partly, for the much lower mortality rate of those wounded in this conflict when compared with those injured in previous wars.

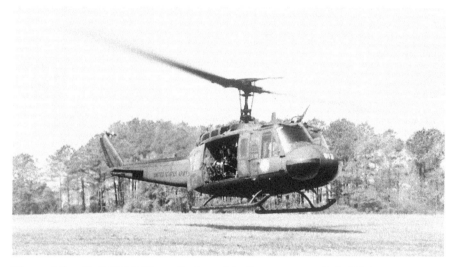

Figure 1.3   Bell UH-1 Huey, first used in the casevac role in Vietnam

Civilian applications

The success of the military approach to casualty evacuation during the Korean and Vietnam wars, and the immediacy of television news coverage, brought the aeromedical helicopter much public attention. It was soon realized that the helicopter might have an important contribution to make in civilian medical practice. Closely following the well publicised wartime successes of helicopters, a dramatic rescue occurred in New York during the summer of 1951. A steeplejack fell on to the roof of St. John's Cathedral and refused to be lowered to the ground by ropes. Captain Gustav Crawford of the New York Police Aviation Bureau landed his helicopter on the roof of St John's and the casualty was strapped to the outside of the aircraft and flown to nearby Riverside Park where he was transported by ground ambulance to hospital.

The helicopter's ability to retrieve the injured from remote, inhospitable or difficult terrain is now well known, but probably the first of all of the world's civilian helicopter air ambulance services was the Swiss Air Rescue Association (known as REGA). REGA was using a piston powered helicopter for limited medical use in 1952 and, in 1968, added turbine powered helicopters to provide better performance in the mountainous terrain.

A later development was the use of helicopters in the rapid retrieval and transportation of the sick and injured in urban environments. Belgium was one of the first countries to realize the importance of helicopter air ambulances in 1963, but they used military helicopters. The same lessons were being learnt in the USA and, by 1965, the Helicopter Emergency Lifesaving Patrol (HELP) project was set up in Philadelphia. At the time, HELP was unique in that its air ambulance service to the Delaware Valley area was achieved by matching medical personnel from a local Hospital (Lankenau) with a commercial (Atlantic Refining Company) traffic reporting helicopter. However, by late 1967, Superior Ambulance Service in Westland, Michigan had started a dedicated commercial helicopter ambulance service using a Bell 47 to support local hospitals.

Two years later, the first combined emergency services helicopter unit was formed in the USA. In 1969, the Maryland State Police and the University of Maryland began a police/rescue/HEMS (helicopter emergency medical service) service covering their entire state. It is said that the helicopters were first introduced to improve patient outcome in what was called the 'neglected disease of modern society'. This phrase was coined in a report by the US National Research Council which revealed that accidents were the leading cause of death in those under 37 years of age. During this time, federally funded projects were conducted through the United States Department of Transportation's National Highway Traffic and Safety Administration to study the feasibility of civilian aeromedical transport programs. Several problems in establishing these services were identified, including tenuous economic viability, the need to dedicate the aircraft to a medical configuration, and the need to integrate the programs into the ground emergency medical systems (EMS). Concurrently, civilian law enforcement agencies and fire departments were developing aviation components to assist in their primary missions. Though not initially designed for air medical duties, these public service programs were occasionally providing the means for such flights.

Europe was following suit and it was the Federal Republic of Germany that was the first country to instigate a major, nationwide service in 1970 (known as ADAC). During the same year the United States Departments of Defense and Transportation began a pilot program called Military Assistance to Safety and Traffic (MAST), first implemented at Houston in Texas, its *raison d'être* was to provide air medical transportation to rural traffic.

The first of the dedicated hospital based helicopter systems (in which the aircraft is leased or owned by a hospital or consortium) was formed at Saint Anthony Hospital in Denver, Colorado in 1972. This service was called 'Flight for Life' and was the model for what ultimately became the largest type of HEMS service in the world. By 1978 there were still fewer than 20 hospital based helicopter programs in the United States. Second generation programs blossomed in the early 1980s amidst increasing governmental interest in aeromedical transport and driven by the cost of aircraft and medical technology. Most programs operated at a loss, and initial data regarding the impact of transport by air began to appear. What had been a predominantly trauma oriented field was expanded to include neonatal, obstetric, and cardiac patients. As a result the number of interhospital flights increased significantly. Since then, there has been a dramatic growth in emergency medical helicopter systems with 170 programs reported in 1992. Collectively, these services have transported 728 000 patients over 92 million miles. A conservative estimate notes that 73 000 patients in the United States owe their lives to helicopters. It has also been estimated that over the past 40 years, a million lives have been saved as a result of all types of aeromedical transport.

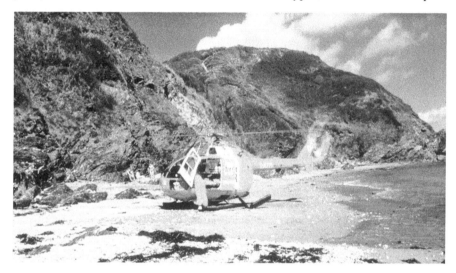

Figure 1.4   Britain's first helicopter air ambulance, *First Air* in Cornwall
(courtesy Cornwall & Isles of Scilly Ambulance Service)

In Europe, too, the lessons learned from battlefield casualty evacuation were put to good use. The Service d'Aide Médicale Urgente (SAMU) was created in the 1960s by French anesthesiologists aware of the high prehospital mortality rate of multiply injured patients. The governments of Switzerland and Germany financed studies to determine the feasibility of incorporating helicopters into emergency medical systems and soon established combined military and civilian networks to cover all major highways and special risk areas such as large cities, coastline and mountainous terrain. In the UK, the 1980s saw the development of, first, a paramedic crewed urban/coastal EMS helicopter (Figure 1.4) in Cornwall, soon followed by the London based Helicopter Emergency Medical Service (HEMS) which carries both a paramedic and doctor on every flight. Despite controversies over efficacy and costs, medical helicopter systems continue to proliferate, with 15 organizations operating in the EMS role in Great Britain in 2005. However, some parts of the country still have no service at all, and in others the coverage is not seven days a week. The Automobile Association (AA) has sponsored a new charity – the National Association of Air Ambulance Services (NAAS) – with an aim to help local charities to upgrade these systems, combined with a rolling programme to provide helicopters for areas not yet covered.

Fixed wing development

The recent history of civilian fixed wing aeromedical transport is more difficult to trace. Often these organizations are hidden from the public view by the media appetite for helicopter operations. However, the growth of international civil aeromedical transportation has been driven by rapid advances in the technology and availability of mass transportation. Larger and faster passenger carrying aircraft have brought cheap, affordable and accessible travel to millions of people throughout the world. Rapid airline growth in the post-war years and commercial exploitation have brought the most exotic corners of the Earth within reach of tourists and business travelers alike. Among these are a number who become ill or injured whilst abroad, some requiring repatriation on compassionate grounds, and others for specialist treatment. Numerous dedicated civilian medical assistance and air ambulance companies now exist (Figure 1.5). In the main, they operate in association with travel insurers, and arrange medical flights, worldwide, using fixed wing aircraft.

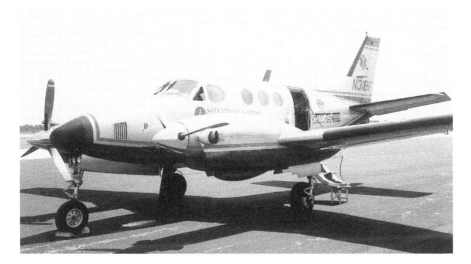

Figure 1.5   Dedicated air ambulance (ShandsCair, Florida)

References

Cook, J.L. (1988) *Dust Off*. Rufus: New York.

Gabram, S.G. and Jacobs L.M., (1990) 'The impact of emergency medical helicopters on prehospital care', *Emergency Medical Clinics of North America*, **8**:85-102.

Holmes, E. (2005) *MEDEVAC Flight in WWII* (Source: US army air forces document obtained from the National Air & Space Museum in Washington, DC.), http://helis.com/stories/burma45.php.

Lam, D.M. (1988) 'To pop a balloon: aeromedical evacuation in the 1870 siege of Paris', *Aviat Space Environ Med.* **59**(10):988-991.

Martin, T.E. (1993) 'Transportation of Patients by Air', in Harding and Mills, *Aviation Medicine* (3rd Ed). BMJ: London.

Meier, D.R. and Samper E.R. (1989) 'Evolution of civil aeromedical helicopter evacuation', *South Med J.* **82**(7):885-891.

National Academy of Sciences, National Research Council (1966) *Accidental Death and Disability, the Neglected Disease of Modern Society*, US Government Printing Office: Washington DC.

Neel, S.H., (1968) 'Army aeromedical evacuation procedures in Vietnam. Implications for rural America'. *J Am Med Assoc.* **204**:99-103.

RAF Strike Command (1982) *Aeromedical evacuation in the RAF*, Ministry of Defence: London.

Royal Flying Doctor Service of Australia (1990) *The Royal Flying Doctor Story*, RFDS: Jandakot.

Chapter 2

Overview

The heterogeneity of aeromedical systems

This chapter aims to introduce the reader to all aspects of aeromedical transportation since, clearly, fixed and rotary wing aircraft can be used in a number of diverse ways. Not only are the missions, and the injuries and illnesses of the patients, widely disparate, but the types of aircraft that can be used will vary accordingly. For instance, there is a great difference between the operations of an urban HEMS helicopter and an air ambulance company which specializes only in long distance repatriations. Also, the transfer of a relatively healthy post-operative patient who may require only a nurse escort from his holiday destination to home, differs significantly from that of a critically injured child who is airlifted, unconscious and bleeding, from the scene of a motor vehicle accident. A wide assortment of aircraft types are therefore used, and each has advantages and disadvantages over the next, depending on the requirements of the mission. Outside of the military and the emergency medical services though, few operators maintain aircraft solely for aeromedical use, relying rather on the adaptation of existing types, as and when the operational requirement arises.

In an attempt to classify types of medical transport missions, previous authors have divided them in to three groups. These are primary, secondary and tertiary responses. A fourth group, the so-called quaternary mission, can also be added. The definitions for these types of aeromedical transfers are simple, and help to explain how different aeromedical organizations work.

Primary retrievals involve recovery of casualties from the scene of their injury or illness, and, in almost all cases, they are undertaken by helicopters (rotary wing aircraft). The helicopter is primarily dispatched to the incident (hence, often called a 'scene flight'). In other words the helicopter and its crew may be the only unit responding to the emergency or, at least, it may be the first to arrive. This often means that there has been minimal (and sometimes no) medical care prior to the arrival of the helicopter. Although flight times are short, the crew faces special challenges in both aviation and clinical terms. The former, because of the dangers associated with landing in uncontrolled and unprepared landing zones, and the latter because of the undiagnosed and untreated major emergencies that they face. Search and rescue (SAR) is a highly specialized variation of primary response.

Secondary transfers involve transport between two medical facilities, usually to a higher (or more appropriate) level of medical care. Thus a patient who has had some degree of stabilization in a small country medical practice or other outlying emergency facility may be transported to the nearest or most appropriate hospital for care which could not be provided at the first facility. As with primary transfers, the patient may not have been fully worked up prior to transport and so re-assessment is a very important part of this process.

A tertiary response occurs when an aeromedical aircraft transports a hospital inpatient to another facility, usually a larger city teaching hospital (or regional centre) for specialist or definitive care.

Quaternary transport is a term commonly used to infer repatriation, usually from overseas, but it might also be within national boundaries in large countries such as the United States or Australia. The transfer might involve the movement of a patient from one major facility to another or, in the recovery phase of an illness or injury, from a higher level of care to a lower one. At the extreme, the patient may even be fit enough to be discharged directly home to the care of his family practitioner. The reason for the transfer is usually social, that is, aimed at returning an injured or ill person to a facility closer to their home and family. This type of mission is typified by the classic travel insurance case where a traveler is escorted back to his home town before he is fit to travel alone. These cases are elective and usually provide enough time for appropriate preparation and planning. The exception is the case whereby a patient requires treatment not available locally before he can be considered fit for the journey home. In this case, he must be moved from one overseas facility to another which can offer the specialist care.

The use of aircraft in the transport of medications, equipment, medical personnel, and human tissues or organ harvest teams to and from airports or institutions represents yet another facet of aeromedical transport.

Helicopters

Search and Rescue

The RAF used amphibious light aircraft during the Battle of Britain (1940) to retrieve aviators who had ditched or parachuted into the cold waters of the English Channel, but fixed wing aircraft have rarely, since then, been used in the patient carrying role in over-sea operations. Both the RAF and the USAAF used light aircraft in early efforts at jungle rescue in the Far East during the latter stages of WWII, but fixed wing aircraft are now almost exclusively used for the search component of SAR. Long range, high endurance, fixed wing aircraft (such as the P3 Orion and Nimrod) are now utilized to locate an incident, drop survival equipment, and to act as airborne rescue coordination centers. Helicopters, with their ability to hover and winch survivors directly on board from any rescue environment (and during all but the most severe weather conditions), are almost exclusively used for actual rescue operations.

In both Europe and North America, the entire coastline, in addition to wilderness areas, are covered by a network of SAR helicopters operated by the national Air

Forces, Navies, and Coast Guard organizations (Figure 2.1). Ninety percent of rescues involve civilian incidents, although the actual *raison d'être* for the SAR network in some countries is the location and retrieval of downed military aircrew and stranded sailors.

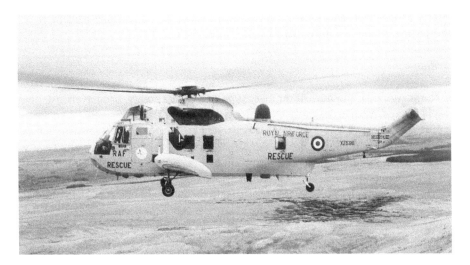

Figure 2.1   Search and rescue helicopter of the Royal Air Force

SAR helicopters are most commonly used in the scoop and run role, and some carry experienced and well equipped paramedic-trained personnel as part of the crew complement. Doctors or flight nurses may also be carried on some missions. In contrast, primary helicopter air ambulances in Australasia commonly also undertake SAR duties, and are almost exclusively staffed by paramedics and trained rescue operatives.

Military helicopters

Over and above the SAR service, other military helicopters may be tasked to aid the civilian community in the event of a disaster or major incident. The Military Assistance to Safety and Traffic (MAST) program operated by the armed forces of the United States is an example. MAST aircraft may participate in the transport of ill or injured patients when no civilian service is able to assist, and when MAST aircraft, equipment, and personnel are not being utilized in pursuit of the unit's primary military mission. However, such action requires approval and organization by the relevant defense department and these helicopters, unlike SAR forces, are not on permanent standby. The time to activate callout may therefore be long, especially at night and weekends, thereby delaying the start of productive service.

Experience in Korea, Vietnam, the Falkland Islands, Israel, the Persian Gulf, FRY (former Republic of Yugoslavia), Iraq, Afghanistan and other recent conflicts has repeatedly shown that helicopters are ideally suited for the rapid collection and removal of battlefield casualties, not only in the tactical situation (that is, from the front line), but also ahead of it (covert operations) and backwards along the evacuation chain through the various echelons of medical care. Helicopters have also proved invaluable in seaborne operations for the transfer of casualties between vessels of the fleet, and from hospital ships to land-based medical centers or to aeromedical staging facilities for onward transportation.

Civilian helicopters

In North America, the most prominent type of civilian rotary wing system is the hospital-based service, designed to transport patients from outlying medical facilities to the base hospital. Helicopters are also operated by public service agencies such as ambulance, fire and police authorities. Aircraft used in these programs are usually multifunctional, and may serve in any combination of emergency roles, including medical, search and rescue, fire suppression, and law enforcement. They are sponsored by national or local government and the costs are borne by the public at large. Other systems may operate under charitable status, or as freestanding private businesses.

Whatever their origin, and from wherever they are tasked, helicopters may be used primarily for transportation directly to and from the accident scene, or they may be utilized solely for the secondary, but urgent, transfer of high dependency patients, medical supplies or organs for donation. In the former (HEMS) role, the responsibility for dispatch and control usually lies with an ambulance authority which will have a local protocol-driven dispatch system to ensure that the EMS helicopter is assigned to the most appropriate missions.

A significant number of flight programs, especially those sponsored by public service agencies, have crews exclusively composed of paramedics, trained to (and often beyond) emergency medical technician – paramedic (EMT-P) standards. There is fervent debate about the need for the expertise of a doctor during the transport of some patients, but it is generally agreed that trained doctors may be of value at the scene of an incident, especially when entrapment or logistic circumstances delay the evacuation of the patient. Although doctors are included as aeromedical crew members in only a minority of programs in North America, many European EMS helicopters (such as the ADAC Notarzt helicopters in Germany and the London HEMS, figure 2.2) routinely carry a doctor who is trained in anesthesiology, emergency medicine or surgery, as well as advanced prehospital emergency care. The major difference between European and North American systems is perhaps the almost exclusively American use of registered nurses.

Helicopters may primarily serve the needs of an EMS agency or accept the role as a secondary function. In either case, a flight program must be fully integrated into the EMS systems in the area it serves. Integration begins with the establishment of geographic service areas. The helicopter system may operate in a rural area where the population is sparse and there is a low density of trauma. In this context, the helicopter is useful to cover large gaps in ambulance cover, especially where few hospitals are scattered over a wide area. Alternatively, an urban based system is likely to operate in an area of large population, yielding a high density of trauma. Although appropriate hospitals may be abundant and nearby, traffic congestion often impairs rapid evacuation by road. Inevitably, operational areas are determined by factors such as aircraft range and speed, location of trauma centers and specialty units, quality of patient care that can be rendered by flight crew, and the location and mission of aeromedical programs in adjacent regions.

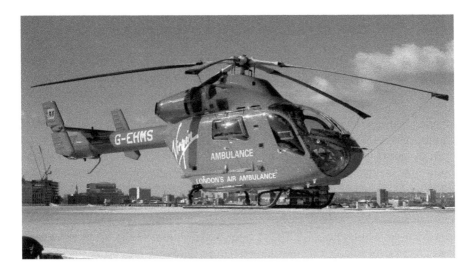

**Figure 2.2   Boeing MD Explorer of the London Helicopter Emergency
Medical Service**

As a modern model of primary care, the Spanish Servicio de Urgencias Médicas de Madrid (SUMMA) was created in the 1980s and carries both a doctor and nurse. The profession of paramedic does not exist, but the pilot is often used as an EMT to help with roadside care as well as lifting and loading. Flight nurses and doctors all receive extensive training in prehospital emergency care and rescue techniques. SUMMA is owned and operated by the Spanish National Health Service, (NHS) but it is financed entirely by public donations. Madrid's EMS helicopters cover the traffic-dense city and suburbs as well as the surrounding rural and mountainous areas. This unique range of missions requires a wide set of skills and capabilities, and EMS operators from other parts of Spain are sending their novice crews to SUMMA for knowledge acquisition and experience. In this manner, the Spanish NHS hopes to have a comprehensive HEMS network in the near future.

Fixed wing aircraft

While helicopter missions attract most publicity and attention, fixed wing flights constitute a significant portion of aeromedical transport operations. Although less expensive to operate than helicopters, conventional aircraft suffer from the single major disadvantage that they require large expanses of open flat terrain in order to collect and deliver their human cargo. Since hospitals are rarely conveniently located near airports, this inevitably requires ground transfers at either end of the flight. In addition, transport time in fixed wing aircraft must take into account the transfer of crew and equipment to the base airport, pilot preparation time, the outbound flight, ground transport to the referring facility, patient pickup, return of the patient and crew to the aircraft, the inbound flight, and return by ground to the home institution from the airport. Fixed wing transports clearly take considerably more time than ground or rotary wing transfers. However, these problems are less significant when the advantages of increased range and duration, greater speed, or increased cabin capacity are required. Fixed wing aircraft are therefore only occasionally used in the primary response role, and usually then, only when distances are great. They are almost exclusively utilized for interhospital transfers and repatriation.

Many air ambulance services are actually brokers or charter organizations which match patients with transport needs to available non-dedicated aircraft, supplies, and medical and flight crew. Fixed wing air ambulance services which provide dedicated medically configured aircraft, top-shelf equipment, regular crew, and strong medical direction are much less numerous than brokers, and may charge more for services rendered, in order to support their more expensive infrastructure. Nonetheless, the improvement in the quality of care which may ensue when using a dedicated service can well offset the disparity in cost. Fixed wing services may be sponsored by private fee-for-service or subscription companies (such as Med-Plane in the United States, Vuelo de Vida in South America, and Medical Rescue International in South Africa), medical assistance companies acting on behalf of travel insurers (such as Europ Assistance and Mondial) or those acting on behalf of corporate clients (such as International SOS), charities (such as Australia's Royal Flying Doctor Service and the former Pacific Air Ambulance), or governmental agencies (such as Life Flight New Zealand, and, again, Pacific Air Ambulance). Commercial airlines are often used for fixed wing aeromedical transfers, but experience with commercial repatriation of patients has been minimally reviewed in the medical literature. The military continues to have extensive experience with fixed wing transport as part of its daily operational scheme.

In terms of innovation and development, the inter-war years are overshadowed by the post-WWII era. The enormous cultural and social changes which succeeded the austere war years saw the introduction of relatively inexpensive and easily accessible air travel, coinciding with a steadily increasing affluence in most societies, and the availability of more leisure time. The inevitable result was a dramatic expansion of tourism which has continued for the past six decades. Where tourism has increased, so, too, has the need to repatriate those unfortunates who have been injured or fallen ill many miles from home. International travel is now so routine, that often little thought is given by travelers to the potential health problems of their destination. Although many will consider vaccination against low risk endemic infectious diseases, they fail to appreciate the impact of such factors as the local hygiene practices, climate, food, the risks of accidental injury and of the medical facilities that exist there. For instance, in 2001, almost 20 per cent (more than 35 000) of British travelers abroad requested some form of medical assistance by means of travel insurance. One company alone repatriated almost 3000 patients; just under half requiring either a medical or nursing escort.

Fixed wing transfers are conducted in all shapes and sizes of aircraft. Ambulant patients may travel in conventional passenger carrying aircraft (airliners) and may need only some form of medical supervision, with the provision of emergency drugs and equipment for the possibility of any untoward problem occurring during the transfer. Patients with minor disabilities might be offered seating with more leg-room (perhaps in upper class), or allocated two seats to allow more lateral space. Stretchers can be carried on many aircraft types, but usually require a block of nine conventional seats (Figure 2.3) in a commercial airliner. This is not only expensive, but can also be the cause of delays and inconveniences to the airline, not just when loading and unloading patients, but also in the time taken for engineering personnel to fit the stretcher frame. It is therefore not surprising that some airlines (such as British Airways, April 2005) have justified stopping their stretcher service.

Airline medical authorities may refuse medical clearance for some types of patient, and critically ill patients are difficult to manage on conventional passenger carrying airliners. These aircraft are not designed to carry the medical equipment that is so often needed in the care of the seriously ill and, despite screening, it is almost impossible to maintain patient privacy. Therefore, whenever possible, small dedicated air ambulance aircraft are used to transport high dependency patients and those who might otherwise be refused carriage by the airlines.

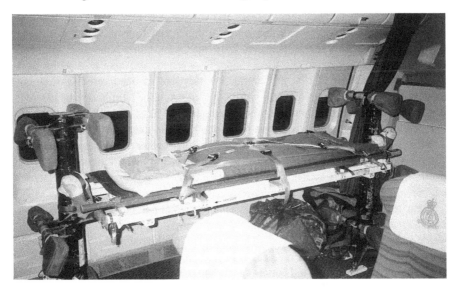

Figure 2.3   Military stretcher fit replacing a block of conventional seats

Different aircraft types are used for different mission assignments. Light aeroplanes are small single or twin engine aircraft. They are typically unpressurized, provide minimal room for patient care, have high noise levels, and travel at slow speeds. Medium range aircraft may be powered by piston engines or turboprops. They are often pressurized and provide adequate working space for patient care. They may have a range of 600 to 1200 miles (1000 to 2000 km) and reach speeds of up to 250 knots. Small jets have the longest range (up to 3000 miles/5000 km), the fastest speed (up to 450 knots), and the least interior noise of all commonly used aeromedical aircraft. Their streamlined shape, however, severely limits cabin space and may interfere with the ability to care for the critically ill patient.

The cost of a dedicated aeromedical flight depends very much on the aircraft type, destination, and on the medical requirements in transit. To retrieve a seriously ill patient from Spain, for example, and deliver him to a hospital in the United Kingdom, is unlikely to cost less than US$12 000. This expense is out of reach of the average traveler, and health insurance is essential. Although reciprocal health agreements are available between some countries (for example, within the European Community), this entitlement covers only the cost of emergency treatment and does not extend to the expense of repatriation.

Fixed wing aeromedical response to disasters

The 12 months up to November 2005 was a remarkable year for the unusually high number of natural disasters that occurred around the world. As 2004 drew to a close an earthquake in Indonesia resulted in a tsunami with tens of thousands of casualties around the rim of the Indian Ocean. There then followed the worst hurricane season in recorded history for the United States and Central America. Hundreds died and thousands were injured or made homeless by hurricane Katrina which destroyed New Orleans and other towns along the US Gulf Coast. Other hurricanes followed to pile more damage on to the places already affected, and also to a wider area of devastation. Lesser storms in Central America had earlier caused widespread flooding and the population had still not recovered when the next hurricane arrived. More lives lost. And then there was the earthquake in Pakistan and Kashmir which flattened towns and villages over a vast mountainous and inaccessible area.

In situations like these, no single country has the resources to manage the mass casualties that need medical evacuation to places of safety where treatment can be given. In the words of one Pakistani doctor '*We don't need money, we need doctors and helicopters, and we need them now!*'

Helicopters have proven useful for evacuating small numbers of casualties from remote areas of devastation where road infrastructure does not exist or where it has been destroyed by the disaster itself. They are also invaluable in the roles of search and rescue, and in delivering medical aid to where it is needed most. But moving large numbers of casualties and patients suffering the effects of disease and exposure is more of a problem. The military is familiar with large scale evacuation, and the establishment of aeromedical staging facilities which link field hospitals to secondary and tertiary referral hospitals. Nevertheless, military strategic evacuation response to disasters can sometimes be slow, especially when requests go through international agencies. One organization has decided to provide a civilian alternative.

The Swedish National Air Medevac (SNAM) project is an ambitious and yet highly successful endeavour which has proven the concept of a civilian rapid response long range aeromedical evacuation and repatriation capability. The project is funded by the Swedish government and is a joint collaborative effort between the Swedish Civil Aviation Authority, the National Board of Health and Welfare, the Swedish national air carrier, Scandinavian Airlines (SAS), two county council health boards, the University Hospital in Umeå, and a large number of enthusiastic volunteer medical and nursing air ambulance personnel.

The project speaks for itself in many ways (Table 2.1), but has one exceptional aspect that should be highlighted – the time taken to generate a mission. This generation time is only six hours. This is the time taken to convert a completely ordinary Boeing 737-800 commercial airliner from the SAS fleet to a flying intensive care unit and air ambulance. The aircraft can be any one from the fleet. It does not require any prior major structural modifications for this role.

All the medical equipment necessary to support the mission is kept in a constant state of readiness in Arlanda airport (Stockholm) so it can be loaded onto the aircraft within six hours of the alert. A roster of volunteer flight and medical crews meet the aircraft whilst it is still being converted and make necessary preparations in time for a departure within the six-hour deadline.

SNAM offers a highly flexible and effective airborne medical facility with critical care and air ambulance capabilities. The system can be generated in well under half a day, and it is staffed by experienced people. This impressive collection of personnel is made up from a large pool of enthusiastic volunteers who have been trained specifically for this task and who work day by day in either the aviation or air ambulance role. This, and the fact that the aircraft requires no prior modification, keeps the cost low. In essence, SNAM is a rapidly deployable, mobile and cost-effective facility which extends the arm of a modern hospital and delivers high technology medical care to where it is needed most.

Table 2.1   Features of the Swedish National Air Medevac Program

- A fully equipped modular airborne intensive care unit with six beds for critical ventilated patients
- Space and equipment for six additional ill or injured stretcher patients
- Seats for 23 walking wounded
- Highly trained and skilled aeromedical crew
  - Doctors (seven)
  - Nurses (11)
  - Medical technician (one)

- Non-medical crew
  - Flight crew (two pilots)
  - Cabin crew (three)
  - Aircraft engineers (two)
  - Operations coordinator (one)

Preventing potential problems

The ultimate solution to the problem of inflight medical emergencies lies in their prevention. There are few clinical reasons for refusal of aeromedical transportation and, although some conditions will require careful thought in the planning stages of the transfer, none is an absolute bar. Since the flight environment is unique, a knowledge and understanding of the physical, physiological and psychological stresses imposed by altitude and the constraints of air travel will allow anticipation, and therefore prevention, of clinical problems that may occur in flight or at any other stage of the transfer. The atmosphere is a hostile place. As air pressure declines with increasing altitude, less oxygen is available for cellular metabolism, and gases trapped within body cavities will expand. There may be problems with motion sickness, vibration, noise, cold or humidity, not to mention the psychological terror felt by some who can imagine nothing worse than being locked in a flying metal tube traveling at 500 mph (430 knots) at an altitude of 35 000 ft (10 000 m)

Beyond purely clinical concerns, the medical crew must be aware of (and should plan for) logistic factors such as the duration of out-of-hospital time, ground transfers, airport formalities, inflight facilities/equipment/skills, airborne sector times, time zone changes, stopovers, changes of aircraft, medical facilities at each stage and the actual time of arrival, and the weather, at the destination facility. The overall aim is to deliver the patient safely from point of origin to destination and causing no further harm. If useful treatment can be started or continued, then so much the better. Essentially, the ideal is that care in the air should be as found on the ground. This is a tall order, but its achievement can be helped by ensuring that adequate medical equipment and medications are available during the transit, and that members of the flight medical team are thoroughly familiar with their usage, and that they have the knowledge and skills to deal with both the predictable and the unexpected.

The aeromedical transport community

Several organizations exist to meet the needs of the aeromedical transport profession. Within the United States, the Association of Air Medical Services (AAMS) serves as the representative of the aeromedical transport industry. Flight physicians and medical directors are linked in the Air Medical Physician Association (AMPA). There are also professional organizations for flight nurses, flight paramedics, pilots and mechanics, and communications specialists. The Commission on Accreditation of Aeromedical Services (CAAMS), comprised of members of the aeromedical transport profession and other interested parties, provides meaningful self-assessment and recognized certification of programs meeting designated standards of excellence. The Aerospace Medical Association is a scientific body which holds a large aviation medicine meeting annually, and which has an active air medical transport group. Other scientific aeromedical organizations include the International Committee of Aerospace Medicine (ICASM) and the Australia and New Zealand Aviation Medicine Society.

In the UK, the CCAT (Clinical Considerations in Aeromedical Transport) training organization represents the interests of doctors, nurses and other health professionals working in aeromedical practice, especially on educational matters and professional advice. Nurses may otherwise be represented by the Inflight Nurses Association of the Royal College of Nursing. The Royal Aeronautical Society has an Aviation Medicine Group, although its interests are mainly directed towards the problems of aircrew and research into current military aviation medicine issues, but an affiliation of physicians working for medical assistance companies meets twice yearly to discuss current issues of common concern.

Similar organizations exist in many other countries with active aeromedical communities. International groups concerned with aeromedical transport include the International Society of Aeromedical Services (ISAS) and the European Aero-Medical Institute (EURAMI).

The world of aeromedical transport is chronicled in two journals specific to the profession. The Air Medical Journal serves as the scientific organ, publishing original research, abstracts, and reviews of interest to air transport specialists. AirMed is the industry's chronicle, and features articles on the growth and development of aeromedical services worldwide. The International Travel Insurance Journal (ITIJ) is another useful publication which has a section on travel health and a useful directory of worldwide travel assistance and air ambulance organizations. Its sister journal, the International Healthcare Journal (IHJ), is a valuable source of information on health issues around the globe for those involved in international repatriations. A selected list of flight services, references, organizations, and Internet sites serving as portals to the aeromedical community is provided at the end of this chapter.

The future

The past 20 years have seen significant growth in the number of aeromedical organizations involved in all types of patient transport missions. The development of new ideas and concepts, and the introduction of new equipment, procedures and guidelines, which help to ensure the safety of patients and crew alike, has accompanied this growth. But technology and knowledge do not stand still. With the expected entry in to service of the Airbus A380 in 2007, larger aircraft will become commonplace. There will inevitably be more potential travelers than ever before. Aircraft will fly faster, perhaps higher, and certainly for longer duration, making even more destinations accessible on single sector passages.

One of the most exciting recent developments is satellite linked remote diagnostic technology, capable of transmitting monitored physiological data such as electrocardiography and blood pressure, as well as video and audio downloads for real-time supervision by ground-based medical experts. The use of other new medical technologies, such as computerized diagnostics and dry-reagent biochemical tests will also make treatment decisions more reliable. Equipment is becoming increasingly miniaturized, reliable and affordable. If small dependable capnographs for detecting misplacement of endotracheal tubes were the prize of the 1990s, then portable blood laboratory analyzers are the must-have items of the new century. Other non-invasive monitoring techniques (such as for cerebral blood flow and cardiac output) are in various stages of investigation, and therapy devices such as intra-aortic balloon pumps are becoming increasingly common in the transfer of cardiac patients.

In the field of training, emergency medical care is now firmly center stage, especially since it is now accepted that trauma is the commonest killer in the young, and that acute cardiovascular disease is a frequent cause of death in the middle aged. The advent of new training courses (such as the CCAT courses) and recognition by examination (the Diploma in Aeromedical Retrieval and Transport) have been universally welcomed. It is popularly felt that every medical practitioner must be able to manage the essential initial stages of resuscitation (the 'golden hour') and that those at the sharp end of emergency care must be educated in the special needs of the prehospital environment (the 'platinum five minutes'). Training, though, is of little value without ongoing research and development of new ideas. As international travel continues to increase, the growth of the aeromedical industry will, doubtless, follow. The application of new ideas and technologies are likely to result in major innovations in the logistics of patient carriage by air and in the development of properly integrated transport systems within national and international medical care programs.

References

Anon (1995) 'Air ambulance services'. Aviation Industry Association of NZ (Inc). *N Z Health Hospital* 47(6): 12-13.

Bingham, K. (1992) 'Clearing the air on inflight health', *Doctor* 8 March 36.

Bricknell, C.M. and T. MacCormack (2005) 'Military approach to medical planning in humanitarian operations', *Br Med J.* **330**:1437-9.

Court, C. (1995) 'Survey highlights risk of foreign holidays', *Brit Med J.* **310**:1287.

Croser, J.L. (2003) 'Trauma care systems in Australia', *Injury* 34(9):649-51.

Crowther, E.S. et al. (1996) 'Mission, staffing, and budget data of flight programs in the United States', *Air Med J.* **15**(3):111-8.

Fairhurst, R.J. (1992) 'Health insurance for international travel', In: Dawood, R. (ed.) *Travellers' Health* (3rd ed.), Oxford University Press: Oxford.

Foster, P. and N. Malick (2005) 'Clock is ticking for those who miss mercy flights', *The Daily Telegraph* 13 Oct 2005, p. 14.

Gilligan, F., Sharley, P. and A. Berry (2004) 'Travel insurance and medical evacuation', *Med J Aust.* **180**(9):486.

Hotvedt, R. et al., (1996) 'Which groups of patients benefit from helicopter evacuation?' *Lancet* **18**:1362-1366.

Lackner, C.K. and Stolpe E. (1998) 'New order of things: an international overview of air medical transport', *Air Med J.* **17**(4): 142-5.

Langhelle, A. et al. (2004) 'International EMS systems: the Nordic countries', *Resuscitation* **61**(1):9-21.

Leggat, P.A. and R. Griffiths (2004) 'Travel insurance and medical evacuation', *Med J Aust.* **180**(9):484.

Martin, T.E. (1992) 'A new concept for a mobile, rapidly responding and versatile aeromedical unit', *Aviat Space Environ Med.* **63**(5):406.

Martin, T.E. (1992) 'Lessons from the Gulf war – aeromedical evacuation', *J Br Assoc Imm Care* **15**(1):2-6.

Porter, J.D.H., Stanwell-Smith R. and G. Lea (1992) 'Travelling hopefully, returning ill', *Brit Med J.* **304**:1323-4.

Swedish National Air Medevac, (2005). www.snam.se

Wilde, H. et al. (2003) 'Expatriate clinics and medical evacuation companies are a growth industry worldwide', *J Travel Med.* **10**(6):315-7.

Further reading

Books

Harding, R.M. and Mills F.J. (1993) *Aviation Medicine* (3rd Ed.), BMJ: London.

Ernsting J. and King P.F. (2006) *Aviation Medicine* (4th Ed.), Arnold: London.

de Hart, R.L. (1985) *Fundamentals of Aerospace Medicine*, Lea and Febiger: Philadelphia.

Martin T.E. (2001), *Handbook of Patient Transportation.* Greenwich Medical Media (now Cambridge University Press): London.

Rayman, R.R. (1990), *Clinical Aviation Medicine* (2nd Ed), Lea and Febiger: Philadelphia.

Dobie, T.G. (1972) *Aeromedical Handbook for Aircrew*, AGARDograph No 154.

McNeil, E.L. (1983) *Airborne Care of the Ill and Injured,* Springer-Verlag: New York.

Journals

Aviation, Space and Environmental Medicine (monthly). Published by the Aerospace Medical Association, 320 S. Henry Street, Alexandria, VA 22314, USA.

Telephone: +1-703-739-2240. Fax: +1-210-342-5670
Email: *ASEMjournal@att.net* Website: *www.asma.org*

Journal of The Emergency Medical Services (monthly).
Air Med (bimonthly).
Air Medical Journal (quarterly).
Prehospital and Disaster Medicine (quarterly)
All published by JEMS Communications, 1947 Camino Vida Roble, Suite 200, Carlsbad, CA 92008, USA.
Telephone: +1-619-431-9797. Fax: +1-619-431-8176

International Travel Insurance Journal (monthly).
International Healthcare Journal (monthly).
Both published by Voyageur Publishing & Events Ltd, Voyageur Buildings, 43 Colston Street, Bristol, BS1 5AX, UK.
Telephone: +44-117-922-6600. Fax: +44-117-929-2023
Email: *mail@itij.co.uk*
Websites: *www.itij.co.uk* and *www.ihj.org.uk*

PART II
Physics and Physiology

Chapter 3

The Atmosphere

T. Martin and M. Glanfield

Introduction

An understanding of the atmosphere and its basic properties is vital in aeromedical practice. The physics of that part of the atmosphere where life can exist (the biosphere) provides the framework upon which a working knowledge of altitude and aviation physiology is based. Perhaps more so than in any other field of environmental science, the twin studies of physics and physiology have grown and developed in concert over the centuries, each leading to new developments and discoveries in the other. Nowhere is this truer than in the study of the effects of flight on the human body.

The nature of atmosphere

Air is a mixture of gases and, like solids or liquids, gases obey the laws of physics. Gravity is the force which attracts objects to each other. Although it is an extremely weak force, over very small distances or when the objects have large mass (or both) the force of gravity becomes measurable. Although it requires a research laboratory to detect the minuscule attraction between two lead spheres each of mass 1 kg spaced a few centimeters apart, two fully laden oil tankers floating side by side will be pulled together with a force of about 5000 newtons, the same as the weight of 500 kg. And even though the surface of the earth is 3200 km from its centre,[1] a mass of 1 kg is pulled downwards with a force of 9.81 N (or in other words it has a weight of 1 kg). Gravity is what gives mass weight. It is immaterial whether the mass of 1 kg is solid, liquid or gas. We are of course more familiar with solids or liquids having weight. But gases have weight too, and it is the weight of air above the surface that gives us *atmospheric pressure.*

The atmosphere extends upwards in excess of 50 miles (80 km), becoming less dense with altitude. Just as the pointer on a set of kitchen scales will show more and more weight as we add coins to a stack in the scale pan, so atmospheric pressure increases if there is a greater height and therefore weight of air above us (Figure 3.1). Conversely if you were to measure the atmospheric pressure at the foot of a tall building and on the roof, the pressure (that is, the weight of air) on the roof would be less than at the base. So it is that atmospheric pressure falls with height. The density

---

1   For the non-mathematically minded, for gravitational purposes the mass of the earth can be considered to be concentrated at a single point at its centre.

of air will vary, being less dense at altitude, so the fall of pressure with altitude is rapid near sea level and less at high altitude. For example a climb from sea level to 1500 ft (455 m) results in a fall in pressure of 44 mmHg whereas an ascent from 46 000 ft to 47 500 ft (also a 1500 ft/455 m difference) results in only an 8 mmHg drop. At 18 000 ft (5486 m) half the weight of air is below and half above, the pressure is half that of sea level, at 33 500 ft (10 210 m) it is one quarter and at 53 000 ft (16 154 m) one tenth.

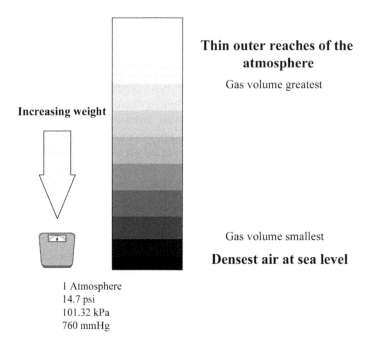

Thin outer reaches of the atmosphere

Gas volume greatest

Increasing weight

Gas volume smallest

Densest air at sea level

1 Atmosphere
14.7 psi
101.32 kPa
760 mmHg

Figure 3.1   The atmosphere as a column

Units of pressure

We are bedevilled with a range of pressure units, none of which seems to easily convert to any others. The S.I. unit of pressure is the *Pascal*, one pascal (newton per square metre) is rather a small pressure and so we have become used to dealing in kilopascals (kPa) and even megapascals (MPa). A conversion table between units of pressure and orders of magnitude can be found at the end of this chapter.

Units of pressure may be based on a force per unit area (pounds per square inch or newtons per square metre), the height of a column of liquid (millimeters of mercury of meters of sea water) or others, such as millibars. Although we should be using kPa in all things medical, mmHg are still used for blood pressure and for convenience in respiratory physiology. The logic behind this is that it is easy to visualise quantities between ten and a hundred (hence miles per hour on a car speedometer); arterial and tissue PO_2 values fall within this range. In the United States of America you will receive a barometric pressure in inches of mercury but in Europe it will be in millimeters of mercury or hectopascals!

Composition and structure

The mixture of gases which surrounds the Earth in a flexible, elastic envelope is called the *atmosphere*; it extends to an upper limit of around 50 miles (80 km). Conventionally there are three layers which are of variable depth, depending where on the Earth's surface the measurement is taken (Figure 3.2). The most important, from an aviation point of view, is the *troposphere*. Reaching about 20 000 ft (6100 m) at the poles and 65 000 ft (19 800 m) at the equator, it is separated from the *stratosphere* by a boundary called the *tropopause*.

The phenomena collectively known as *weather* (activity such as clouds, precipitation, turbulence and winds) occurs within the troposphere, but temperature, pressure and humidity can be measured throughout the atmosphere. Most conventional passenger aircraft fly predominantly in the troposphere, and this layer is characterised by the presence of water vapour, a constant rate of decrease of temperature with increasing altitude (the *adiabatic lapse rate*), and the presence of large scale vertical air currents. Above the tropopause temperature no longer falls with increasing height.

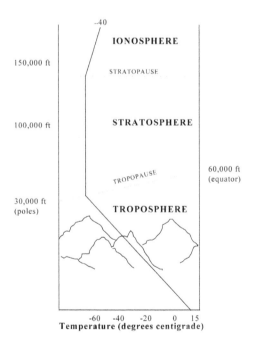

Figure 3.2   The three layers of the atmosphere

Air consists of matter. It therefore has the properties of mass and density (mass per unit volume) and, being a gas, it can be compressed. The major components are oxygen (21 per cent) and nitrogen (78 per cent). For practical purposes, the remaining minority gases can be ignored because they play no part in normal respiratory physiology. The gas proportions are kept constant throughout the troposphere because of the mixing actions of the vertical air currents. The content of water vapour will vary depending on location, altitude, and temperature, since warm air has a higher capacity to carry water vapour compared with cold air. Since the temperature is lower at altitude, air compressed and carried into the aircraft cabin is inevitably of low humidity.

The Gas Laws

The Gas Laws relate the physical properties of *Temperature Pressure* and *Volume* in a fixed mass (quantity) of gas. If you heat up a gas without allowing expansion its pressure will rise. If you increase the volume of (expand) a gas at constant temperature its pressure will fall. The laws that govern this behaviour are Charles Law and Boyle's Law:

Charles Law relates pressure to (absolute) temperature at constant volume:
$$P \propto T_{abs}$$
Boyle's Law relates pressure to volume at constant temperature and is illustrated in Figure 3.3:
$$P \propto \frac{1}{V}$$

Combining these:
$$PV \propto T_{abs}$$

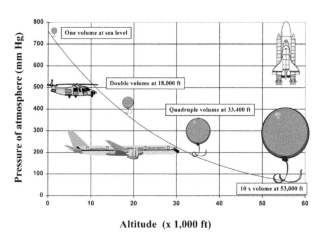

Figure 3.3   The pressure-volume relationship with altitude (dry gases)

Dalton's Law of Partial Pressure ('known to many, understood by few')

A fluency in the application of Dalton's Law is necessary for the understanding of altitude physiology, for it describes how the effects of a fall in pressure are reflected in a reduction in oxygen availability. Dalton's Law – first described over two hundred years ago – relates the ambient pressure (in whichever units you wish to measure it), the percentage by volume of your chosen gas in a mixture of gases, and the partial pressure of your chosen gas (in the same units in which it was measured). So for dry air at sea level, with percentages rounded off:

Gas	Composition % by volume	x total pressure	= partial pressure
Nitrogen	78%	760 mmHg	592.7 mmHg
Oxygen	21%	760 mmHg	159.4 mmHg
Inert gases	1%	760 mmHg	7.6 mmHg
Carbon dioxide	0.035%	760 mmHg	0.3 mmHg
All gases	100%	760 mmHg	total pressure

Put another way, the total pressure of a gas mix is the sum of the partial pressures of the constituents.

Dalton's Law is important because gases are dissolved in fluids in proportion to the partial pressure at the fluid/gas interface, and because the distribution of gases throughout the body is by diffusion down a partial pressure gradient.

Both Boyle's and Dalton's law are summarised in Figure 3.4.

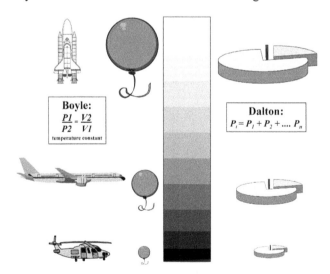

Figure 3.4   Boyle's and Dalton's Laws

Temperature and altitude

Solar radiation reaching the Earth's surface supplies approximately 1-2 kW per square metre (5 million horsepower per square mile). This is despite some losses due to reflection (as some energy is radiated back into space), and to absorption in the troposphere by the relatively dense air and clouds. The energy which reaches the surface causes it to warm up and allows further radiation back out to space. A balance is struck, so that atmospheric loss equates to solar gain and prevents the surface from continuously heating up.

Above the surface, temperature falls steadily with increasing altitude throughout the troposphere with a lapse rate of approximately 2°C (3.6°F) every 1000 ft (305 m). This is called the adiabatic lapse rate, since adiabatic cooling occurs as gases expand (a phenomenon which can be felt at the outlet of a gas cylinder as gas is released). Equilibration of atmospheric loss and solar gain cause temperature in the stratosphere to be constant. Since the tropopause is higher at the equator, stratospheric temperatures are lower here than at the poles.

Figure 3.5 shows how the position of the sun relative to the Earth's surface will concentrate or spread the solar energy. The subsequent uneven heating results in a vertical circulation pattern of air movement from the equator to the poles (Figure 3.6) forming the basis of the world's weather.

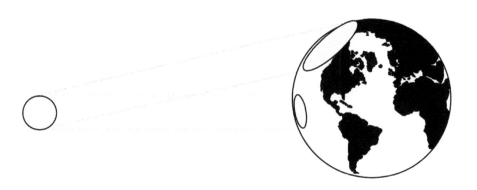

Figure 3.5   The position of the sun relative to the Earth's surface

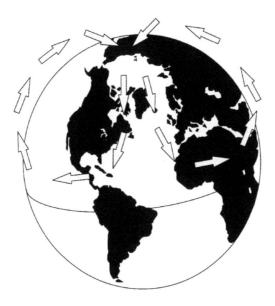

Figure 3.6   Patterns of air movement caused by vertical air currents

Turbulence

The amount and intensity of turbulence depends on the stability of the air mass in which the aircraft is flying. It may be caused by thermal activity (convective currents of warm air rising from an area of surface which is warmer than its surroundings), wind shear (a change in wind speed at different heights), the lifting of warm air over cold (a weather front), downdrafts from large cumulus type clouds (especially cumulo-nimbus), and the uplift of air over hills, mountains and other irregular terrain. The wake of other aircraft can also cause turbulence, occasionally enough for following small aircraft to lose control. Turbulence is also related to wind speed and gust strength; even small obstacles near the ground can generate turbulence in inclement weather.

Ionising radiation

Cosmic radiation is composed of energy sources which originate from outside the solar system (galactic radiation) and from our own sun (solar radiation). The former is of much higher energy and produces a steady predictable flow of particles. The Earth's magnetic field offers considerable protection at the equator by deflecting much of the radiation, but this effect diminishes to zero at the poles. Further protection is offered by absorption of low energy particles and secondary cosmic rays (produced from the collision of high energy particles with gas molecules) by atmospheric molecules. Background radiation therefore increases with altitude. At a high cruising altitude (60 000 ft/18 300 m), background radiation is about twice that of conventional aircraft flying at 40 000 ft/ 12 200 m. The total dose received, though, is likely to be less because of the much faster ground speed, and therefore shortened flight time, of flight at high altitude.

Production of solar radiation is increased by sun spots (solar flares) and, although generally of lower intensity than galactic radiation, is less predictable and can occasionally be intense. However, expert opinion considers there to be negligible risk to aircrew, let alone to occasional flyers. The annual maximum recommended dose for passengers (1 mSv) equates to about 100 hours of flight in an aircraft such as the supersonic Concorde, or long-haul transpolar travel (where atmospheric protection is minimal), or about 200 hours of subsonic transequatorial flying. Aircrew are limited to 20 mSv (the recommended total annual dose for workers exposed to ionising radiation). This is highly unlikely to be exceeded by aeromedical crew.

Ozone

When ultra-violet rays from solar radiation hit the atmosphere, ozone (triatomic oxygen, O_3) is formed from normal molecular oxygen (O_2). This occurs above 50 000 ft (15 240 m), with maximal concentration found at about 100 000 ft (30 480 m). Ozone, even in small quantities, is a highly toxic oxidising agent. Fortunately, it is extremely unstable and is rapidly dissociated by heat; in effect, it is largely converted back to diatomic oxygen as it passes through the engine compressors en route to the interior of the pressure cabin. Although it is not considered to be a significant hazard to aviators, recent studies have demonstrated cabin concentrations in excess of the exposure standards, and future aircraft may well be fitted with catalytic converters.

Conversion between units of pressure

One atmosphere:

760 millimeters of mercury (or Torr)	mmHg
29.92 inches of mercury	inHg
10 meters of sea water	msw
1013.2 millibars	mb
1013.2 hectopascals	hPa
101.32 kilopascals	kPa
14.7 pounds per square inch	psi

Orders of magnitude

pico	nano	micro	milli	(ten)	kilo	mega	giga
10^{-12}	10^{-9}	10^{-6}	10^{-3}	10	10^{3}	10^{6}	10^{9}

References

Birch, N.H. and Bramson, A.E. (1979) 'Meteorology', in *Flight Briefing for Pilots 4 (Associated Ground Subjects)*, Pitman: London.

Boyes, L. (1981) *Pilot's Weather Guide*, TAB Books: Philadelphia.

Campbell, R.D. (1981) 'Aviation Meteorology' in *Ground Training for the Private Pilot Licence (Manual Two)*, Granada: London.

Fitzgerald, B.P. (1973) *Weather in Action*, Methuen Educational: London.

Harding, R.M and F.J. Mills (1993) 'Special Forms of Flight', in *Aviation Medicine (3rd Ed.)*, BMJ: London.

Chapter 4

The Physiological Effects of Altitude

T. Martin and M. Glanfield

The important effects of altitude

On climbing through the atmosphere, although the composition of air remains constant, both pressure and density decline. Effectively this means that fewer oxygen molecules are available for physiological use. More than 90 per cent of oxygen used by the body is required for the production of energy-rich adenosine triphosphate (ATP). The oxidation of carbohydrates in the glycolytic pathway and carboxylic acid (Kreb's) cycle yields 38 molecules of ATP per molecule of glucose. Other molecules (fats and proteins) are oxidized in associated pathways. Without oxygen, ATP is produced by anaerobic catabolism with the subsequent production of lactic acid. This is an inefficient process resulting in only two molecules of ATP per molecule of glucose. In addition, accumulation of lactic acid in most tissues limits cellular activity. Beyond 10 000 ft (3005 m), without acclimatization, the paucity of oxygen becomes problematic. This deficiency of oxygen is called *hypobaric hypoxia*. At the same time, gases trapped within body cavities will expand. The effects of increasing volume cause stress on biological tissues. Normal passengers and crew may feel some discomfort, but serious complications are rare. Patients with injured tissues, or gas in ectopic locations or in excessive amounts, may suffer painful and even life-threatening complications unless measures are taken to minimize or alleviate the volume change.

Finally, for completeness, *aviator's decompression illness* (DCI) must be mentioned even though it is extremely rare below 25 000 ft (7620 m). Like caisson disease in divers, the clinical features are thought to be due to the formation of nitrogen gas bubbles which lodge and cause symptoms in either the joints (*the bends*), the lungs (*the chokes*), the skin *(the creeps)* or in the spinal cord or other parts of the central nervous system *(the staggers)*. DCI is highly unlikely to be experienced during aeromedical transportation unless the aircraft suffers a rapid decompression emergency above 25 000 ft (7620 m) or extra nitrogen has been loaded into the tissues as would occur with recent compressed air (SCUBA) diving.

Normal respiratory physiology

Alveolar air

Alveolar gas is air saturated with water at body temperature and contains carbon dioxide (CO_2). Since CO_2 is soluble and diffuses readily, the partial pressure of CO_2 in blood leaving the pulmonary capillaries is effectively in equilibrium with that of alveolar gas.

Pulmonary ventilation (the depth and rate of breathing) is automatically regulated to keep pace with CO_2 production and under normal circumstances the alveolar partial pressure of CO_2 ($PACO_2$) is constant at around 5.3 kPa (40 mmHg). In contrast, because of normal physiological ventilation/perfusion inequalities, the arterial partial pressure of oxygen is slightly lower than that of alveolar gas. The partial pressures of the components of the alveolar gas mixture at sea level are:

Nitrogen	76.0	kPa	570	mmHg
Oxygen	13.7	kPa	103	mmHg
Carbon dioxide	5.3	kPa	40	mmHg
Water	6.3	kPa	47	mmHg
Total *(ambient pressure)*	101.3	kPa	760	mmHg

The total ambient pressure at 8000 ft (the maximum equivalent altitude in a pressurized aircraft) is 75.3 kPa (565 mmHg) and the partial pressure of oxygen in dry air would therefore be 21 per cent of 75.3, that is, 15.8 kPa (119 mmHg). However, within the alveoli, the partial pressures are:

Nitrogen	55.4	kPa	416	mmHg
Oxygen	8.7	kPa	65	mmHg
Carbon dioxide	4.9	kPa	37	mmHg
Water	6.3	kPa	47	mmHg
Total *(ambient pressure)*	75.3	kPa	565	mmHg

Since alveolar gas is fully saturated, the vapour pressure of water remains a constant 6.3 kPa (47 mmHg) at body temperature at all altitudes. The partial pressure of CO_2, however, is reduced because of the hypoxic drive to increase pulmonary ventilation, effectively washing CO_2 out of the lungs.

Confusion often arises over the difference between alveolar and arterial partial pressures (also called tensions). Figure 4.1 shows how the partial pressure of oxygen (PO_2) varies between the ambient atmosphere and delivery to the tissues.

Oxygen carriage

Although some oxygen is dissolved within the plasma, most is carried in combination with hemoglobin (Hb) in erythrocytes. The maximum amount of oxygen that can be combined with 1 g of Hb is 1.39 ml. Assuming 15 g Hb per 100 ml of blood, the oxygen carrying capacity is:

$$1.39 \times 15 = 20.8 \text{ ml} / 100 \text{ ml blood.}$$

The ratio of the actual quantity of oxygen combined with Hb and the oxygen carrying capacity is called the *oxygen saturation* of Hb, where:

$$\text{oxygen saturation} = \frac{\text{amount of oxygen combined with Hb}}{\text{oxygen carrying capacity}} \times 100\%$$

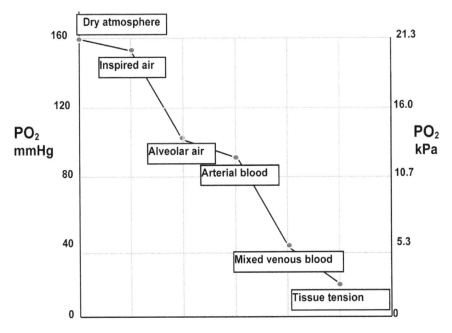

Figure 4.1   The oxygen partial pressure gradient from dry atmosphere to minimum pressure level

The relationship between oxygen saturation and oxygen tension (partial pressure of oxygen in the blood) is described by the sigmoid shaped oxygen dissociation curve (Figure 4.2). This characteristic shape is of great importance. The flat upper portion ensures that moderate variations of alveolar oxygen tension around the norm of 13.7 kPa (103 mmHg) at sea level, and in particular a small degree of hypoxia, have little effect on the amount of oxygen combined with Hb in arterial blood (that is, its saturation). The steep portion at lower oxygen tensions ensures optimal dissociation (delivery) of oxygen from Hb into the tissues. A large drop in saturation (as a large quantity of oxygen is given up to the tissues) results in only a small fall in tension. This is important in maintaining oxygen tension at an appropriate level for normal tissue function.

The shape is not influenced by the concentration of Hb, but the position of the curve may be shifted left or right by disturbances in acidity (pH), arterial CO_2 tension ($PaCO_2$), and temperature. Tissue that works hard will produce hydrogen ions, CO_2 and heat. A fall, therefore, in pH, and/or a rise in $PaCO_2$, and temperature will shift the curve to the right and thereby increase the amount of oxygen given up by the blood at a given oxygen tension. The net effect is improved oxygen delivery to the tissues.

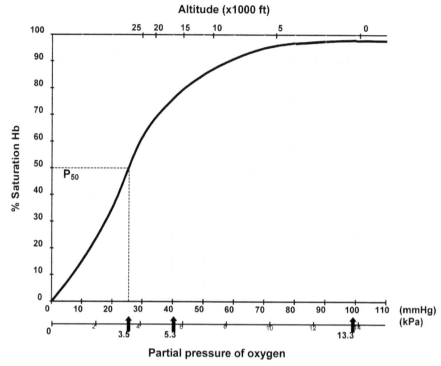

Figure 4.2   The oxygen dissociation curve at 37°C and pH 7.4

Hypoxia

Hypoxia is oxygen deficiency in body tissues sufficient to cause impairment of physiological function. The most relevant type of hypoxia in the flight environment is *hypobaric (hypoxic) hypoxia* which may become apparent in normal individuals above 10 000 ft (3050 m), in the so-called physiological deficient zone. Without supplemental oxygen, blood oxygen saturation at sea level of 98 per cent will decline to about 90 per cent at 10 000 ft (3050 m) and 65 per cent at 20 000 ft (6100 m). Although hypoxic hypoxia is caused by an inadequate partial pressure of oxygen in inspired air (and inadequate gas exchange at the alveolar-capillary membrane), it is also experienced by those with a ventilation/perfusion defect, or with an airway obstruction. Since these patients are hypoxic at sea level, they will clearly be at increased risk of hypoxic damage during flight.

Other forms of hypoxia will also exacerbate the complications of hypobaric hypoxia. *Hypemic (anemic) hypoxia* is caused by a reduction in the oxygen carrying capacity of the blood. This may be due to anemia, hypovolemia, carbon monoxide poisoning, heavy smoking, or congenital or drug induced methemaglobinemia. *Stagnant (circulatory) hypoxia* is oxygen deficiency due to reduction in tissue perfusion, as occurs when cardiac output fails to satisfy tissue requirements (cardiogenic shock), after long periods of positive pressure breathing, or from venous pooling, arterial spasm, or occlusion of a blood vessel. *Histotoxic hypoxia* is the inability of the body tissues to utilize available oxygen, for instance with cyanide poisoning which uncouples oxidative phosphorylation.

Signs and symptoms of hypoxia

There is considerable variation in the effects of hypoxia between individuals; the speed and order of appearance of signs and symptoms, and their severity, depend on the intensity of the hypoxic stimulus. The most important factors determining this intensity will be the altitude to which the individual is exposed, the rate of ascent, and the time at that altitude. In addition, extremes of ambient temperature and physical activity of the individual may make demands on available oxygen, as will a number of other personal factors. Over and above pathological conditions (even minor infections), there are many influences on an individual's tolerance to hypoxia. These include personal fitness, previous acclimatization, metabolic rate, diet, nutrition, emotions, fatigue, some medications, and alcohol. Transport in a pressurized cabin will reduce the potential for hypoxic complications but medical crew must be aware of predisposing medical conditions which can exacerbate hypoxia at altitude. These pre-existing conditions include any which interfere with gaseous exchange, or oxygen carriage, delivery, or demand. In addition consideration must be given to the effects of the mild hypobaric hypoxia in a pressurized cabin of an aircraft at altitude upon 'organs at risk' such as ischemic myocardium, a poorly healing lower leg wound, or brain tissue in the aftermath of a cerebrovascular accident (CVA).

In the aeromedical transport scenario significant hypobaric hypoxia should not occur in a fit person as the cabin altitude will normally be maintained below 10 000 ft (3050 m). Indeed the cabin altitude in commercial passenger carrying aircraft should not exceed 8000 ft (2440 m). However cabin depressurization can occur, and all those involved in inflight care must be able to recognize the symptoms and signs of hypoxia, which are likely to be insidious in onset. These signs and symptoms in otherwise healthy individuals can be predicted from knowledge of the sensitivity of different tissue to a reduction in oxygen tension:

Central nervous system   Neurones are extremely sensitive to lack of oxygen, especially in the so-called higher areas of the brain (those responsible for judgement, self-criticism, concentration and mental tasks). Signs of cerebral hypoxia may begin when the alveolar PO_2 falls to 6.7-8 kPa (50-60 mmHg). Cerebral blood flow is affected by the partial pressures of both oxygen and carbon dioxide. Hyperventilation (a normal response to hypoxia) will induce hypocapnia sufficient enough to cause cerebral vasoconstriction and decreased perfusion. A shift in pH from 7.4 to 7.1 will reduce the cerebral blood flow by half. When arterial PO_2 falls to 6 kPa (45 mmHg), a hypoxically driven vasoconstriction also occurs. Below 6 kPa the reverse happens, and increased cerebral blood flow results from the vasodilatory effects of extreme hypoxia attempting to offset the vasoconstriction caused by hyperventilatory response (hypocapnia).

Initial central nervous system (CNS) signs and symptoms may not be recognized. Early signs include loss of attention, reasoning skills and judgement, a sense of detachment and deterioration in visual fields and colour vision. A feeling of warmth is common as are paraesthesiae of the hands, feet or lips resulting from the inevitable respiratory alkalosis. The ability to perform fine motor tasks is also impaired. Progressive mental confusion, diminished sensory input, and unconsciousness will supervene if exposure to hypoxia remains untreated. The arterial PO_2 at which unconsciousness occurs varies between 2.7 and 4.7 kPa (20 and 35 mmHg), depending on cerebral perfusion (that is, on the balance of hypercapnia and hypoxia). Neuronal death begins when tissue PO_2 reaches 2 kPa (15 mmHg). The degree of brain damage to the individual, and whether or not it is reversible, will depend on the extent and location of areas exposed to sub-critical oxygen tensions.

Respiratory system At about 5000 ft (1524 m), the initial respiratory response to hypoxia is an increase in the rate and depth of respiration. The maximum response occurs at 22 000 ft (6710 m) when minute volume (MV) will be almost doubled. Most of this increase is secondary to changes in tidal volume rather than respiratory rate and is, in effect, a balance between the increase in MV caused by the chemoreceptor response to hypoxia and the decrease in MV caused by inhibition of the respiratory centers. Although an overall increase in MV will increase oxygen demand and lead to production of excess CO_2, hyperventilation will result in a gross reduction of the partial pressure of carbon dioxide. This, in turn, causes a respiratory alkalosis and a shift of the oxygen dissociation curve to the left, increasing the affinity of hemoglobin for oxygen. The net effect is impaired oxygen delivery to the tissues, since a lower PO_2 is needed to bind a given amount of oxygen (that is, it remains bound at the lower oxygen tensions found at tissue level).

Hypoxia significant enough to lower saturation below 80 per cent will cause vasoconstriction of the pulmonary vascular bed, resulting in an elevation of pulmonary arterial pressure and an increased workload on the right side of the heart. Acidosis is also a potent pulmonary vascular vasoconstrictor. Supplemental oxygen may relieve hypoxia, but may simultaneously decrease alveolar ventilation, thereby increasing acidosis and worsening pulmonary vasoconstriction.

Cardiovascular system The cardiovascular system is relatively resistant to hypoxia compared to the respiratory and central nervous systems. Heart rate will increase at altitude, rising to 15 per cent greater than the sea level value at 15 000 ft (4570 m), and will approximately double at 25 000 ft (7620 m). Although stroke volume (SV) remains unchanged, cardiac output (SV × heart rate) will increase accordingly.

Vasodilation occurs in most areas, resulting in a fall in peripheral resistance. Physiological reflexes will maintain or elevate the systolic pressure, and pulse pressure will therefore widen. Mean arterial pressure remains constant.

As these effects continue, the increase in cardiac activity will demand more oxygen and, if these needs are not met, the already hypoxic myocardium will respond with a decrease heart rate, failure of contractility (reduction in SV) and dysrhythmias.

Physiological stages of hypoxia

Up to 10 000 ft (3050 m)   Sometimes called the *indifferent stage*, typically the oxygen saturation will range from 90-98 per cent in normal individuals. Although there will be no awareness of symptoms and no noticeable impairment, at 5000 ft (1520 m) a 10 per cent reduction in night vision may be detected and performance at novel tasks may be impaired.

10 000 – 15 000 ft (3050 – 4550 m)   Oxygen saturation in an uncompromised person will be between 80-90 per cent. An increase in respiratory rate, heart rate, and systolic blood pressure help to offset the decrease in oxygen carriage. These effects have led to this phase being called the *compensatory stage.* Normal individuals may remain asymptomatic, but many will begin to experience nausea, dizziness, lethargy, headache, fatigue, and apprehension. Poor judgement, decreased efficiency, impaired coordination, and increased irritability may become obvious after a 10 to 15 minutes exposure at 12 000 – 15 000 ft (3660–4550 m).

15 000 – 20 000 ft (4550 – 6100 m)   Oxygen saturation will be between 70-80 per cent. Physiological mechanisms can no longer compensate for the oxygen deficiency and even individuals at rest are aware of the hypoxic symptoms. This is sometimes called the *disturbance stage,* during which subjective symptoms of air hunger, headache, amnesia, decreased level of consciousness, and nausea are more pronounced. The senses are diminished with impairment of visual acuity due to blurring or tunneling of vision, and loss of color clarity. There may be weakness, numbness, tingling and decreased sensation of touch and pain. Reaction time, short-term memory, speech and handwriting may be greatly impaired, and slowed mentation makes calculations unreliable. Behavior may appear aggressive, belligerent, euphoric, over confident or morose, and impaired muscular coordination makes delicate or fine movements impossible. Despite a noticeable increase in respiratory rate, central cyanosis may be obvious and muscular spasm and tetany may result from hypocapnia. Any physical exertion at this stage will markedly exacerbate the signs and symptoms, and may lead rapidly to unconsciousness.

Above 20 000 ft (6100 m)   Oxygen saturation drops to 60-70 per cent in this *critical stage.* Previous symptoms that may have been overlooked can no longer be ignored as higher mental functions and neuromuscular control decline rapidly. In addition to the features of the disturbance stage, objective findings now escalate to include myoclonic jerking of the upper limbs, grand-mal type seizures, and, often with little or no warning, unconsciousness. Unless the hypoxia is relieved immediately, irreversible cerebral damage will increase, and death will shortly follow.

Treatment of hypoxia

In planning aeromedical missions, prevention of hypoxia must always be regarded as of paramount importance. A thorough understanding of the patient's clinical condition and of the demands made upon him by the flight will help medical crew to evaluate oxygen and pressure requirements for the journey. Recognition of signs and symptoms is the next priority. The ability to adequately monitor the patient during transport (for example, electrocardiography, pulse oximetry and end-tidal capnography) may be critical. It is also advisable for aeromedical personnel to monitor cabin altitude, or at least to be in communication with the flight crew, so that any drastic changes do not go unnoticed.

Supplemental oxygen remains the key to treatment. If, despite additional oxygen, evidence of hypoxia persists, the aeromedical escort must consider depletion or malfunction of the onboard oxygen system, deterioration in the patient's condition, or that the patient cannot tolerate the change in barometric pressure. The latter may require aircraft descent, or an increase in cabin pressurization.

Supplemental oxygen

The goal of oxygen therapy is to increase the alveolar concentration of oxygen to meet the demands of tissue metabolism. Portable pulse oximetry can give medical crew valuable information about the response to oxygen therapy, but its limitations must be understood. One such limitation is that oximetry gives no information on oxygen carriage. Taken to the extreme, if a patient had only one red blood cell, and that cell was 100 per cent saturated, every time it passed the oximetry probe, the machine would read 100 per cent! Clearly this patient is not carrying enough oxygen (since the carriage mechanism is deficient) but this is not reflected in the saturation measurement. For this reason, it is inadvisable to base the FiO_2 and/or ventilator settings strictly upon pulse oximetry. It is essential to calculate the patient's individual oxygen requirements.

Nonetheless, pulse oximetry can be invaluable. Sensible practice is to measure the patient's oxygen saturation (SpO_2) at point of collection, whether in the overseas hospital or, in the case of an out-patient, wherever the patient is staying. This will serve three functions. It will be a baseline reading against which inflight oxygen delivery can be titrated. Used in conjunction with other information it will give a useful indication of the likelihood that inflight supplemental oxygen will be needed. And finally (in particular for those cases escorted by a nurse on a scheduled flight) it may give a timely warning that the case should not be transported at that time or by that means.

To ensure maximum oxygen carriage at all altitudes, one might ask why not deliver 100 per cent FiO_2 throughout the entire journey? Quite simply, as well as being uneconomical, and the weight penalty incurred by carrying unnecessary oxygen cylinders, 100 per cent inspired oxygen over long periods is irritant and may be toxic to the respiratory tract. It may also contribute to delayed otic barotrauma.

These complications are irrelevant during primary missions, but for long haul flights 100 per cent FiO_2 should be used only when clinically necessary.

The minimal acceptable oxygen concentration might arguably be that which would give an alveolar PO_2 equivalent to that found at 8000 ft (2440 m), since normal individuals are unaware of any symptoms at that altitude. However, patients will generally have higher oxygen demands because of their pathology or treatment. The aim must therefore be to maintain alveolar PO_2 at their sea level equivalent, probably in the range 10.7 - 13.3 kPa (80 - 100 mmHg).

For patients who are hypoxic at ground level, a recent blood gas result is useful to help calculate altitude equivalence. Using Figure 4.3, the patient's arterial PO_2 can be used to find the equivalent altitude (for normal individuals). If the patient's location is significantly higher than sea level, the height should be deducted from this equivalent altitude.

The resultant final figure (the sea level compensated equivalent altitude) can be plotted on Figure 4.4 to give the fractional inspired oxygen needed to maintain an alveolar PO_2 of 13.3 kPa (100 mmHg).

When an arterial PO_2 is not available, clinical acumen and an understanding of the symptoms and signs of hypoxia will be the best guide. A knowledge of the FiO_2 at the time the arterial sample was collected is essential and, even then, this calculation can only be approximate. Medical crew must err on the side of caution. Constant reappraisal of the patient is essential, and FiO_2 should be titrated to match clinical and monitored responses.

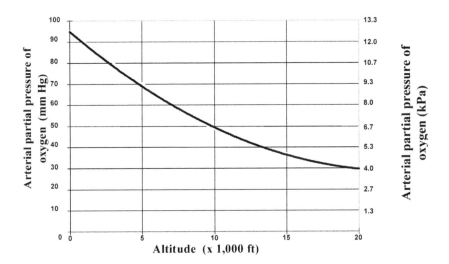

Figure 4.3 **Arterial PO_2 up to 20 000 ft (6100 m), breathing air**

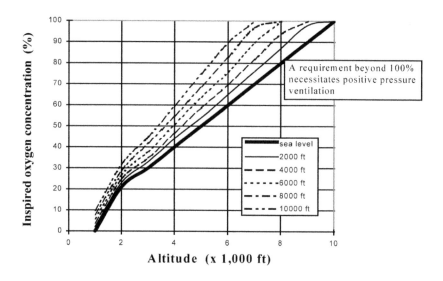

Figure 4.4   The concentration of oxygen required in the inspired gas to maintain alveolar PO$_2$ of 13.3 kPa (100 mmHg)

Gaseous expansion

There are several organs in the body which contain some form of gas. They may be filled with saturated air (in the middle ear cavities and paranasal sinuses), alveolar gas (saturated air enriched with carbon dioxide in the lungs) or a mixture of air and gases generated by digestive processes (in the gut). These cavities communicate with the ambient atmosphere with varying degrees of efficiency and the gas contained within them obeys Boyle's Law, that is, they expand as the ambient pressure decreases (Figure 4.5 shows the ideal relationship for dry gas).

However, Boyle's Law relates to dry gas. Gas in body cavities is saturated with water vapor at body temperature which exerts a constant vapor pressure of 6.3 kPa (47 mmHg). The net effect is that the greater the altitude, the greater the magnitude of gaseous expansion, as described by the modified Boyle's equation:

$$RGE = (P_i - 47) \div (P_f - 47)$$

where
RGE = relative gas expansion
P_i = initial pressure (mmHg)
P_f = final pressure (mmHg)

If there is unrestricted communication between the gas filled cavities and the outside atmosphere, expansion will cause no difficulty or discomfort. Conversely, if the increase in volume cannot be vented, stretching of the walls of the cavities causes a local rise of internal pressure which may be significantly painful.

This takes on a new significance when gas is ectopically located, such as in postoperative patients, or in those who have had gas or air introduced after an injury or as part of a diagnostic procedure. Medical crew should also consider the effects of gaseous expansion on patients with ileus or gastric distension, and on items of medical equipment .

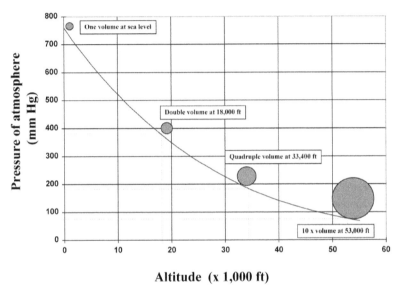

Altitude (x 1,000 ft)

Figure 4.5   Relationship between gas volume and pressure at altitude

Barotitis media (Otic Barotrauma)

The middle ear is connected to the nasopharynx and external atmosphere via the eustachian tube and is separated from the outer ear by the tympanic membrane. The eustachian tube usually functions as a one way valve allowing gas to escape, but not return to the middle ear. Gas expands in the middle ear behind the tympanic membrane as altitude increases. It escapes through the eustachian tube every 500–1000 ft (1525–3050 m), or when there is a pressure differential of approximately 2 kPa (15 mmHg). This equalization of pressures between the middle ear and the surrounding atmosphere is felt as a 'popping' as air passes out of the eustachian tube. On descent from altitude, the gas within the middle ear contracts, creating a negative pressure within the middle ear and pulling the tympanic membrane inward. Under normal circumstances, the eustachian tube will not allow the passive movement of air into the middle ear. However, the eustachian tube can be actively opened, allowing equalization with the middle ear by elevating the pressure in the nasopharynx, such as by swallowing or the Frenzel maneuver ('pinch the nose and blow'), or by moving the jaw to open the normally collapsed entrance to the eustachian tubes.

Any inflammation of the mucosa, such as an upper respiratory tract infection, allergy, or sinusitis, may cause obstruction, and equalization may be impossible. This is especially important in children who have small diameter tubes which easily obstruct with minor inflammation. The severity of symptoms will depend upon the individual's initial condition, the rate of ascent or descent, and individual compensatory mechanisms. A sensation of fullness in the ears may occur as equalization takes place during ascent. If pressures are not equalized, hearing loss will occur as a result of decreased vibration of the eardrum and severe pain, tenderness, vertigo, nausea, perforation of the eardrum and bleeding can occur during either the climb-out or approach, although problems are most often encountered on descent because the tympanic membrane is drawn inwards by the reduction of gas volume in the middle ear.

Treatment is directed toward the equalization of pressure between the middle ear and the atmosphere before symptoms become severe. Equalization may be accomplished by yawning, swallowing, or performing the Frenzel maneuver. A topical vasoconstrictor (decongestant) nasal spray may be beneficial when used about 15 minutes before descent. Sleeping patients should be awakened five minutes before descent, so they can swallow more frequently, and infants may be given a bottle during take-off and landing. However, while this reduces the likelihood of barotitis media, it may increase the incidence of gastrointestinal distress after take-off due to increased swallowing of air.

A slow descent from altitude will minimize the incidence and severity of symptoms. If descent is too rapid, the pilot may have to increase altitude again to allow equalization of pressure in the middle ear before attempting to descend again.

Barosinusitis (Sinus barotrauma)

Normally air can pass in and out of the sinus cavities freely and the only evidence of equilibration is a slight tickling sensation. If the mucous membrane lining of the sinuses is swollen, air may be trapped and will expand as altitude increases. The Frenzel maneuver is not effective in opening the blocked sinuses and symptoms soon develop. These may include severe pain in the cheek or forehead, lacrimation, and epistaxis. The treatment for barosinusitis is similar to the treatment of barotitis media, with the most effective being the use of a decongestant nasal spray and returning temporarily to a higher altitude.

Barodontalgia

Air trapped in dental fillings, decay, abscesses or crowns may result in a severe toothache, most commonly experienced during ascent. Management, although probably impossible for the urgent aeromedical transport patient, should primarily be preventative dental care. The only treatment, if it occurs in flight, is analgesia. Descent to lower altitude when pain is severe may be considered, if logistically possible, and will certainly alleviate symptoms while waiting for analgesic medication to take effect.

Abdominal distension

The stomach and intestines normally contain up to a liter of gas. Carbonated beverages, gas-producing foods, large meals, air swallowing and pre-existing gastrointestinal problems (especially gut infections) may all increase the amount of gas in the gut. As gas expands on ascent, an individual may experience feelings of abdominal pressure, pain referred from diaphragmatic irritation, shortness of breath or hyperventilation from diaphragmatic splinting, nausea or even vomiting. Significant distension may result in venous pooling. In addition, tachycardia, hypotension, and syncope may result from a vasovagal response to severe pain.

Prevention is the key to avoiding these problems. Both patients and crew would be wise to avoid gassy drinks and large meals prior to flight, especially those containing gas-producing foods. In general the most notorious gas-producers are dried peas and beans, pulses, cabbage, cauliflower, cucumber, turnip, sprouts and high roughage foods such as celery and bran. Loose non-restrictive clothing may also be of benefit, and sufferers should not be modest at venting expanding gas to relieve discomfort. Patients with a bowel obstruction, ileus, or recent abdominal surgery must have a patent free-draining nasogastric tube in place prior to transport.

The respiratory system

The lungs freely communicate with the ambient atmosphere and, except in the rare circumstance of emergency rapid decompression, no problem will be encountered with pressure equalization. However, special attention should be paid to the patient with suspected or proven pneumothorax. Unless adequately vented, expansion of the ectopic gas will cause further collapse of pulmonary tissue at altitude. Patients can be safely transported once a patent chest drainage tube is in place. However, careful monitoring for evidence of hypoxia or occlusion of the chest tube throughout the journey is essential. Any patient who is artificially ventilated must be closely monitored for the possible development of a tension pneumothorax.

A pulmonary bulla will usually communicate with the (open) respiratory tract, but often through a narrow opening. Adverse distension or possible rupture of the bulla will therefore depend upon the rate of reduction of pressure as well as the ratio between the size of the bulla and the diameter of its opening. This should be considered when transporting a patient with chronic lung disease.

Cabin pressurization

An ideal aircraft cabin might be expected to have an internal pressure set to one atmosphere (101.3 kPa, 760 mm Hg), but the penalties (weight of the cabin, and pressurization equipment, the power requirements, and the risks of large pressure differentials across the cabin wall) would be insurmountable. A compromise cabin pressure between 6000 and 8000 ft allows the occupants to breathe air in comfort, and with minimal risk of explosive decompression due to structural failure.

Pressurization is made possible by the indrawing of air from the outside. It is compressed by engine-driven compressors or tapped upstream of jet combustion chambers. It is then delivered to the cabin where the pressure is maintained by controlling flow out of the aircraft. Air delivery is automatically controlled so that the cabin pressure differential usually remains at a constant value over a range of aircraft altitudes (*differential control*). The air delivery system also allows thermal regulation and humidity control.

Rapid decompression

Rapid decompression is an unusual event in civilian aircraft, but may occur if the cabin wall is breached, or with malfunction of the pressure control system. Pressure initially falls rapidly, and then more slowly as internal pressure equilibrates with the lower ambient pressure outside. The rate of decompression is affected by the volume of the cabin, the size of the defect, and the difference between the initial cabin pressure and the outside air pressure. The injurious effects on the aircraft occupants are:

Air blast　Until air pressures equilibrate, the velocity of air flow around the defect will be great. Dust, debris and loose articles will be sucked by the wind flow. If the defect is large enough, or the pressure differential great, even large items and people not securely strapped to their seats may be moved. Once equilibration occurs, if the defect is large, occupants sitting nearby may suffer wind burns, as was seen in the Aloha Boeing 727 incident in 1988.

Cold　The eventual cabin temperature will depend on the size of the defect, the outside air temperature, and the aircraft's altitude and speed. The rapid expansion of air as it equilibrates to a lower pressure also reduces its temperature.

Fogging　Cold air holds less water vapor than warm air. Sudden cooling of air as it expands therefore causes fogging as water vapor condenses out of the cooling air mass. This condensation fog clears quickly once equilibration of pressure is reached.

Gaseous expansion If emergency decompression occurs while the glottis is closed, the lungs may suffer barotrauma as trapped gas expands rapidly. This may result in simple or tension pneumothorax or, more seriously, arterial gas embolisation.

Decompression illness (DCI) The incidence of DCI is insignificant below 30 000 ft and is virtually unheard of in civilian aircraft. However, its occurrence is more likely in occupants who are ill, have been recently injured, or who are overweight.

Hypoxia Hypoxic effects are likely to be rapid in onset with catastrophic hypoxemia occurring within seconds if rapid decompression equilibrates above 30 000 ft. Above this altitude, alveolar PO_2 is lower than venous PO_2 with the result that oxygen passes out of the blood into the lungs and is expired with each breath. It is therefore essential for crew, passengers, and patients alike to access an emergency oxygen supply as soon as possible. Although unconsciousness may supervene within half a minute (Table 4.1), mental impairment will occur even more quickly, and sensible reasoned actions may become impossible.

Table 4.1   The time of useful consciousness up to 36 000 ft (10 930 m)

Altitude (ft/m)	Time of useful consciousness (s)
25 000/7620	270
30 000/9100	145
36 000/10 930	71

Source: 'Hypoxia and Hyperventilation', in Ernsting J., Nicholson A.N. and D.J. Rainford (eds) *Aviation Medicine* (3rd Ed.), Arnold: London.

The need for sea level cabin altitude

For an aircraft, especially a jet, to travel at or near sea level there is a great penalty in range, comfort, fuel burn and speed. In order to maintain cabin pressurization at the sea level equivalent, the aircraft may have to fly at 15 000 ft instead of 35 000 ft. However, there are certain medical conditions in which any depressurization may have a severe effect. Mention has already been made of a high FiO_2 requirement at sea level, and of inadequately drained pneumothorax. Ectopic gas in the cranial cavity or eye will be unable to expand with a fall in pressure, with consequent compression of adjacent tissue. Finally decompression illness, unless fully resolved, may recur at altitude. The advice of a diving medicine specialist should be obtained if there is any doubt about the wisdom of repatriation by air.

References

Blumen, I.J. (1995) 'Altitude physiology and the stresses of flight', *Air Med J.* **14** (2):87-99.

Dobie, T.G. (1972) *Aeromedical Handbook for Aircrew*, AGARDograph No 154.

Harding, R.M. (2003) 'Hypoxia and Hyperventilation', in Ernsting J., Nicholson A.N., and D.J. Rainford (eds) *Aviation Medicine* (3rd Ed.), Arnold: London.

Gradwell, D.P. (2003) 'Prevention of Hypoxia', in Ernsting J., Nicholson A.N., and D.J. Rainford (eds) *Aviation Medicine* (3rd Ed.), Arnold: London.

Harding, R.M. and F.J. Mills (1993) 'Problems of Altitude', in Harding R.M. and F.J. Mills (eds) *Aviation Medicine* (3rd Ed.), BMJ: London.

Lumb, A.B. (2000) 'Oxygen', in *Nunn's Applied Respiratory Physiology* (5th Ed.), Butterworth-Heinemann: London.

Macmillan, A.J.F. (2003) 'The Pressure Cabin', in Ernsting J., Nicholson A.N., and Rainford D.J. (eds) *Aviation Medicine* (3rd Ed.), Arnold: London.

Chapter 5

The Biodynamics of Flight

T. Martin and M. Glanfield

The effects of acceleration

Life within the gravitational envelope of the planet exposes us all to an acceleration directed towards the center of the Earth which has a magnitude of 32 ft/s² (9.81 m/s²). This gravitational pull, when acting on a mass, gives rise to the force we know as weight.[1] All life forms have evolved to operate in this '1 G' environment. However, modern means of transport can expose us to much greater accelerations which may have either physiological or pathological effects, depending on the duration and magnitude of the acceleration, its direction, and rate of application. Short duration accelerations (less than one second duration) may result in injury or death. Examples include forces experienced during crashes or ditching and, for the military pilot, operation of ejection seats, carrier deck catapults, and the opening shock of parachutes.

Long duration acceleration

Long duration accelerations in excess of 1 G add to the weight of objects and result in physiological changes as body organs and fluids obey Newton's third law of motion and respond with an equal and opposite reaction to the applied acceleration.

Under normal circumstances, occupants of passenger aircraft are likely to experience only mild or moderate accelerations compared with the aircrew of modern agile military aircraft. But, like fast-jet pilots in combat, two types of acceleration may be experienced:

Linear acceleration   Linear acceleration results from an increase or decrease in the rate of movement along a straight line (Figure 5.1). In minor form this will be encountered on take-off, and is also felt as the thrust of jet engines is reversed during the landing run of large passenger aircraft. No physiological consequences occur in the normal seated individual when the force is applied across the anteroposterior axis of the body (the actual direction depending on which way the occupant is seated).

---

1 One rotation of the earth takes almost 24 hours and the gravitational effect on everything on the planet depends on the centrifugal force experienced at the location of the object. Hence, an object weighs less at the equator than at the poles.

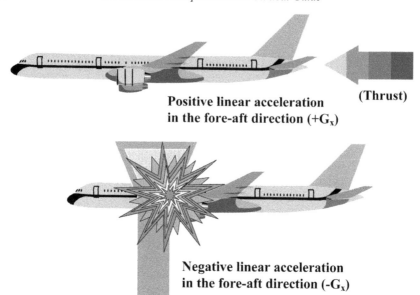

Positive linear acceleration   **(Thrust)**
in the fore-aft direction (+G$_x$)

Negative linear acceleration
in the fore-aft direction (-G$_x$)

Figure 5.1   Linear acceleration

Stretcher patients lying parallel to the long axis of the aircraft are at risk of shift of body organs and fluid volumes in response to the inertial forces of linear acceleration. There is some evidence that blood movement towards the lower extremities incites baroreceptor reflexes with subsequent transient tachycardia in normal subjects. It may be sensible to position patients with cardiac disease or hypovolemia with the head towards the back of the aircraft to improve myocardial perfusion as acceleration causes pooling of blood in the upper part of the body. For patients with fluid overload or head injury, it may be advantageous to position the patient's head toward the front of the aircraft so that acceleration acts to pool the blood in the lower extremities. For the head injured patient, this may reduce the risk of a transient increase in intracranial pressure (ICP) during take-off, but hard evidence for this speculation has not been demonstrated and some would argue that a foot first position is safer from a crash restraint point of view. In any case, the consequence of any short-term acceleration on take-off may be trivial in comparison with the longer duration 'nose up' or 'nose down' attitude of the aircraft during the climb-out or descent and approach to land. This attitude will vary with aircraft type. As it is usually impractical to change either the orientation of the patient in flight, or the tilt of the aircraft stretcher, careful consideration must be given to the 'head forward or feet forward' choice of position.

Buffeting is a sequence of irregular linear accelerations operating in the long axis of the seated occupant. It is often experienced when flying at high speed in turbulent conditions, especially through or under storm clouds, but it can be just as bad at low level, in hot climates and when flying over mountains. These rapidly alternating vertical accelerations may reach a magnitude of up to 3 G and will cause fatigue for all and anxiety to those who are apprehensive of flying. The buffeting may be sufficient to throw unsecured occupants against the cabin wall or furniture, and injuries may occur.

Clear air turbulence (CAT) is difficult to predict. It occurs above 30 000 ft (9100 m) in, as the name implies, clear skies, with none of the cloud warnings that are customary at lower altitudes. It is caused by vortices at the boundaries of the jet streams. These are winds that travel around the Earth in the upper troposphere and lower stratosphere at speeds in excess of 100 miles per hour (161 kph). CAT has been severe enough to cause structural failure of aircraft, and it is essential that crew and patients alike are firmly restrained in their seats or stretchers. Every effort must be made to reassure patients throughout this experience, which some will find most terrifying.

Radial acceleration   A change in direction of motion of the aircraft will result in a radial acceleration, effectively due to rotation about a distant point (Figure 5.2). The force acts outward from the center of a circular path but is perceived as an increase in weight by the occupant (that is, as an acceleration forcing the body into the seat or towards the aircraft floor). This feeling of 'heaviness' as an aircraft turns steeply is familiar to most travelers.

Acceleration is measured in G units (multiples of g, the acceleration due to gravity) which, by convention, is labeled G_z when the force acts in the long axis of the seated body, G_x when it acts anteroposteriorly across the body, or G_y when it acts laterally across the body. Positive acceleration with the head directed towards the center of rotation ($+G_z$) is the force most commonly experienced. Although some military aircraft are able to withstand accelerations of $+12G_z$, passengers and crew of transport aircraft are unlikely to experience any more than $+2G_z$, except in an emergency (for instance if the pilot is required to take urgent maneuvering action to avoid a collision).

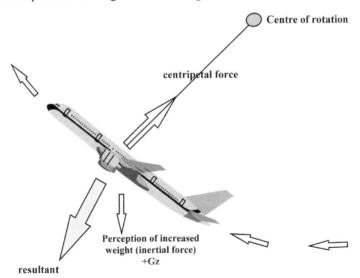

Centre of rotation

centripetal force

Perception of increased weight (inertial force) $+Gz$

resultant

Figure 5.2   Radial acceleration

At these low levels of acceleration, the hydrostatic effects of positive G are minimal and unlikely to be a serious cause for concern. Any patient with impaired circulation is already likely to be lying supine on a stretcher (with the acceleration now acting across the anteroposterior axis of the body).

If $+G_z$ is sustained, the hydrostatic pressure in vessels below the level of the heart is increased and venous return is impaired. By Starling's Law a reduction in cardiac output will follow, setting in train physiological responses resembling those seen in hypovolemic states. Reflex tachycardia and selective vasoconstriction ensue in an attempt to maintain adequate blood pressure.

Medical crew should be aware that this effect on weight is experienced by everything in the aircraft, not just by its occupants. Consequently traction weights, and monitors or equipment boxes resting on the patient, will become heavier as the aircraft maneuvers. Latched shelves above the patient must be firmly secured; it is not unknown for them to become detached and fall onto the patient during sudden aircraft maneuvering. In addition, repeated fluctuating maneuvers are stressful, fatiguing, and likely to increase the risk of motion sickness.

Vibration

The term *vibration* implies alternating or oscillating forces of such frequency and amplitude that they can be felt by the aircraft occupants. Vibration during transportation is inevitable, but the features of vibration from aircraft are somewhat different from those experienced in land-based ambulances. Aircraft designers aim to minimize vibrations and ensure that any that can not be prevented will minimally affect the passengers and crew. The main sources of vibration in fixed wing aircraft are the engines and turbulence, from whatever cause. Helicopters are a special case with vibration frequencies associated also with main and tail rotors, and the gearbox.

With respect to adverse effects on the body, the most significant frequency range lies between 0.1 and 40 Hz. All body parts have characteristic *natural frequencies* and therefore oscillate at distinct frequencies within the spectrum. For instance, the head resonates at about 6 Hz and the forearm at around 40 Hz. The result is discomfort and fatigue as the victim uses muscular effort to stabilize the body. Low frequencies can also cause blurred vision, shortness of breath, motion sickness, and chest or abdominal pain. Exposure to moderate vibration results in a slight increase in metabolic rate. Aircraft vibration may interfere with normal body thermoregulation, causing vasoconstriction and a decreased ability to sweat. The hyperthermic patient may therefore have impaired cooling ability. Conversely, vibration may also worsen the hypothermic patient's condition.

Medical crew must also be aware of effects on equipment. Vibration may interfere with invasive and non-invasive electronic patient monitoring, not least that sensors, electrodes and leads may become disconnected. Similarly, tenuously placed endotracheal tubes and intravenous lines may be dislodged. Inflight vibration has also been shown to cause malfunction of activity-sensing pacemakers.

Little can be done to eliminate or reduce vibration which is a function of the design and maintenance of the aircraft. However, to minimize the harmful or uncomfortable effects, it is advisable to avoid or reduce direct contact between the patient and the airframe. Adequate energy absorbing cushions, mattresses, or padding should be used for the stretcher and seats, and both patients and crew members should be firmly but comfortably restrained when vibration levels are high.

Noise

The vibration of air (sound), like the vibration of the aircraft structure, can be one of the most irritating factors encountered by aeromedical personnel. Noise is generally considered to be sound which is loud or otherwise unpleasant. There is great individual variation in tolerance to the effects of noise, and to what is considered to be unpleasant, but the longer the exposure, and the more intense the noise, the greater the annoyance and inconvenience, as well as being a cause of potential damage. Prolonged or intense exposure may also result in ear discomfort, deterioration in performance of tasks, headaches, fatigue, nausea, visual disturbances, and vertigo.

Excessive noise may interfere directly with patient care. Noise is generated by aircraft engines, propellers, helicopter rotors, airflow within the cabin pressurization system, the friction of air as it passes over the aircraft fuselage, radios, and medical monitoring equipment, not to mention the babble generated by other passengers and crew trying to communicate over this cacophony. Such a background level of noise negates the use of a stethoscope. It is therefore important for medical crew to use other means to monitor the patient. Blood pressure can be palpated or monitored by invasive or noninvasive devices. Visual observation for a variation in respiratory rate, chest expansion, level of consciousness, and discomfort may all suggest a change in the patient's respiratory status, and confirmation should be sought from pulse oximetry and end tidal capnography.

During helicopter operations, and in some military transport aircraft, hearing protection should be worn by both the medical crew and patient. Simple ear plugs or ear defenders will usually suffice, but headsets and helmets offer better noise attenuation and will improve communications between crew members or between the patient and the medical team. Active noise reduction headsets are available for aircrew and might be considered for patients with extreme sensitivity to noise. It should be remembered, though, that the space between the noise attenuator, whatever is used, and the patient's tympanic membrane will become an external 'cavity' and, as such, will be subject to changes in gas volume with altitude. Headsets and the like must therefore be moved away from the ears from time to time during climb-out and descent.

Motion sickness

Air sickness is just one form of motion induced nausea and emesis, all of which have similar clinical features. As with other flight stressors, individuals vary in their response to motion stimuli and, although some may be very tolerant of the provocation caused by aircraft movement, if the stimulus is intense enough and of sufficient duration, all will eventually succumb. Air sickness is a very common complaint; even aircrew (especially trainees) are not immune. Surveys have indicated that as many as 60 per cent of pilot candidates have suffered from air sickness at some time.

It is not entirely clear why animals have evolved a nauseogenic response to motion (most vertebrates can be induced to vomit). The mechanisms underlying the condition in man are not well understood, but it is known that functioning labyrinths are essential for the response to occur. Motion sickness tends to happen when visual and vestibular evidence of motion are in conflict, or when signals from the semicircular canals and otoliths do not conform to expected patterns (*the sensory conflict theory*). This helps to explain the nausea that is experienced by some when watching implied movement on wide cinema screens, during flight simulator training, or while immersed in virtual reality.

Air sickness appears to be no different in its physiological origin to other forms of motion sickness. Low frequency oscillatory motion in the frequency range of 0.1 to 0.8 Hz, as experienced in turbulent flight conditions, is a particularly offensive provocation, but there is no obvious reason why higher frequencies do not induce the same response.

Infants are rarely air sick, but the incidence reaches a peak in late childhood, and thereafter declines moderately with maturity. Women are more affected than men, and a number of factors are known to worsen or precipitate the symptoms. Paramount among these is the anxiety that may be induced either by a fear of flying or, indeed, a fear of being air sick. Some aircraft maneuvers are more provocative than others, and unintentional unexpected motion, such as during turbulence, may provoke both nausea and an anxiety overlay. In addition, an overly warm or stuffy environment, the sight or smell of food (or of others vomiting) can be enough to turn even the strongest of stomachs. Any patient with pre-existing nausea, gastric distension, ileus, or who is taking nauseogenic medications is obviously at increased risk. The signs and symptoms are, almost certainly, familiar to every reader of this book. Motion sickness is truly a debilitating experience. Sufferers may describe an increased 'stomach awareness', nausea, retching, or frank vomiting. They may feel apathetic, malaised, fatigued, or even exhausted. Feelings of overwhelming warmth, headache, pallor and diaphoresis (sweating) are common.

For the normal individual, prevention can be helped by ensuring a sensible diet prior to flight and antiemetics for those known to be most susceptible. Many classes of drugs have been used, but none has been shown to be significantly more effective than hyoscine (scopolamine), and most have undesirable side-effects that limit their use. Indeed, hyoscine causes drowsiness which is not avoided when taken by transdermal route (skin patch). The doctor or nurse must ensure that any medication which they take does not adversely affect their ability to care for their patient.

Special care must be taken with patients whose condition may be worsened or compromised in the event of emesis (see chapters 11 to 16). Patients and passengers who succumb may receive some comfort if their anxieties can be allayed, and if they are able to concentrate on an activity (although not reading, which tends to worsen the symptoms). Relief may also be achieved by reducing further sensory conflict, either by fixing the gaze outside of the aircraft if the horizon is clearly visible, or by lying flat with the head still and the eyes closed.

References

Hepper, A.E. (2003) 'Restraint systems and escape from aircraft', in Ernsting J., Nicholson A.N. and D.J. Rainford, (eds) *Aviation Medicine* (3rd Ed.) Arnold: London.

Benson, A.J. (2003) 'Motion Sickness, in Ernsting J., Nicholson A.N. and D.J. Rainford, (eds) *Aviation Medicine* (3rd Ed.) Arnold: London.

Blumen I.J. (1995) 'Altitude Physiology and the Stresses of Flight', *Air Med J.* **14** (2):8,7-99.

Glaister, D.H. and Prior A.R.J. (2003) 'The Effects of Long Duration Acceleration', in Ernsting J., Nicholson A.N. and D.J. Rainford (eds) *Aviation Medicine* (3rd Ed.) Arnold: London.

Harding, R.M. and F.J. Mills (2003) 'Acceleration', in Harding R.M. and F.J. Mills, (eds) *Aviation Medicine* (3rd Ed.) BMJ: London.

Rood, G.M. and James S.H. (2003) 'Noise and Communication', in Ernsting J., Nicholson A.N. and D.J. Rainford (eds) *Aviation Medicine* (3rd Ed.). Arnold: London.

Stott, J.R.R. (2003) 'Vibration', in Ernsting J., Nicholson A.N. and D.J Rainford, (eds) *Aviation Medicine* (3rd Ed.) Arnold: London.

Chapter 6

Transmeridian and Long Haul Flights

The world and its time zones

The Earth can be considered as a sphere covered by a grid of lines called meridians of longitude and parallels of latitude. These lines are overlaid on maps of the planet's surface to aid navigation. Parallels of latitude are all lines encircling the Earth, parallel to the equator (the parallel with the greatest diameter), from zero degrees (at the equator) to 90 degrees north (north pole) and 90 degrees south (south pole). Meridians are semicircles (each of the same radius) which connect the north and south poles. Opposite meridians form a complete Earth circumference, unlike the parallels of latitude. Longitude is measured up to 180 degrees west and east from the zero meridian (*prime meridian*) which passes through the Greenwich observatory in London.

By convention, international travel and other worldwide matters are based on *Coordinated Universal Time* (UTC), which is the current time on the prime meridian, also known as *Greenwich Mean Time* (GMT). UTC/GMT is always given in 24 hour notation and referred to by the term 'zulu' during radio transmissions and in flight planning.

Standard Time is the local time adopted by a certain area, for instance across an entire country, or part of a wide country spanning several lines of longitude (Table 6.1).

A potential source of confusion is that the United Kingdom (UK) is in the Western European Time Zone. Western European Standard Time (WET) is therefore the same as GMT and UTC.

Most countries adopt the time of the zone in which they are (predominantly) situated. Each zone is 15° longitude wide (extending 7½° longitude either side of its central meridian), and differs from UTC/GMT by a whole number of hours:

$$24 \text{ (hours)} \times 15 \text{ (degrees)} = 360 \text{ (degrees)}$$

The zones are therefore numbered 1 to 11 east (−), and 1 to 11 (+) west. This is often remembered as *'east is least and west is best'*. Each zone represents an hour difference from that either side of it. Zones zero and 12 are common to both − and +, with the *International Date Line* (IDL) being 180° longitude away from the prime meridian. In practice it would be possible to collect a patient from the eastern side of the IDL and transfer him to a hospital on the western side on a date one day before his departure!

Table 6.1   American Standard Times

Zone	Difference to UTC (hours)
Eastern	- 5
Central	- 6
Mountain	- 7
Pacific	- 8
Alaska	- 9
Hawaii	- 10

When planning complicated long haul aeromedical flights, medical personnel should consult time zone maps (for example, Figure 6.1), such as those found in airline inflight magazines. Note that many countries adopt a different local time during the summer months (e.g. BST – *British Summer Time* – is GMT plus one hour), and that the dates these local times change are not consistent worldwide. As an example, a European Community (EC) directive designates the start and end dates of summer time as the last Sundays in March and October respectively. Hence, at 1.00am GMT/ UTC, the clocks go forward one hour on Sundays 26 March 2006 and 25 March 2007 (at the start of BST), and are put back again on Sundays 29 October 2006 and 28 October 2007 (at the end of BST).

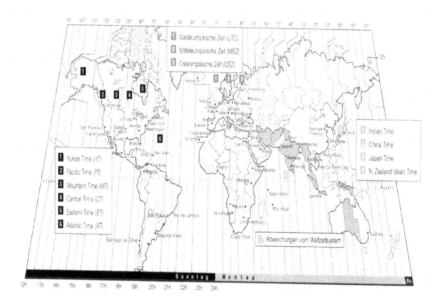

Figure 6.1   Example of time-zone map
Source: Lufthansa.

Circadian rhythms

Overnight flights and journeys that cross time zones are of particular importance in aeromedical transportation. Transmeridian travel causes the normal sleep-wake cycle to be disrupted with wake periods being at abnormal and often inconvenient times. Furthermore, the sufferer will complain of excessive tiredness (over and above the fatigue caused by the flight), loss of appetite and general malaise. Adequate and good quality sleep is essential for medical personnel to adapt to irregular work schedules. This is especially so, since alterations in circadian rhythms reduce effectiveness and can impair psychomotor performance. All animals possess biological clocks which regulate physiology. In humans, circadian rhythms exert a pattern of sleep and wakefulness which is closely related to the 24 hour day-night cycle. The most important influence on circadian rhythms is the daily alternation between light and dark. Other influences include temperature, activity and artificial or social synchronizers called *zeitgebers* ('time-givers'), such as clocks, meal-times and radio/TV programs, etc. In the absence of external time cues, the individual is said to be free-running, that is, no longer entrained. Under such circumstances the period of the biological clock lengthens beyond 24 hours.

Over 50 circadian rhythms are known to exist. Almost all homeostatic functions oscillate in this manner, and the overall pattern of circadian rhythmicity can be measured by such indices as body temperature, plasma cortisol release, and melatonin. Melatonin plays a key role in the function of the clock mechanism (the 'oscillator'), but the seat of clock activity appears to lie in the suprachiasmatic nucleus (SCN) of the hypothalamus. The SCN appears to control plasma growth hormone secretion, skin temperature, calcium excretion and slow wave sleep. It receives neuronal projections from the retina which may provide the major light-dark cues. A second oscillator is known to exist, although its location is unclear. It controls plasma corticosteroid levels, potassium excretion, body core temperature, and rapid eye movement (REM) sleep. The ability to sleep varies with the phase of the temperature cycle and, because the oscillator is slow to change, it is difficult to adjust sleep patterns rapidly after a time zone change ('jet lag') or after a shift in the work-rest cycle.

Transmeridian flights

Sleep after transmeridian flights is influenced by the timing of the flight and the direction of travel. Westward flights, say from London to Washington with a sleep period delay of five hours, enable individuals to fall asleep quickly and sleep more soundly in the first rest period after the flight. The only detrimental effect is likely to be less restful sleep during the latter part of the night as one tries to extend sleep toward the local time of rising (which, in this example, approximates to midday in the home time zone). By the third night, normal sleep patterns have usually been established and adaptation to the new time zone will have occurred.

If sleep can be avoided during an eastbound flight (that is, if the 'natural' rest period is ignored), once the immediate effect of sleep loss is overcome, the first sleep after the journey will be of better quality than after a westbound sector. Paradoxically, though, quality of sleep is likely to deteriorate over the next few days and adaptation may take longer.

The difference in adaptation between easterly and westerly flights may be a reflection of the longer natural free-running cycle. When environmental cues are removed, we have a tendency to lengthen our day. This is not such a problem with a westbound journey (which, because of the delayed sleep period, lengthens the first day), whereas an eastbound journey requires a shortening of the day (that is, the sleep period is brought forward).

The majority of long haul aeromedical flights will require medical crew to collect the patient and return in a relatively short period. It is expensive to allow medical personnel time to adapt to the new time zone, and it would be senseless, since the crew will, in most cases, be returning to the time zone from whence they came. The main problem for crew with return transmeridian flights is therefore coping with, rather than adapting to, time zone changes. As described above, sleep after a westbound sector is usually restful, at least for the first half of the night. However, the timing of the return flight is of great importance. Most authorities agree that it is better to stay on the home time zone; maximum alertness will therefore occur earlier than if the rhythm was fully synchronized with the western time zone. On the day of the return flight, suboptimal alertness will occur in the western afternoon and evening. However, if the flight is delayed until the evening, medical crew can take a rest sleep in the late afternoon which will help to advance the sleep-wakefulness cycle and will avoid excessive tiredness during the latter half of the journey.

Jet lag

Jet lag occurs when travel across time zones takes the human body rapidly into another phase of the 24 hour day-night cycle at a speed which exceeds the ability of synchronizers to entrain physiological rhythms. The subsequent desynchronization may lead to generalized discomfort and malaise, sleep disturbance, disruptions of feeding pattern and bowel habit, and suboptimal levels of performance at important times of the day. These symptoms diminish gradually after arrival at the final destination as circadian rhythms take a finite time to re-entrain to local time.

There is great individual variation in how the effects of jet lag are perceived. To some it is essential to be on top form immediately after arrival at the destination (for instance, when going directly to collect a patient for a return flight). Others may need to be at peak performance a day or so later. It is now well established that sleep after transmeridian flights is influenced by both the timing of the flight and the direction of travel. In a recent study of aircrew flying eastward and westward long haul routes, it was shown that the lowest levels of alertness tended to occur at the end of the outward flight (for the earlier westward departures) and at the end of the return flight (for the eastward and later westward departures). On almost all flights, levels of alertness were higher at the end than at the beginning of a rest period, and the improvement was related to the amount of sleep obtained.

There have been many suggested treatments for jet lag, and some airlines have produced advice and guidelines for their passengers. Simple measures have been advocated, such as sleeping on the aircraft (which, of course, is not practicable for single medical crew escorting patients, but may be possible during the staging flight), and the avoidance of heavy meals and alcohol. For some travelers, simply the knowledge that performance is likely to be impaired for a day or two allows planning of a suitable work schedule. Mild hypnotics, such as zopiclone and temazepam, may help to ensure adequate rest but have no direct influence on the rate at which re-entrainment occurs.

Many travelers now advocate melatonin, a naturally occurring hormone which is secreted by the pineal gland and retina under the influence of cyclical sympathetic drive. Its production is maximal at night and suppressed by light of sufficient intensity and it appears to advance the next sleep epoch. Hence, it has been proposed as a remedy for jet lag and is said to be most efficacious when taken close to the destination target bedtime when five or more time zones are crossed. Taken in this way, melatonin appears to advance the circadian cycle, possibly by acting directly on the suprachiasmatic nucleus, although there is recent evidence that melatonin tends to encourage sleep by lowering body temperature.

There is little evidence of the best dose and dosing schedule, although there are a few papers which describe doses between 0.1 mg and 3.0 mg as being optimal. Studies of adverse effects show that they mostly occur in doses of 10 mg and over, and there seems to be no particular advantage of doses greater than 1.0 mg. Anecdotal reports suggest taking melatonin when you should be asleep at your destination, for instance, on a west to east flight from New York to the UK, departing at, say, 15:00 Eastern Standard Time, the melatonin should be taken three hours into the flight (that is, at 23:00 GMT/UTC). To speed normal entrainment, melatonin may then usefully be taken at bedtime for a few days after return.

However, long-term use has its drawbacks. One notable finding is that withdrawal of melatonin after using it for two weeks, causes further disruption of circadian rhythms and therefore has the potential to worsen the effects of jet lag. Although there is little evidence, it is clear that melatonin derived from bovine brain is likely to be associated with risk of transmission of disease. Hence melatonin is now synthesized, but, there is scant information available on its long-term safety. Some have therefore suggested taking melatonin by the traditional Indian yogi practice of 'amaroli'. This involves drinking your own urine (but not the early morning sample which is far too concentrated)!

Aromatherapy also has its proponents. Virgin Atlantic Airways offers an aromatherapy kit to its Upper Class passengers (Figure 6.2), but no benefit has been proven.

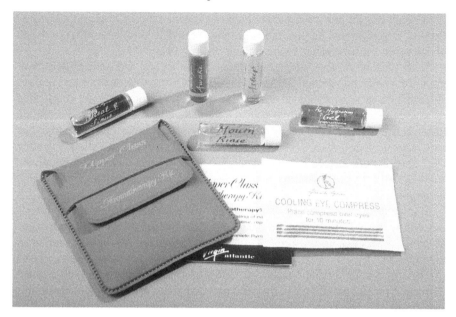

Figure 6.2   Virgin Atlantic Airways aromatherapy kit

Figure 6.3 gives an extreme example of a long haul flight. It records the sleep epochs immediately prior to and after flights between London Heathrow (LHR) and Auckland (AKL). Both flights have two sectors staging through Los Angeles (LAX). The first is westbound from UK to NZ, and the second is the return journey, eastbound from NZ to UK. It is a useful exercise to plan how you would deal with both jet lag and fatigue assuming you need to be able to work at optimal performance one day after arrival in both directions.

North-South long haul flights

Many north-south flights are scheduled overnight. Since few or no time zones are crossed, the predominant problem is one of sleep deprivation unless crew members are already stabilized on a night shift pattern. To some extent, fatigue can be prevented by adequate sleep prior to departure. Napping may also appear to help tiredness, but tests show that alertness and performance deteriorate despite most individuals subjectively feeling less tired after the nap.

Some aspects of flight common to all long distance journeys are also likely to worsen fatigue. These include the mild hypoxia experienced at altitude, low humidity, extremes of temperature, vibration, noise, boredom, and relative inactivity.

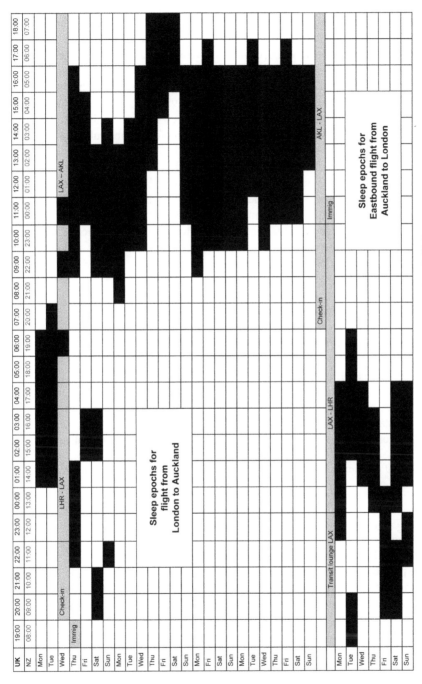

Figure 6.3   Sleep epochs either side of westbound and eastbound long haul flights

Performance and time on duty

Aircrew are well protected, under statute, from the fatiguing effects of long duty periods. In 1944, the Convention on International Civil Aviation recommended limitations to flight crew work periods. Individual countries have endorsed this recommendation and established national laws which govern these duty times. In the UK, this entered the statute books in the 1950 Air Navigation Order and was re-emphasized by the Civilian Aviation Authority in their CAP 371 publication in 1990. This publication also makes recommendations for the specific requirement of aircrew flying air ambulance missions (Table 6.2), but there is no such guidance or regulation for air medical personnel.

A similar situation exists in the USA where the Federal Aviation Administration regulates flight time limitations for all commercial flight crew. It has been suggested that those medical personnel who undertake frequent and long distance aeromedical missions should adopt the recommendations made for cabin attendants (also in CAP 371). Several other authorities have made similar suggestions (summarized in Table 6.3). The air ambulance industry has been slow to see the importance of adequate rest for its medical personnel, but medicolegal concerns are now driving some organizations to look critically at this issue.

Table 6.2   Flight time limitations for air ambulance flight crew

- Dedicated air ambulance flights may be extended by up to a maximum of four hours
- Medical escort must be onboard
- Occupants are limited to crew, patient(s) and relative(s). No other passengers
- At least 48 hours must elapse between the end of one extended mission and the start of another
- A pilot may only extend three air ambulance missions in any consecutive 28 days

Source: Civil Aviation Authority (1990) *CAP 371. The avoidance of fatigue in aircrews* (3rd Ed.) CAA: London.

Planning medical crew duty times

Fatigue is the body's normal response after a long or arduous waking period. Workload may be physical or mental, and tiredness may result also from boredom and inactivity. The combination of irregular work patterns and sleep disturbance can greatly impair alertness and performance. This is especially true if time zones are crossed and if duty periods are long. Furthermore, the adverse affects of sleep disturbance and deprivation are cumulative, and care must be taken to ensure that frequent flyers are allowed sufficient rest between journeys. Chronic fatigue requires a prolonged period of rest.

Performance during long shifts is influenced by four main factors:

1. Time elapsed since start of duty.
2. Time of day.
3. Adaptation to local time zone.
4. Time since last sleep.

When an individual is fully rested at the start of a duty period performance improves on task over the first five hours. It then tends to drop precipitously and falls to a plateau at about 16 hours of time-on-task.

An individual who is adapted to the local time zone, and is therefore entrained in normal circadian rhythms, will perform best in the afternoon. Whatever time the duty shift started, performance then declines until it reaches a trough at about 0500 in the morning (that is, the nadir of the circadian cycle).

Table 6.3   Summary of proposals for flight time limitations for aeromedical personnel

British Aeromedical Practitioner's Association	• Maximum 32 hours' continuous duty without rest. • No single member of crew continuously responsible for patient for more than 16 hours. • Or more than four hours for critical care transfer. • Rest period should be at least 1½ times the preceding duty period plus one hour for every time zone crossed.
Medical assistance organizations	See chapter 19.
Civil Aviation Authority (rules relating to cabin attendants)	• A flying duty period can be one hour longer than permitted for aircrew. • Minimum rest periods can be one hour shorter. • Maximum duty hours must not exceed 60 hours in one week, 105 hours in any two consecutive weeks, or 210 hours in any four consecutive weeks.

Medical personnel and those who organize aeromedical schedules would be wise to avoid situations which might lead to the superimposition of the low plateau of time-on-task and the circadian nadir. Performance under these circumstances could be expected to be significantly worse than at either of the low points independently. Unfortunately, the situation is further compounded by insufficient or poor quality rest prior to the start of duty, and when time zones are crossed. In the worst case, individuals might be unable to stay awake during the final sector of a long flight. The consequences for patient care are obvious. If such circumstances are unavoidable, it will be essential to have more than one member in the medical team, and proper division of labour should be organized with adequate rest periods for all concerned.

Clinical and logistic problems of long haul travel

The discussion, so far, has centered on the problems of fatigue, alertness and performance of the medical team. However, in planning aeromedical missions, the consequences to the patient must be taken into consideration. These must cover the entire journey and therefore should include the flight duration, departure time, and time zone passage and ground transfers at either end. Least at risk will be those who are already sedated and those being transferred on stretchers. Paradoxically, it is usually the ambulant patient who has most to suffer. Often postoperative, and sometimes cardiac, these patients are already stressed before they arrive at the airport. This is worsened by the busy and chaotic environment as they pass through the tedious but essential formalities necessary before boarding. Most normal individuals feel stressed even before the flight. Patients have the added anxieties of their illness; they may also be leaving relatives behind, and may seem disproportionately worried about seemingly less important matters, such as ensuring that baggage has been checked in, and so on.

All these apprehensions may cause or worsen sleep disturbance and exacerbate general feelings of lack of wellbeing. More specifically, though, careful thought must be given to timings of drugs, meals and treatments. In particular, some drugs are time-dependant, such as insulin, thyroxine, antibiotics and the progestin *nonstop* or *minipill*. The simplest answer is to maintain the patient on the local standard time of the point of departure throughout the journey. Drugs, treatments and meals should continue to be given at the expected times, and the patient's watch should not be changed to the destination time zone. This information must be passed on to the handover team at the destination hospital.

Similarly, drugs which need to be evenly spaced (for example, antibiotics six hourly) should continue to be given as planned before departure. It must be clearly documented in the patient's transfer notes that drugs and treatments were given at local times. To avoid confusion later, it is advisable to include the new time zone in parenthesis, for example,

Penicillin V 250 mg I/V given at 1730 Eastern Std Time (2230 GMT).

Finally, the medical team is responsible for ensuring that the patient is appropriately dressed for the destination environment and also for any stopovers en route. Departing Florida during an early evening in April, the weather is likely to be comfortably warm; arrival eight hours later in the early morning in Edinburgh, and the patient will encounter a much colder ambient temperature, which is also likely to be wet and windy. Warm clothes are important if the patient is to spend anything more than a few seconds exposed to the elements while transferring to a terminal building or waiting to be moved into a ground ambulance. Several thin layers are preferable to single bulky items. Waterproof garments, umbrellas, hats and gloves may also be needed. Patients on stretchers will need extra blankets; these should also be insulative and lightweight. Very special care must be taken of those with spinal injuries, and also the unconscious, who may be unable to control their own body temperature or unable to notify the medical crew when thermally uncomfortable. Infants are also extremely sensitive to extremes of ambient temperature. An incubator may be required to maintain the necessary thermal range.

References

Anon. (2005) 'History of legal time in Britain', http://www.srcf.ucam.org/ ~jsm28/ british-time/

Anon. (2005) 'World time zones', http:// www.timeanddate.com/worldclock/

Arendt, J. and S. Deacon (1997) 'Treatment of circadian rhythm disorders – melatonin', *Chronobiol Int* **14**(2):185-204.

Avery, D., Lenz M. and C. Landis (1998) 'Guidelines for prescribing melatonin', *Ann Med.* **30**(1):122-130.

Herxheimer, A. and K.J. Petrie (2001) 'Melatonin for preventing and treating jet lag', *Cocharane Database Syst Rev.* **1**:CD001520.

Kapur, R. (2002) Discussion topic: 'Melatonin', on Drs. Net aeromedicine forum (www.doctors.net.uk) 25 September.

Karasek, M., Reiter, R.J., Cardinali, D.P. and M. Pawlikowski (2002) 'Future of melatonin as a therapeutic agent', *Neuro Endocrinol Lett* **23** Suppl **1**:118-21.

Martin, T.C. (1995) 'Adverse effects of rotating schedules on the circadian rhythms of air medical crews', *Air Med J.* **14**(2):83-6.

McFarland, R.A. (1974) 'Influence of changing time zones on aircrew and passengers', *Aerospace Medicine.* **45**:648-658.

Neil, S. (2002) Discussion topic: 'Melatonin', on Drs. Net aeromedicine forum (www.doctors.net.uk) 12 December.

Nicholson, A.N., (2003) 'Disturbed sleep in aircrew', in Ernsting J., Nicholson A.N. and D.J. Rainford (eds) *Aviation Medicine* (3rd Ed.), Arnold: London.

Nicholson, A.N. and B.M. Stone (1987) 'Sleep and wakefulness handbook for Flight Medical Officers' (2nd Ed.), AGARDograph No 270.

Nicholson, A.N. and P.A. Pascoe et al. (1988) 'Sleep after transmeridian flights', *Lancet,* **ii**:1205-8.

Pascoe, P.A. (1992) 'Jet Lag', in Dawood R. (ed.) *Travellers' Health* (3rd Ed.), Oxford University Press: Oxford.

Petrie, K., Conaglen J.V., Thompson L. and K. Chamberlain (1989) 'Effect of melatonin on jet lag after long haul flights', *Brit Med J.* **298**:705-7.

Sack, R.L., Hughes R.J., Edgar D.M. and A.J. Lewy (1997) 'Sleep-promoting effects of melatonin: at what dose, in whom, under what conditions, and by what mechanisms?', *Sleep* **20**(10):908-915.

Skene, D.J., Lockley S.W. and J. Arendt (1999) 'Use of melatonin in the treatment of phase shift and sleep disorders', *Adv Exp Med Biol.* **467**:79-84.

Stone, B.M. et al. (2004) 'Alertness of aircrew on long eastward and westward flights', Paper 575, Aerospace Medical Association Annual Scientific Meeting, Anchorage, Alaska.

UK Civil Aviation Authority (1990), *CAP 371. The avoidance of fatigue in aircrews* (3rd Ed.), CAA: London.

UK Civil Aviation Authority (1998). CAA Aeronautical Information Circular AIC25/1998, CAA: London.

UK Civil Aviation Authority (2004). CAA Aeronautical Information Circular AIC 99/2004 Pink 72, CAA: London.

Zhdanova, I.V., Wurtman R.J., Morabito C., Piotrovska V.R. and H.J. Lynch (1996) 'Effects of low oral doses of melatonin, given 2-4 hours before habitual bedtime, on sleep in normal young humans', *Sleep* **19**:423-431.

PART III
Operational Considerations

Chapter 7

Operational Aspects of Aeromedical Transport

Mission profiles

Aeromedical assignments may be described as primary, secondary, tertiary or quaternary responses. Primary responses are commonly known as 'scene flights' and are usually of short duration. The aircraft may enter as the first responder or at the call of a ground prehospital care provider. Aircraft involved in secondary responses transport patients from outlying emergency departments where some degree of stabilization has been performed; the patient is then delivered into the care of a higher level facility. A tertiary response occurs when an aeromedical aircraft transports a hospital inpatient to another facility for definitive care and a quaternary mission is when an aircraft is used to repatriate patients from overseas. Aeromedical aircraft may also be requested to perform search and rescue, public relations, fire suppression, or law enforcement missions. The use of aircraft in the transport of drugs, medical supplies, and human tissues or organ harvest teams, represent an additional facet of aeromedical care.

Aeromedical aircraft

No single aircraft is ideal for the needs of all these aeromedical roles or is suitable for the care of all types of patients requiring transportation. The needs of the program must mesh closely with the capabilities of the aircraft. The aircraft may be owned by the sponsoring agency (for example, hospital or ambulance service) or leased from a vendor. Likewise, pilots and mechanics may be employed by the sponsor or vendor. Medical crew are typically employed directly by the sponsoring institution and must meet training, skill, and experience requirements established by their employers.

It is the joint responsibility of both vendors and program sponsors to ensure that all applicable governmental regulations are being followed in regards to aircraft operation and maintenance.

The aircraft itself must be capable of lifting with a full complement of crew, equipment, supplies, and the fuel required for the duration of the mission. An adequate reserve of fuel and other consumables (such as oxygen) must be carried at all times. The range of the aircraft is defined by the rate of fuel consumption and its ground speed. Clearly, more fuel will be required on longer missions, and the aircraft must be able either to tolerate an increased load or to trade fuel for crew or equipment. The envelope defining the aircraft's center of gravity must be large enough to account for differing weights of its occupants, the varying seating patterns, and movements of crew, patients, and equipment within the aircraft. The center of gravity must not be upset by inflight medical care. Cruising speed must be high enough to ensure that use of the aircraft provides a clear advantage over ground transport. This is especially true when responding in urban areas and when hospitals are nearby. At high altitudes, issues such as cabin pressurization, supplemental oxygen for flight crew members and passengers, and service ceiling become important. The electrical system of the aircraft must provide enough power to allow failsafe function of all onboard medical equipment, unless it has its own autonomous supply, as well as provide power to the aircraft's essential avionic and communications systems.

All-weather capability and the ability to fly at night are extremely important considerations in aircraft selection. Most helicopter programs permit flight only under visual flight rules (VFR) conditions; but safety dictates that all aeromedical aircraft should be equipped for instrument flight rules (IFR) conditions to ensure safe return and landing in the event of deteriorating weather. The increased margin of safety provided by the addition of IFR capability clearly increases cost and weight to the aircraft and may require the carriage of a second pilot. Strictly IFR operations may be of limited use in helicopter-only organizations, but is essential for the majority of fixed wing missions. IFR flight is optimally used in conjunction with instrument landing systems (ILS) found at appropriately equipped airports, but global positioning (GPS) navigation systems have application in primary missions where ground-based landing and navigation aids are not available. GPS is also fast becoming the most used general navigation system, although it is not licensed as such in all countries.

Several major ergonomic issues must be considered in selecting an aircraft for aeromedical use. Ease of loading is always important, and especially vital in aircraft which will be used in primary responses. Loading should be accomplished with a minimum of patient maneuvering and lifting. Essentially, doors must allow access for stretchers and, when evaluating helicopters, loading must be possible and safe when blades are turning. The rotor disc must therefore be high.

Inside the aircraft, space is a prime consideration. A minimum of the head and chest of the patient must be accessible to ensure that adequate care can be provided in the worst-case scenario (that is, during cardiopulmonary resuscitation). Aircraft equipped to carry two patients during routine operations must have enough space to access the head and chest of both patients simultaneously. Space and seating requirements must allow for stowage and for use of equipment and supplies within the cabin. A comfortable working environment for the crew, and a means to adequately restrain patients and crew during take-off and landing, and in turbulent flight, are also necessary.

While the exterior characteristics of similar aircraft types may seem identical, it is important to note that interiors may be configured differently depending on the intended function of the aircraft. The suitability of an aircraft to meet the needs of a particular assignment is highly dependent on the internal design. Any discussion of the optimal aircraft for aeromedical transport yields a generous mix of fact, anecdote and opinion. However, some aircraft are clearly more appropriate for certain kinds of missions. The more appropriate aircraft is not always the least expensive, and to base decisions on price alone ignores the potential risks and benefits to the patient. The following case study illustrates this principle.

The Lear 24 business jet is fast and can land on short runways. However, it is not fuel efficient, and therefore its range is limited. An aircraft vendor may offer a price estimate for a Miami to New York mission in a Lear 24 because it will be less expensive than the larger Lear 35. However, the vendor may not realize that the Lear 24 may not comply with certain noise restrictions and that a fuelling stop may be required, negating any speed advantage (if the stop is omitted, the aircraft will reach New York without fuel reserves). The larger, more expensive, Lear 35 will fly from Miami to New York without incident.

Even given that a less expensive aircraft may be appropriate for the patient, it may not always result in the less expensive mission. A US$1000 per hour turboprop that requires five hours to complete a mission is more expensive than a US$1500 per hour jet that completes the task in three. The proper way to compare cost is not by comparing hourly rates, but rather by comparing the total mission cost for a specific itinerary.

Clearly, there is no single solution to finding a general, all-embracing, multi-purpose aeromedical aircraft. The wide variation in roles, the great difference in patient types, the distances to be covered, and the urgency (and therefore speed) required, all complicate the best choice of aircraft. Aircraft design is always a compromise, but cost, alone, must not be allowed to overrule inadequate range, speed, access, working space, interior design or any other feature essential to the safe conduct of the mission. Characteristics of representative aircraft used for aeromedical transport are given in Tables 7.1 and 7.2. Although the manufacturers advertised specification data are useful, they often lack detail necessary for aeromedical decision making. For instance, some aircraft such as the Cessna Caravan are marketed for their ruggedness and performance when operating out of small ill-prepared landing strips; the Caravan data list therefore mentions its short field and obstacle clearance performance. On the other hand, this information is lacking in data sheets for the Fairchild Metroliner because this aircraft is designed for the commuter airline market and operates only out of lengthy prepared runways (see Table 7.1). Cabin work space dimensions are also important and have a vital impact on aeromedical capability (Table 7.2). Figures 7.1 to 7.4 illustrate some typical fixed wing air ambulances.

Table 7.1   Performance data for commonly used fixed wing air ambulances

Specification	Cessna Caravan	Fairchild Metroliner
Flight Ceiling	25 000 ft / 7,620 m	27 428 ft / 8360 m
Cruise Speed at 10 000 ft	184 kt /341 kph	248 kt / 460 kph
Range at 10 000 ft	907 nm / 1679 km	575 nm / 1065 km
SL Rate of Climb	975 fpm / 297 mpm	2632 fpm / 720 mph
Stall Speed (landing)	61 kt / 113 kph	80 kt / 148 kph
Take-off SL ISA		
Groundroll	1365 ft / 416 m	
50 ft obstruction	2420 ft / 738 m	
Landing SL		
Ground roll	950 ft / 290 m	No STOL performance data
50 ft obstruction	1795 ft / 547 m	available
Maximum Useful Load	4500 lb / 2041 kg	5300 lb / 2404 kg
Maximum Weights	8785 lb / 3985 kg	14 502 lb / 6577 kg
Standard Empty Weight	4285 lb / 1944 kg	9181 lb / 4164 kg
Wing Loading	31.3 lb/sq ft	46.95 lb/sq ft
Power source	Single Pratt & Whitney PT6A-114A engine	Twin 809 shp TPE 331 11U engines

Table 7.2   Typical fixed wing air ambulance cabin dimensions

	Beechcraft Super King Air B200	Raytheon Hawker 125/700	Gates Learjet 35A	Cessna Citation 1
Cabin length	22 ft 0 in	21 ft 4 in	17 ft 1 in	15 ft 8 in
Cabin width	4 ft 6 in	5 ft 11 in	4 ft 11 in	4 ft 9 in
Cabin height	4 ft 9 in	5 ft 9 in	4 ft 4 in	4 ft 9 in
Door height x width	4 ft 3 in x 2 ft 3 in	4 ft 3 in x 2 ft 3 in	5 ft 2 in x 2 ft (optional 3 ft wide door)	4 ft 3 in x 1 ft 11 in
Passenger capacity	12 (5 plus stretcher)	5-6 plus stretcher	5 plus stretcher	10-12 (3-4 plus stretcher)
Notes	High cruise speed, comfortable.	Spacious and comfortable.	High cruise speed, long range, fuel efficient, comfortable.	Low profile, but small interior.

Aeromedical helicopters

The same arguments can be applied to the choice of helicopter used for primary or secondary air ambulance missions. In effect, the role of the helicopter defines its performance. For instance, it may need long range (for SAR work), rapid start-up and response time (for HEMS work), large cabin capacity (for interhospital transfers), good fuel and maintenance economy (for charitable organizations), or good performance at altitude (for work in mountainous areas). The abilities to hover and to get in and out of confined landing areas safely are clearly of key importance. These capabilities are defined by the helicopter's published HOGE (hovering out of ground effect) and HIGE (hovering in ground effect) performance data.

In ground effect (IGE) is a condition where the downwash of air from the main rotor is able to react with the ground and give a useful reaction to the helicopter in the form of more lift force available for less engine power requirement. In effect, the rotor downwash impacts with the ground and causes a small build up of air pressure in the region below the rotor disk. The helicopter is then 'floating' on a cushion of air. This means that less power is required to maintain a constant altitude hover. IGE conditions are usually found within heights about 0.5 to 1.0 times the diameter of the main rotor. So if a helicopter has a rotor diameter of 10 m, the IGE region will be about 5 to 10 m above the ground. The actual height varies depending on the type of helicopter, the slope and nature of the ground, and any prevailing winds.

Out of ground effect (OGE) is the opposite, where there is no hard surface for the downwash to react against. As an example, a helicopter hovering 50 m above the ocean surface will be in an OGE condition and will require more power to maintain a constant altitude than if it was hovering at 5 m. Therefore a helicopter will always have a lower OGE ceiling than IGE due to the amount of engine power available.

Published performance figures for a given helicopter may state something like:

Hover ceiling at max weight = 4000 ft OGE and 6000 ft IGE

This means that the fully loaded helicopter can hover at 4000 ft above the ocean, and can hover at 6000 ft above a tall mountain top where the ground is within 0.5 to 1.0 rotor diameters below.

Hovering out of ground effect (HOGE) is important when considering *Category A* take-offs (vertical and/or rearward flight out of ground effect) and SAR involving winching, which is almost always done OGE.

Hovering in ground effect (HIGE) is important when considering whether or not a helicopter can take off and land at altitude. This is essential because the normal helicopter flight profile at both the beginning of the take-off and at the end of the landing involves coming to a hover a few feet above ground level (AGL). A number of important factors affect the helicopter's ability to hover at altitude. The most important are aircraft weight and the density of the air. The heavier the aircraft or the greater the density, the lower its hover-ceiling.

Examples and comparison of typical helicopter air ambulances are illustrated in Table 7.3 and Figures 7.5 to 7.8.

Table 7.3   Comparison of typical helicopter air ambulances

	Agusta A109	Boeing MD Explorer	Eurocopter EC135	Eurocopter EC145
Empty weight	2850 kg	2835 kg	2835 kg	3,585 kg
Useful Load (internal)	1265 kg	1304 kg	1375 kg	1,713 kg
Pilot/passengers (max)	1/7	1/7	1/7	1/9
Number of stretchers (max)	2	2	2	2
Length, rotor turning	13.04 m	11.84 m	12.9 m	13.03 m
Rotor diameter	7.78 m	10.31 m	10.2 m	11.0 m
Capable of 'Category A' take-off	Yes	Yes	Yes	Yes
Internal cabin dimensions				
Length	2.10 m	1.91 m	2.50 - 1.45§ m	N.A.
Height	1.28 m	1.24 m	1.26 - 1.15Φ m	N.A.
Width	1.61 m	1.45 m	1.50 m	N.A.
Speed and response time				
Time from start to lift-off	< 1 min	< 1 min	< 1 min	< 1 min
Max cruise speed	285 kph	250 kph	260 kph	246 kph
Time to fly 50 km	10.5 min	12 min	11.5 min	12 min
HOGE/HIGE capability				
HIGE	5060 m / 16 600 ft	3719 m / 12 200 ft	3045 m / 10 000 ft	2925 m / 9600 ft
HOGE	3597 m / 11 800 ft	3170 m / 10 400 ft	2255 m / 7400 ft	770 m / 2530 ft
Endurance and range				
Endurance	4 hr 01 min	2 hr 54 min	3 hr 24 min	3 hr 35 min
Maximum Range	787 km	543 km	620 km	680 km
Main and tail rotors				
Main rotor tip-ground clearance	2.45 m	approx 3 m	2.4 m	approx 3 m
Tail rotor/anti-torque system	Two blades (exposed)	NOTAR	Fenestron (shrouded)	Two blades (exposed)

§ 2.5 m includes baggage compartment. 1.45 m is main cabin length

Φ 1.26 m at front of cabin and 1.15 m at rear. Baggage space 0.7 m high

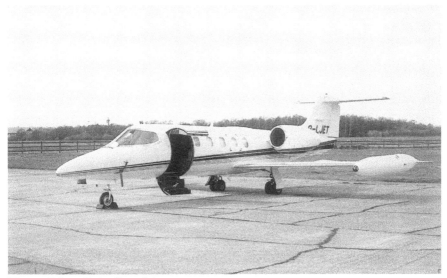

Figure 7.1   Gates Learjet

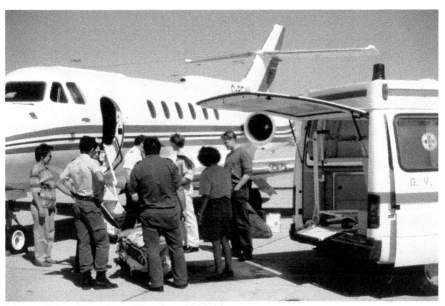

Figure 7.2   Raytheon Hawker 125/700

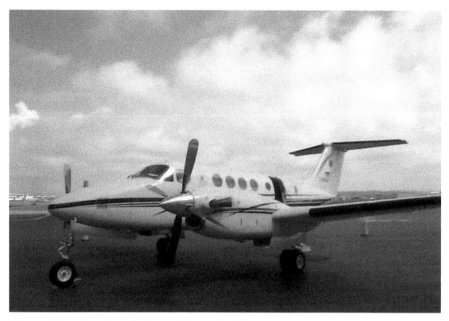

Figure 7.3   Beechcraft Super King Air B200

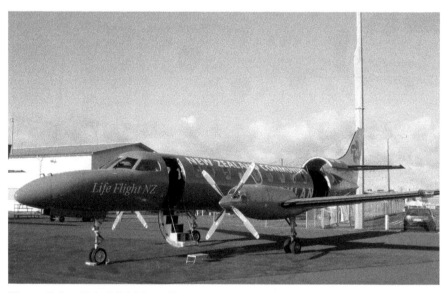

Figure 7.4   Fairchild Metroliner

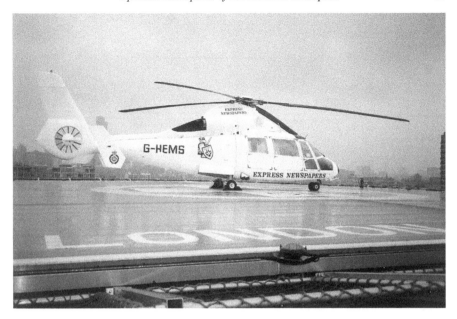

Figure 7.5   **Eurocopter (Aerospatiale) Dauphin**

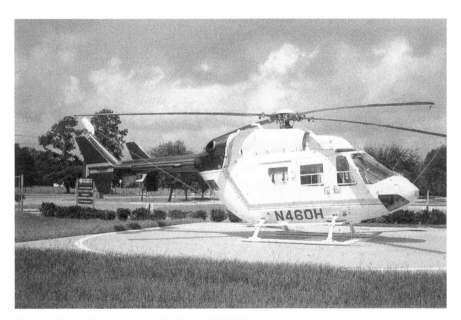

Figure 7.6   **Eurocopter (Bolkow) BK117**

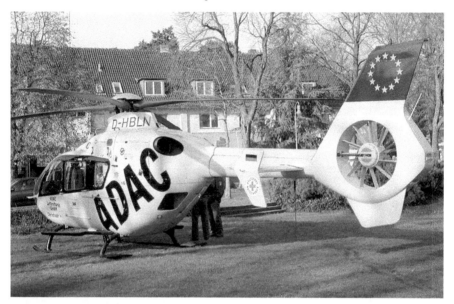

Figure 7.7   Eurocopter EC135

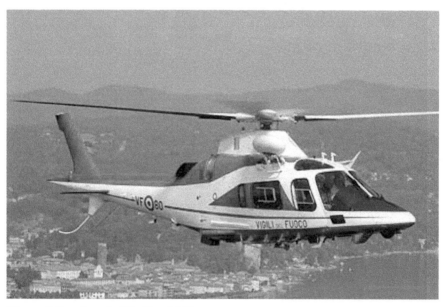

Figure 7.8   Agusta Westland 109

Safety

The growth of civilian aeromedical transport services has been paralleled by an increasing number of EMS related aircraft incidents. In 1986 alone, there were 13 accidents and 18 fatalities involving hospital-based EMS programs in the United States. As a result, the US National Transportation Safety Board (NTSB) reviewed all EMS related accidents in its database. Fifty nine incidents over eight years were identified. More recently, in a ten-year study period up to 2002, there were 84 medical helicopter accidents with 72 fatalities and 64 injured survivors. The NTSB concluded that EMS related accidents were almost twice as frequent (and four times more likely to be fatal) than accidents of non-EMS commercial operators. The final report, entitled, *Safety Study - Commercial Emergency Medical Service Helicopter Operations*, revealed a number of disturbing trends involving aeromedical operations. The rapid increase in EMS helicopter systems in the United States had resulted in a focus on volume of transport and patient capture, rather than safety. Pilots had felt pressured by management to accept flights despite marginal operating conditions. Crew rest was given scant attention, and some items of standard equipment in military helicopters were considered doubtful, at best, for civilian EMS programs. Pilot training was often deficient in interpretation of weather conditions and instrument flight procedures. Only one out of 15 pilots involved in accidents where reduced visibility was considered a factor was actually current in instrument ratings at the time the accident occurred.

Following publication of the NTSB report in 1988, aeromedical programs in the United States made substantial efforts to correct the problems. Among these were the development of safety committees, improved pilot instrument flight training, increased availability of weather information, a drive towards empowering pilots to accept or refuse flights in an unbiased environment, and improvements in onboard safety-related equipment. Accident rates did decrease, and in 1990 no EMS aircraft accidents were reported. Unfortunately, accidents did occur in following years, and incident rates were still unacceptably high at the time of writing.

Single-pilot fixed wing aeromedical operations are permitted in some countries under certain circumstances. In view of the permissible extension in crew hours on aeromedical missions, and the pressure on pilots not to divert to an alternative airport when weather is marginal, the wisdom of allowing single-pilot aeromedical flights (with the exception of short distance and duration missions) is open to question.

Helicopter accidents are clearly a high profile safety issue for the aeromedical transport industry. But while much attention is focused on major aviation accidents and incidents, non-aviation occurrences, minor incidents, and near misses are often not represented in databases. It is the responsibility of everyone in the aeromedical industry to be aware of safety related issues and accident mitigation techniques.

The medical aviation environment

Prehospital aeromedical crews work in a hazardous environment but they also bring a hazard (the aircraft) to the scene whenever they respond. Arrival at the incident site often involves establishing a landing zone in an area with which the pilot is unfamiliar or on terrain not specifically arranged as a landing site. Scene calls often occur at dusk or at night, and may involve distractors such as other public safety agencies, news media, and bystanders. One third of the American EMS helicopter accidents between 1982 and 1991 occurred during take-off or departure. This type of accident often involved a wire strike or impact with trees or objects around the landing zone.

On the ground, there is a danger of rotor strikes involving personnel or equipment, and aircraft damage or personal injuries may occur as rotor wash forces debris into the air. Inappropriate contact with the aircraft also presents a problem. Heated pitot tubes may cause burns if touched immediately after flight, and damage to the tubes themselves may impair function of airspeed and other pressure related instruments. Radio antennas often look like handles or bars; damage to these structures may interfere with essential communications. They are also capable of high energy dissipation and can cause shocks if touched during transmission.

Aeromedical crew may be exposed to extremes of climate and terrain as a part of daily operations. Selection of uniforms and other protective equipment must include consideration of the aviation, safety, and infectious disease aspects of aeromedical operations, as well as exposure to extreme environments. In addition, many organizations operate more than one type of aircraft. Emergency procedures and safety issues vary between aircraft and often even between different configurations of the same aircraft.

The safety program – principles and development

Safety must represent the top priority for medical personnel and aircrew alike. Four basic principles must guide the development of safety programs for aeromedical operations. The program must be comprehensive in scope and time, multidisciplinary in conduct, and applicable to all aspects of flight operations at any given point in time.

Haddon's matrix model for injury prevention provides an excellent basis for developing a safety management program. Development of a matrix to deal with an identified problem may highlight weaknesses not previously considered. Management of safety issues involves consideration of all the matrix sections (Table 7.4).

Table 7.4   Safety matrix: factors in crash prevention and survival

	Pilot/crew	Aircraft	Geography/ Weather	Organization
Pre-crash	Uniforms and protective equipment; Training	Selection; Maintenance	Flight following; Weather updates; IFR status	Flight acceptance protocols; Mission profile; Flight following
Crash	Correct use of protective equipment	Crashworthiness; Loose equipment secured	Terrain; Weather	Notification
Post-crash	Physical condition; Evacuation procedures; Injuries	Access to emergency exits; Fuel leaks	Terrain; Weather	Search and rescue; Post-incident plan; Trauma system; Debriefing

Role of the medical director

The medical director must take an active role in the safety program and be involved in the drafting and regular review of protocols and standard operating procedures. As a doctor, he must recognize that when delivery of medical care and safety come into conflict, the latter must always take precedence. It is important not to interfere with aviation operations, but to fully understand them in order to participate in creating and maintaining a safe environment. Although medical directors are not expected to be experts in aviation, at an absolute minimum they must strive to be intelligent consumers. Every effort must be made to create an integrated medical and aviation team with identical objectives, intimate cooperation and respect for each other's professional decisions.

Prioritization of safety issues has a significant impact on the role of the medical director. Budgeting and training for medical equipment and procedures is occasionally superseded by safety requirements. An aeromedical escort who functions in an unsafe manner despite demonstrating superb good care skills must be subject to guidance and remedial education. At times, the quality of patient care may seem to suffer as flights are aborted, turned down, or rerouted due to safety concerns. It is important to remember that medical concerns must always take a back seat to safety issues, and that unsafe flight operations equates to poor quality patient care.

Accident survivability

An aircraft accident is termed 'survivable' if the forces upon the occupants are compatible with life. Not all survivable crashes have survivors. To a significant degree the chances of surviving a survivable crash depends on crew training and the use of safety equipment. Four major factors help to determine whether a crash is survivable or not. These are the degree of energy absorption within the aircraft structure, occupant restraint, the cabin environment, and crashworthiness.

Crashworthiness describes the relative ability of the aircraft and its components to withstand crushing or rupturing forces, and also considers the functional integrity of such systems as the seat-floor interface, and fuel and oil systems.

The use of occupant restraints clearly increases survivability. With a lap belt restraint, the human body can tolerate only 4 G of vertical force. This increases to 25 G with three and four-point restraints.

Within the cabin environment, the correct placement of medical equipment, the security of heavy items, and interior design are significant factors in minimizing injury. Special attention should be paid to the head strike envelope (the area through which the head moves during a crash impact even if the occupant is restrained).

Finally the degree of energy absorption (the progressive yielding of the airframe upon impact) can diminish the energy of impact transmitted to occupants. Post-crash factors which affect the ability of occupants to leave the aircraft expeditiously include the presence of fire, availability of functional and accessible exits, and maintaining cognitive and locomotor ability to escape from the wreckage.

Pilot factors

In selection of EMS pilot recruits, attention is often focused on the number of hours flight experience the candidate has acquired, but the type of experience, his flight ratings, and level of training are also important. Weather phenomena constituted a significant portion of EMS helicopters accidents in the 1988 NTSB report. Aeromedical pilots should be both IFR rated, and current. IFR qualification and currency are not the same. Under FAA rules, the latter signifies that the pilot has flown a minimum of six hours actual or simulated IFR in the previous six months, including six IFR instrument approaches. Similar rules apply in other countries. Pilot training should also include initial and recurrent programs in *aeronautic decision making* (ADM) and *cockpit resource management* (CRM). CRM and ADM training is aimed at assisting pilots to recognize and correct unsafe and dangerous flight conditions. Courses also review risk assessment and its effect on decision making in the high stress environment of EMS aviation. As aeromedical organizations operate in varied meteorologic, geographic, and sociologic settings, orientation of new pilots must include adequate exposure to, and familiarity with, the organization, the region, and the local EMS environment.

Operationally, the interior configuration of an aeromedical transport vehicle must provide adequate lighting for patient care while not illuminating the flight deck area (to avoid loss of night vision by the pilot). The pilot should be able to isolate himself from the rear portion of the aircraft, when necessary, in order to avoid distractions. Stretchers must be situated in a manner to avoid contact with the pilot or flight controls and instruments. Medical crew often require access to radio or telephone communications separate from that used by the aircrew.

Fatigue affects inflight performance and has been identified as a major contributing factor in EMS accidents. Flight hours should be closely monitored, and pilots who are 'timed out' before their shift is over must be allowed to discontinue flight duties.

Crew considerations

Appropriate training and equipment are essential if medical crew are to work safely in the air transport setting. Medical crew members need to be able to relate the effects of altitude, pressure, vibration, noise, fatigue, and extremes of temperature to their own performance. Problems associated with factors such as recent illness, medications, increase in personal stressors, dental work, alcohol consumption and SCUBA diving, should be addressed both in training sessions and in written policy. Crew members should be able to identify scene situations in which heat stroke, hypothermia, or frostbite present risks, and take steps to mitigate or avoid these dangers.

A thorough familiarization with the aircraft is essential. This includes location and operation of radios and other communication equipment, fire extinguishers, emergency exits, restraint systems, fuel and oxygen shut-off valves, and the emergency locator transmitter. There should be theoretical training and practical experience in emergency procedures and post-crash survival. The program's *raison d'être* determines the content of additional training requirements. Flight crew members must learn to separate medical and aviation concerns in accepting a mission, and they must realize that the latter has priority.

Selection of uniforms and personal safety equipment for aeromedical crew members is often a source of controversy. However, the NTSB report of 1988 recommended that aeromedical flight crews use helmets, protective footwear, and flame resistant flight suits.

Administrative issues

The mission profile of an aeromedical organization describes both the physical environment (including terrain and climate) and activities in which the organization will be involved. While safety related policies will vary with the program and its mission profile, written consensus should exist between the aviation operator, program administrator, and medical management on several key issues (Table 7.5).

Table 7.5   Essential issues of agreement between the aviation and medical components of an aeromedical transport system

- Separation of the medical and aviation decisions to fly
- Responsibility of all personnel to be active participants in the safety program
- Ability of any participant to stop an activity if an unsafe situation is perceived
- Importance of safety related protocols/standard operating procedures
- Serious nature of violations of these protocols and procedures
- Strict adherence to drug and alcohol policies

The medical director should address the question of which prescription and over-the-counter drugs may be used by crew members while on duty. Examples of safety related areas for the development of program policy and standard operating procedures are provided in Table 7.6.

Although adjacent programs often compete with one another, safety related issues represent common ground. Examples of areas of cooperation and mutual benefit include the establishment of standard protocols to prevent 'shopping around' after weather related refusals, coordination of multiple program response to the same incident, assistance with flight following procedures, and coordination in search and rescue.

Table 7.6   Safety related policies/standard operating procedures

- Transport of agitated or violent patients
- Carriage of family members and observers
- Patient loading/unloading with rotors turning
- Use of designated and undesignated landing areas
- Chemical contamination and hazardous (HAZMAT) incidents
- Search and rescue operations
- Transport of prisoners
- Transport of individuals with weapons
- Multi-organizational response to same incident
- Potential interference with flight operations from bystanders

Landing zones and airport ramps

Helicopter landing zones are inherently dangerous places. The most obvious risk is of injury from impact with rotor blades and tail rotors. This danger is heightened while on the scene or at the receiving facility, as blades dip lowest to the ground at the slower rotor speeds associated with start-up and shutdown of the engines (especially when the wind speed is high). Injuries may also occur as debris, dust, sand, snow or spray are propelled through the air by rotor wash. These dangers are exacerbated by increased noise levels (with subsequent difficulty in hearing warnings), and slippery surfaces found on exposed landing pads. All personnel who may interact with aeromedical aircraft must be properly educated in patient transfer techniques and landing zone safety, or should keep well clear. It is policy on many airfields and airports that groundcrew wear high visibility clothing when operating in the vicinity of maneuvering aircraft, and so aeromedical organizations have followed suit.

Some hospitals have designated landing areas that may be appropriately lit and secured. In many countries, these sites have fixed coordinates and are marked on aviation charts and listed in landing site directories. Often they will have assigned approach and departure procedures. The majority of primary responses, however, will occur at unmarked sites and it will be up to the aircrew themselves, or local EMS personnel, to find the best landing site near to the scene of the incident. In an ideal situation, landing zones should be at least 60 ft (approximately 20 m) square, but the actual space requirement will, of course, be dependent on the helicopter rotor disc diameter (some military helicopters are very large, especially twin rotor types such as the Boeing-Vertol Chinook). At night, for safety, the landing site should be a minimum of 100 ft (approximately 30 m) square, with the corners marked by lights, and a flare placed upwind. The area should be smooth and flat, and must be clear of all wires, poles, trees, vehicles, animals and people. Once on the ground, crowd control is paramount. Prehospital care providers may approach the aircraft only at the discretion and direction of the flight crew, and never from the rear, where there is a danger of tail rotor strikes in most helicopter types. After landing, the pilot must spend some time on the ground inspecting the landing site and departure path for undetected hazards to lift-off.

Airport ramps are no less hazardous, and indeed may be even more so because access is often not controlled by the presence of law enforcement or prehospital care personnel. Spinning propeller blades of other aircraft may be invisible and cause serious injury or death on strike, and prop wash or jet blast may hurl items into the air.

Risks are not only to bystanders and crew. Aircraft themselves may be damaged by careless behavior at a landing zone or on an airport ramp. Loose objects on the ground can be sucked into turbine engines with disastrous effect, or may impact with vital flight hardware or avionic attachments. Ambulances and other vehicles have been known to impact the aircraft, usually in the enthusiastic desire to assist with expeditious patient loading and carriage.

Communications

Aeromedical transport services require the ability to communicate with a variety of individuals and agencies under a multitude of circumstances. Proper coordination of communications is vital for safe and efficient patient care. Mobile or standard (land line) telephones are the most commonly used means of access to aeromedical systems. In most countries, a free emergency telephone service (for example, *999* or *911*) is the primary means of access to EMS helicopters but, especially in the

USA, many organizations have dedicated toll-free lines which run directly into the communications center.

On the other hand, radio is undoubtedly the most common operational mode of communication. The most powerful radios in aeromedical transport systems are usually located at the base site or communications center. Mobile systems yield lower outputs over smaller distances and are often linked to repeaters (base stations which reinforce and retransmit the signal) to enhance capabilities. Least powerful are portable radios, with very limited range. With all systems, transmission is greatly enhanced by flat surroundings and attenuated by hills, mountains, foliage, and large buildings. As was tragically discovered during the King's Cross fire in London, most do not work underground. Radios may be equipped to provide simplex (one voice on the channel at any one time) or duplex modes, depending on their operating frequency. The radio spectrum has been divided into bands, each of which has its own official designation and characteristics (Table 7.7).

A well functioning communications center is a critical element of a successful aeromedical system. Guidelines established by the Association of Airmedical Services (AAMS) suggest that all communications center personnel be trained to basic life support level, and should receive training in dispatch and communication procedures. Dispatchers must be trained to process and triage calls from outside agencies and notify flight crew of missions without delay. They must also be skilled in internal communications, and be able to convey flight information, medical orders, and patient status reports to doctors, nurses, and other relevant staff. Communications specialists must also be able to establish links with surrounding EMS and aeromedical programs to provide a means for accessing additional equipment and personnel. The base site must have the capability to be in constant and continuous communication with the aircraft and referring agents. Flight following, with frequent position reports and the accurate determination of direction, distance, and coordinates to scenes and institutions, is a further essential function of the communications center.

Similarly, the aircraft must have good communications capabilities with the base site, ground EMS services, police and fire services, fixed base operators, air traffic control centers, and other air traffic. Redundancy in the communications system allows the pilot to concentrate on aircraft operations while medical crew take patient information, give reports, or provide landing zone instructions to ground personnel.

The communications specialist is usually the individual who initiates the post-accident incident plan. This describes the response of the program to a variety of emergency situations. It includes notification processes, communications procedures, current lists of phone and pager numbers, initial actions to be taken upon activation of the plan, and other specific responsibilities. Situations which call for initiation of the plan should include unexpected flight diversions, emergency landings, suspected or confirmed accident or incident, and when the communications center is unable to locate the aircraft. All members of the flight program must be familiar with the plan and their role in it. Currency is maintained by regular review and annual drill.

Table 7.7   Radio frequency band characteristics

Band	Advantages	Disadvantages
VHF Low	• Long range • Greater mobile-mobile range • Least foliage attenuation • Follows curve of earth	• Skip interference • Few channels • No frequency coordination • Noise interference • Crowded • No repeaters • Frequent dead spots • Simplex mode only • Building interference
VHF High	• Better audio quality • Lowest price • Medium range • Less skip interference • Less noise interference • Low foliage attenuation • Reflects around buildings	• Few channels • No frequency coordination • Very crowded • No repeaters • Poor mobile-mobile range • Simplex mode only • Inside building interference
UHF	• Many channels • Frequency coordination • Very clear audio • Limited skip interference • Repeaters available • Good building penetration	• Short range • Co-channel interference • Higher cost • High foliage attenuation
800 MHz Cellular	• Trunked system available • Almost no skip interference • Very little noise • All systems have repeaters • Good fill in and around buildings in urban areas	• Highest cost • Shortest range • Highest foliage attenuation

References

Bledsoe, B.E. and Smith, M.G. (2004) 'Medical helicopter accidents in the United States: A 10 year review', *J Trauma Inj, Infect,Crit Care.* **56**(6): 1325-9.

Bottner, J. and T. Schiera (1994) 'Aircraft capabilities for air medical transport', in Blumen I.J. and H. Rodenberg (eds), *Air Medical Physician's Handbook*, AMPA: Salt Lake City.

Davis, E. (1994) 'Communications in air medical transport', in Blumen I.J. and H. Rodenberg (eds), *Air Medical Physician's Handbook*, AMPA: Salt Lake City.

Dodd, C. (1994) 'The cost-effectiveness of air medical helicopter crash survival enhancements: An evaluation of the costs, benefits, and effectiveness of injury prevention interventions', *Air Med J.* **13**:281-93.

Fenn, J., Rega, P., Stavros, M. and N.F. Buderer (1999) 'Assessment of U.S. helicopter emergency medical services planning and preparedness for disaster response', *Air Med J.* 18(1):12-15.

Fisher, J., Phillips E. and Mather J. (2000) 'Does crew resource management training work?', *Air Med J.* 19(4):137-9.

Fox, R. (1988) 'Crash survivability', *Air Med Safety Quarterly* 1:23-5.

Gilbert, C. (1994) 'Aviation safety for the air medical physician', in Blumen I.J. and H. Rodenberg (eds), *Air Medical Physician's Handbook*, AMPA: Salt Lake City.

Lackner, C.K. and E. Stolpe (1998) 'New order of things: an international overview of air medical transport', *Air Med J.* 17(4):142-5.

MacDonald, E. and J. Heffernan (2002) 'Safety above all: an Air Medical Safety Advisory Council update', *Air Med J.* 21(4):15-16.

Maguire, B.J., Hunting, K.L., Smith, G.S. and N.R. Levick (2002) 'Occupational fatalities in emergency medical services: a hidden crisis', *Ann Emerg Med.* 40(6):625-32.

Martin, T.E. (2004) 'HMFC – Radio Comms', pre-course reading for Helicopter Medical Flight Crew course, www.ccat-training.org.uk.

Wuerz, R. (1994) 'Integration of ground and air EMS', in Blumen I.J. and H. Rodenberg (eds), *Air Medical Physician's Handbook*, AMPA: Salt Lake City.

Chapter 8

The Medical Flight Crew

Crew configuration

Few topics in aeromedical transport circles excite more passion and debate than the optimal configuration of medical flight crew. Flight teams are both selected and limited by factors such as patient type, patient mix, aircraft capabilities, finances, local resources, marketing, and cultural considerations. Although some fixed wing services may fly with a crew of one while transporting a single stable patient on a routine repatriation or interfacility transfer, most high dependency aeromedical transport services use two medical crew members. However, situations may occur where flight conditions such as heat, humidity, altitude, or fuel load necessitate flying with a single crew member. On the other hand, services may fly with three or more crew members such as when there is a need for specialized team members to accompany standard crew, or when several patients are transported on the same flight.

Homogenous and heterogenous teams

The first step in determining a program's crew configuration is to decide whether to use flight teams in which each member has the same training or to use crews of differing background. Both may offer advantages.

Homogenous crews (in which both members of the crew are of the same professional group) provide for an absolute understanding between team members of the capabilities and limitations of each other. While this understanding may come with time in any medical team, a more innate, intuitive, and immediate understanding is present when both team members have experienced the same type of training. Team work and efficiency are therefore enhanced. Homogenous teams also ease scheduling conflicts by providing complete interchangeability between all members on the roster. Continuing education and on-site training is also more easily accomplished. These are important considerations for smaller services with few personnel.

The most common type of homogenous team in the USA is the dual nurse pairing. Given the large number of interfacility transfers performed by aeromedical services and the number of advanced treatment modalities used, the dual nurse team is a reasonable choice (Figure 8.1). The requirements for employment usually include critical care experience as well as advanced training and certification in aeromedical care. The nurse crew may be scheduled into other in-house services during 'down' time, thereby maximizing efficiency and they often enhance their prehospital skills by cross-training at the advanced life support level. Ongoing ground EMS experience can improve cooperation and credibility with local EMS systems while strengthening skills and confidence. Clearly, continuing education focused on the particular problems faced by flight nurses, along with ongoing inpatient critical care experience, maximizes crew efficiency.

The dual paramedic crew is a reflection of aeromedical transport's roots in military casualty evacuation. Generally, these teams are used by services that primarily provide emergency rather than elective transport, or by public service agencies that maintain a dual role (that is, law enforcement, fire, or military operations). The unique mixture of field experience and advanced skills that paramedics provide may make them ideal crew members. Paramedics are familiar with uncontrolled out-of-hospital scenes and initial stabilization, and are likely to be accustomed to working independently, yet under the guidance of protocols and on-line medical supervision, that is, as part of a team. Continuing education focusing on the particular problems of interfacility critical care transports may maximize the confidence and proficiency of dual paramedic crews, enabling extension of their prehospital role.

In contrast to crews made up of similarly trained personnel, heterogenous crews utilize mixed pairings. In this configuration crew members have dissimilar core training, though later cross-training may be an ultimate goal. In the United States, the paramedic/nurse combination is widely used. The paramedic has expertise, training, and experience in handling the uncontrolled scene and the unstabilized, unpackaged patient, whereas the critical care flight nurse has experience in caring for unstable patients with multiple advanced monitoring and treatment modalities. A team with diverse strengths allow for the efficient management of a wider variety of patients. Teams constructed of personnel with different strengths leads each to enhance his or her knowledge, skills, and abilities through the influence of the other. In these teams, the whole may exceed the sum of the parts.

This same argument can be applied to the inclusion of a doctor as a member of the flight team (Figure 8.2). The in-depth knowledge, education, and advanced skills of the flight physician represent a positive addition which compliments the experienced paramedic or nurse who offer a dimension to patient care overlooked in medical school education (see Chapter 16). Having a doctor on board may also solve problems with communications, distance, dialogue with referring physicians, and rapidly deteriorating patients. It may also deflect criticism and questions over issues of continuity of care, responsibility, and compliance with patient transfer regulations. In some cases there may also be a marketing benefit and, in international operations, there is often a cultural advantage to the presence of a doctor. However, the increased costs of having a flight physician on board may outweigh these somewhat intangible assets. The flight physician, as a minimum, should be qualified to act as an on-line medical supervisor. In other words, he must have a thorough knowledge of flight physiology, of the unique problems and limitations of the aeromedical setting and, if working in the primary role, of the prehospital and interfacility referral systems.

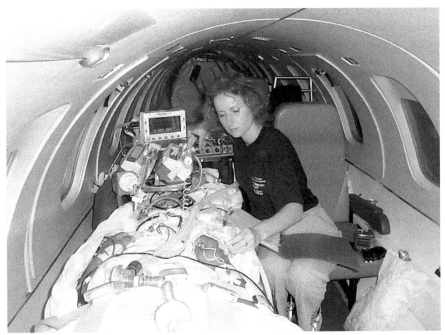

Figure 8.1   Flight nurse and patient during a repatriation mission

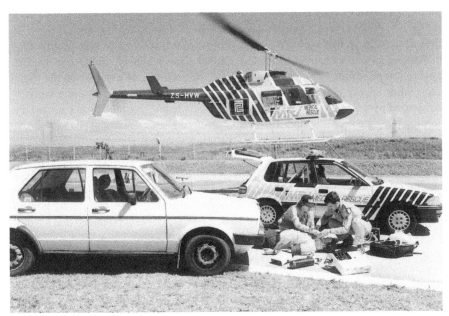

Figure 8.2   Flight physician and paramedic team
Source: Medical Rescue International (SA)

An important and expanding role for aeromedical systems is the transfer of the specialty patient. Such patients are those who are best served by a specialist medical team with training and experience distinct from that of standard flight medical crew. Examples include the patient on an intra-aortic balloon pump who may require a perfusionist's care, the unstable neonate for whom a pediatrician or neonatal nurse might be essential, or the unstable ventilated patient who could benefit from the care of an anesthesiologist or respiratory therapist. At larger medical centers, some organ harvest and transplant teams utilize rapid response air transport services, although this is usually for delivery of the team, or retrieval of an organ. Specialty patients can increase the utilization of transport services, enhance revenue, and provide valuable positive promotion for the flight program. All of these attributes can be important for the flight manager trying to justify the maintenance of an expensive service when faced with an administration committed to cost control.

Many services utilize a system where primary air crews are available on-site for immediate response to emergency calls and specialty crews are available on-call or standby for flights requiring special services. Specialty crew members who may be unfamiliar with the aviation environment are often accompanied by a primary crew member for assistance and logistic support. This arrangement allows the flexibility to respond to special transport needs without sacrificing efficiency and safety.

Flight crew efficacy

Little is known about the efficacy of different flight crew configurations, and those studies which have been reported have often been questioned because of flaws in study design, the lack of a 'gold standard', the use of subjective data, and the difficulty of drawing firm conclusions from the limited data available. Subjective studies provide mixed results regarding the need for the presence of a doctor on the flight team, while recent objective works reveal no difference between trauma patients transported by a doctor/nurse and nurse/paramedic team. One study has compared a German doctor/paramedic and American nurse/paramedic team and found that the former offers an advantage in the care of the trauma patient. However, differences in the structure of both EMS systems, the patient demographics, and the EMS response times make the validity of this study difficult to interpret. Objective work delineating the efficacy of varied crew configurations is scarce and inconclusive. However, a British government funded study of the London Helicopter EMS, comparing ground (paramedic-based) and helicopter (physician-based) transport concluded that a small number of patients do benefit.

Several subjective studies in the pediatric literature suggest that the presence of a pediatrician during critical care transport is preferred or even required in certain patients, but accurately identifying these patients beforehand has proven difficult. Little study comparing the other types of flight crews in use has been attempted to date, although one work showed no difference in the care of trauma patients between dual-certified nurse/paramedic and one dual-certified/one paramedic crew member.

Clearly, it remains for the individual flight program to identify the elements which define its patient population and to make a decision on the composition of medical flight crew based on the factors unique to its individual mission and circumstances.

Flight crew education

An educational scheme for flight medical crew must address clinical and operational issues unique to aeromedical transportation. Educational efforts should expand on the knowledge and skills already possessed by the flight team, and focus on principles that will enable flight medical crew to better assess, stabilize, treat, and transport critically ill patients in the flight environment. Thresholds for action should correlate with the degree of acuteness, taking into account the benefit to the patient versus the risk of the intervention. As the severity of the patient's illness escalates, the aeromedical escort must learn to appropriately escalate the degree of intervention. Optimal educational models consist of a mixture of didactic, clinical, and procedural experiences, such as exemplified by the American College of Surgeons ATLS (Advanced Trauma Life Support) course and introduced into aeromedical care by the UK-based international CCAT (Clinical Considerations in Aeromedical Transport) course.

Educational techniques

Adults do not learn in the same way as children. The following educational principles may be valuable when designing educational programs for medical flight crew:

1. A generous mix of short duration lecture format material with small-group reinforcement and frequent checks of understanding enhances information retention better than long and tedious (boring for the student) lecturer-led presentations.
2. Practical hands-on sessions should be used as often as possible to further reinforce theoretical teaching. It is better to train aeromedical personnel on aircraft and with the equipment that they will use rather than cover the material in a lecture.
3. Similarly, in terms of audiovisual materials, it is true that 'the real thing is more relevant than a model, and a model is better than a picture'.
4. The use of interactive scenarios is a useful educational tool which enables the student to unify and synthesize an approach to clinical situations.
5. Instructors should ask open-ended, thought provoking questions during the teaching process in order to stimulate discussion, develop logical thinking processes, and prompt further questions and study.
6. Direct questions to named individuals keeps the whole class on the ball! However, it never helps to belittle or embarrass an individual who cannot anwer a question. Praise is always due when students give a satisfactory

response, but it behoves the instructor to develop techniques to facilitate understanding and learning for those students who have failed to comprehend important points.

7. Emphasis should be placed on self-education by reading, attendance at meetings, and taking part in web-based or other electronically available educational material. Asking questions of peers and consultants should also be encouraged.

If every member of the flight medical team understands his individual strengths and deficiencies he can be motivated and encouraged to pursue education in areas of weakness and to teach others in areas of expertise.

Evaluation of the individual aeromedical escort's judgement and performance can be accomplished by written tests, oral examinations, case reviews, scenario training, and field observation. It must be understood by supervisors, and emphasized to crew, that these evaluatory techniques will not be used as disciplinary tools, but as ways to identify areas for improvement. The optimal means for medical directors and supervisors to both evaluate flight team performance and enhance team cohesiveness is by flying with the team as often as aircraft and patient commitments allow.

Areas of emphasis

Every member of the flight medical team must possess a thorough knowledge of the medical care policies and protocols used by the system. Clearly, operational considerations require specific instruction in flight physiology, safety, communications, and the means of delivering optimal patient care within the aeromedical environment.

Training in marketing techniques is an area that may also be of great value to aeromedical services. Specific instruction for doctors, nurses, other hospital staff, and EMS providers might be added as an integral part of flight team education. Knowing how to respond to uncomfortable situations (such as suspected patient mismanagement by the referring medical team) can spare ill feelings that operate to the detriment of the flight program and the patients who might benefit from its services. The importance of quality assurance (QA) and continuous quality improvement (CQI) programs in maintaining standards and improving patient care must also be conveyed to the team. The flight crew should receive specific instruction on medicolegal issues, especially on proper medical documentation. Accurate charting will not only improve documentation and decrease medicolegal risk, but also ensure an audit trail for QA and CQI purposes.

All aeromedical crew members should receive currency training based on individual and program needs. Recurrent training should emphasize those cognitive and procedural skills which are significant to each system's typical missions (patients and flight operations). Accrediting organizations or regulatory bodies may require recurrent training at fixed frequency intervals and therefore training schedules must reflect these realities.

Although each aeromedical service must consider its own individual needs for training, a model curriculum and training manual has been developed for the US Department of Transportation under the title Air Medical Crew National Standard Curriculum. A sample curriculum based on these guidelines is presented in Table 8.1.

In the UK, although flight nurses had been trained by the Royal College of Nursing for many years, doctors were poorly represented until the 1990s. An international multi-disciplinary course called CCAT (*Clinical Considerations in Aeromedical Transport*) was established in 1997. It was originally intended for budding flight physicians, but soon opened its doors also to flight nurses, paramedics and aeromedical managers. Its success and international reputation has led to the development of a two- stage (basic and advanced) aeromedical course for fixed wing flight medical crew, plus additional linked courses for the specific benefit of *Helicopter Medical Flight Crew* (HMFC) and those who wish to know more about passenger *Medical Emergencies in Flight* (MEF). Information on these courses can be found on *www.ccat-training.org.uk*

Similar courses are bound to follow, but one postgraduate center (University of Otago, Wellington School of Medicine, New Zealand) has adopted a novel approach and now teaches the theory of aeromedical retrieval and transport medicine using distance learning and web-based teaching techniques (*www.otago.ac.nz/aviation_medicine*).

Table 8.1   A model curriculum based on the *Air Medical Crew National Standard Curriculum* (USA)

i.   **Flight physiology**
    1. Pressure, volume, and temperature relationships of gases.
    2. Composition, pressure, and temperature of the atmosphere.
    3. Effects of noise, vibration, and acceleration.

ii. **The emergency medical services**
    1. Local, regional, and national disaster plans.
    2. Identification, assessment, triage, and routing of patients.
    3. Communication and the local incident command structure.

iii. **Search, rescue, and survival**
    1. Air and ground search and rescue.
    2. Wilderness survival techniques appropriate to the area.
    3. Map reading and use of a compass.

iv. **Hazardous materials**
    1. The meaning of common placards.
    2. Information sources on hazardous materials.
    3. Containment and medical management after exposure.

v.   **Equipment**
    A. Aviation and aircraft related equipment
      1. Master switch and fuel shut off valve.
      2. Emergency locator transmitter.
      3. Rotor brake (where applicable).
      4. Oxygen shut off valve.
      5. Fire fighting and emergency egress systems.
    B. Medical equipment
      1. Oxygen supplies and mechanical ventilators.
      2. Infusion pumps.
      3. Pacemaker generators.
      4. Cardiac monitors and defibrillators.
      5. Manual, doppler, and automatic blood pressure cuffs.
      6. Pulse oximetry.
      7. Immobilization equipment.

vi. **Policies and procedures**
    1. Infection control and prevention.
    2. Operational policies and procedures.

vii. **Patient care**
    A. Neurological disorders
      1. Increased intracranial pressure.
      2. Closed and open head injuries.
      3. Spinal cord injuries.
      4. Cerebrovascular accidents.

B. *Cardiovascular Disorders*
    1. Acute myocardial infarction.
    2. Ventricular and supraventricular dysrhythmias.
    3. Left ventricular failure and shock.
    4. Malignant hypertension.
    5. Aortic dissections/aneurysms.
    6. Cardiopulmonary arrest.

C. *Respiratory Disorders*
    1. Respiratory arrest.
    2. Pulmonary edema.
    3. Pulmonary embolism.
    4. Bronchospasm and obstructive airway disease.
    5. Pneumothorax and hemothorax.
    6. Upper airway problems.
    7. Use of mechanical ventilation.

D. *Trauma*
    1. Splinting of fractures and spinal immobilization.
    2. Airway management of the trauma victim.
    3. Management of hemothorax and pneumothorax.
    4. Management of shock.
    5. Management of orthopedic trauma.
    6. Assessment and management of abdominal injury.
    7. Trauma scoring systems.
    8. Management of the burn victim.

E. *High Risk Obstetrical and Neonatal Patients*
    1. Pre-eclampsia and eclampsia.
    2. Pregnancy induced hypertension.
    3. Normal vaginal delivery and preterm labor.
    4. Obstetrical hemorrhage.
    5. Neonatal hypoglycemia.
    6. Respiratory distress syndrome and cyanotic heart disease.
    7. Meconium aspiration and tracheo-esophageal fistula.
    8. Myelomeningocele.
    9. Gastroschisis and omphalocele.
    10. The APGAR scoring system.

F. *Pediatric Disorders*
    1. Croup and epiglottis.
    2. Child abuse and neglect.
    3. Infectious diseases common to childhood.
    4. Psychosocial development during childhood.

References

Association of Hospital Based Emergency Air Medical Services (1988) *Air Medical Crew National Standard Curriculum*, US Department of Transportation, National Highway Safety Administration, Washington.

Baxt, W.G. and P. Moody (1987) 'The impact of a physician as part of the aeromedical prehospital team in patients with blunt trauma', *J Am Med Assoc.* **257**:3246-50.

Burney, R.E., Hubert, D., Passini, L., R. Maio (1995) 'Variation in air medical outcomes by crew composition: a two-year follow-up', *Ann Emerg Med.* **25**(2):187-92.

Burney, R.E., Passini, L., Hubert, D. and R. Maio (1992) 'Comparison of aeromedical crew performance by patient severity and outcome', *Ann Emerg Med.* **21**(4):375-8.

CCAT (2005) Clinical Considerations in Aeromedical Transport. Aeromedical courses website, *www.ccat-training.org.uk.*

Fonne, V.M. and G. Myhre (1996) 'The effect of occupational cultures on coordination of emergency medical service aircrew', *Aviat Space Environ Med.* **67**(6):525-9.

Fromm, R.E. (1994) 'Training of the air medical flight crew: practical applications', in Blumen, I.J. and Rodenberg, H. (eds), *Air Medical Physician's Handbook*, AMPA: Salt Lake City.

Gabram, S.G., Hodges J., Allen P.T., Allen L.W., Schwartz R.J. and L.M. Jacobs L.M. (1994) 'Personality types of flight crew members in a hospital-based helicopter program', *Air Med J.* **13**(1):13-7.

Gryniuk, J., National Flight Paramedics Association (2003) 'The role of the flight paramedic in air medical safety and crew resource management', *Air Med J.* **22**(4):12-4.

Hamman, B.L., Cue J.I., Miller F.B. et al. (1991) 'Helicopter transport of trauma victims: does a physician make a difference?', *J Trauma* **31**:4990-4.

High, K. and M. High (2001) 'Strategies for becoming a flight crew member', *Emerg Med Serv.* **30**(3):53-5.

Hutchison, T. (1994) 'Training of the air medical flight crew: general concepts', in Blumen I.J. and H.,Rodenberg (eds), *Air Medical Physician's Handbook*, AMPA: Salt Lake City.

Krohmer, J.R., Hunt, R.C., Benson, N. and R.B. Bieniek (1993) 'Flight physicians training program – core content', *Prehosp Disast Med.* **8**(2):183-4.

Macnab, A.J. (1991) 'Optimal escort for interhospital transport of pediatric emergencies', *J Trauma.* **31**:305-9.

McCloskey, K.A. and C. Johnston (1990) 'Critical care interhospital transports: predictability of the need for a pediatrician', *Pediatr Emerg Care.* **6**:89-92.

McCloskey, K.A. and C. Johnston (1990) 'Pediatric critical care survey: team composition and training, mobilization time and mode of transport', *Pediatr Emerg Care.* **6**:1-3.

Myers, K.J., Rodenberg H. and D. Woodard (1995) 'Influence of the helicopter environment on patient care capabilities: flight crew perceptions', *Air Med J.* **14**(1):21-5.

Poultan, T.J., Gutierrez, P.J. and D.J. Schwabe (1987) 'Physicians' role in aeromedical transport questioned', *Ann Emerg Med.* **16**(12):1412-3.

Rhee, K.J., Strozeski, M., Burney, R.E. et al, (1986) 'Is the flight physician needed for helicopter emergency medical services?', *Ann Emerg Med.* **15**:174-7.

Schmidt, U., Frame, S.B. et al, (1992) 'On-scene helicopter transport of patients with multiple injuries – comparison of a German and an American system', *J Trauma.* **33**:548-55.

Shaner, S., Brooks C., Osborn R., Hull M. and R.E., Falcone (1995) 'Flight crew physical fitness: a baseline analysis', *Air Med J.* **14**(1):30-2.

Sibold, H. (1994) 'Crew configuration', in Blumen I.J. and H.Rodenberg (eds), *Air Medical Physician's Handbook*, AMPA: Salt Lake City.

Stohler, S.A. (1998) High performance team interaction in an air medical program. *Air Med J.* **17**(3):116-20.

Topley, D.K., Schmelz, J., Henkenius-Kirschbaum, J. and K.J.Horvath (2003) Critical care nursing expertise during air transport. *Milit Med.* **168**(10):822-6

University of Otago (2005) Aeromedical Retrieval and Transport courses website, *www.otago.ac.nz/aviation_medicine.*

Williams, K.A., Rose, W.D. and R. Simon R. (1999) 'Teamwork in emergency medical services', *Air Med J.* **18**(4):149-53.

Wynn, J.S. (2001) 'Leadership strategies for a stronger industry', *Air Med J.* **20**(4):18-9.

Chapter 9

Aeromedical Equipment

General requirements

There is a wide choice of equipment available to medical personnel, but not all is compatible with the aviation environment. Furthermore, given that the costs are high, it is vital to ensure that correct choices are made before purchase is confirmed. Essentially, in addition to the need for accuracy and reliability (usually only one item of each type of equipment can be carried), equipment for use in aircraft must be compact, lightweight, and rugged enough to be able to withstand the stresses of accelerations, vibration, and the possibility of rapid decompression. In addition, the equipment must continue to work dependably without loss of accuracy in conditions of prolonged hypobaric pressure, thermal extremes, and variations in humidity.

The exact nature of the medical equipment carried on board will depend on both the type of aeromedical mission and on the specific problems of the patients being transported. Although some equipment found in hospitals may also be utilized for air transfer work, such equipment must comply with extra safety and performance requirements before it can be used in aircraft. This chapter discusses equipment that is commonly used in air ambulance and medical retrieval work and emphasises how the aviation and prehospital environments might affect functionality. The equipment can be conveniently categorised as follows:

1. Equipment required for patient carriage
2. Equipment required for patient care

Equipment required for patient carriage

This includes such items as stretchers, vacuum mattresses, splintage, spine boards, restraint systems and loading devices.

Stretchers

Stretchers to be used in an aviation environment must meet a number of standards. These include the ability to be securely and effectively mounted to the floor or body of the airframe. In many jurisdictions the stretcher and mountings have been designed and tested to ensure that they can withstand a significant impact force – commonly a 20 G crash. Stretcher bridges are used to mount medical equipment to prevent it lying loosely on or around the patient. These must also be crash rated but also portable and useable. They may need to fit a variety of stretchers and will need independent power and oxygen options.

Spinal support

The vacuum mattress has almost completely replaced the spinal turning frame. It is extremely useful for long flights as, with suitable internal padding (such as a sheepskin blanket), it can greatly increase patient comfort whilst minimising the risk of pressure areas. Pressurization changes in flight necessitate checking and adjusting the state of the vacuum within the mattress as residual gas volumes increase with altitude. Spine boards, spinal extrication devices, cervical collars, and so on, need to be compatible with ground-based ambulances. Ideally the aircraft should have its own equipment even if the main role is to handover to a ground-based ambulance crew. The equipment already applied to the patient can then be exchanged for fresh equipment from the ground ambulance.

Limb splintage

Similarly, a wide range of compatible splints and tractions devices should be available to the medical crew. Traction devices should not be reliant on external weights because of the effect of acceleration and vibration (G) forces on increase of weight. Pneumatic splints will be affected by pressure changes on climb to altitude and the subsequent descent.

Loading systems

Loading systems and devices have been designed for specific aircraft, for specific stretcher-bridge systems, and for fleet-wide use by individual aeromedical organizations. Some systems have been adopted for wheelchair carriage and others make use of non-specific cargo or catering lift devices (Figure 9.1).

Equipment required for patient care

Nursing care materials

For any transfer, the flight nursing bag must hold all that will be required for the entire journey. No reliance can be placed on the availability of essential supplies from the referring hospital (especially when overseas), nor from the aircraft operator or airline. Doctors escorting patients without the benefit of a nursing colleague would be wise to seek advice as soon as patient details are available before setting out on the mission. Every aspect of patient care must be considered, from blankets, pillows and special mattresses (egg-shell, spenco, vacumat, anti-allergy, sheepskin, and so on) to feeding aids and utensils, toiletries, disposable bedpans, and urinals.

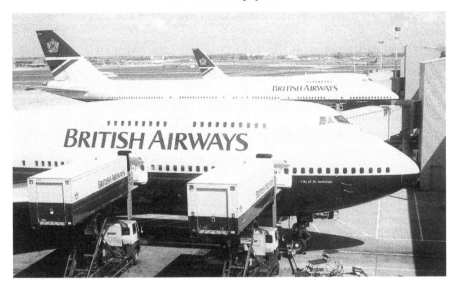

Figure 9.1   Using a cargo lift for stretcher access to a commercial airliner

In addition, although it is best to avoid exposing or touching wounds in flight, extra dressings and other wound care products may still be required. Personal protection items should include sterile and non-sterile gloves, masks, aprons, a container for used 'sharps', and plastic bags for the collection and disposal of clinical waste.

Helicopter air ambulances

HEMS primary transfer missions   The range of equipment depends on the type of mission. For instance, in primary 'scoop and run' missions, little may be required apart from oxygen and oxygen delivery devices, measures for haemorrhage control, intravenous cannulation and basic monitoring such as noninvasive blood pressure (NIBP) and electrocardiogram (ECG). In many HEMS missions the air ambulance may be responding in support of ground crews. In this case some standard ambulance equipment may not be carried, but rather 'borrowed' from ground crews as required. This might apply to simple items like bandaging and so on. If, however, the aircraft is required to respond independently, then all basic ambulance equipment as well as advanced items must be carried. A typical list of HEMS equipment might include the items specified in Tables 9.1 and 9.2.

Table 9.1   HEMS typical onboard medical equipment and specialist kit

Onboard equipment	Specialist kit
• defibrillator	
• capnograph	• paediatric pack containing:
• ventilator	- airways, endotracheal (ET) tubes
• piped oxygen	- masks
• syringe pumps	- cannulae, and so on.
• pressure infusers	
• spare IV fluids	• burns pack containing:
• protective helmets	- burns dressings
• protective gloves	- clingfilm
• identification tabards	
• mass casualty triage cards	• communications:
• extrication device	- mobile telephone
• bolt cutters	- VHF radio

Table 9.2   HEMS typical portable medical equipment

Portable equipment	Thomas pack containing
• multimodal monitor	• stethoscope
• pulse oximeter	• sphygmomanometer
• ventilator and oxygen	• torch
• cervical collars	• intubation equipment
• suction device	• bag-valve-mask system
• traction splint	• needle cricothyroidotomy set
• MAST garment	• surgical airway set
• scoop stretcher	• chest drain set
• Vacumat stretcher	• IV administration sets
• drugs pack containing:	• central venous cannulae
- resuscitation (ALS) drugs	• sterile surgical pack
- opiate analgesics	• aortic cross clamp
- anaesthetic agents	• Gigli amputation saw
- muscle relaxants	• dressings
- bronchodilator	• warmed IV fluids:
	- crystalloid solution (for example, Ringers)
	- colloid solution (for example, Gelofusine)
	- mannitol 20%

In addition to obvious diagnostic and therapeutic medical machinery and matériel, items needed by HEMS operators will include personal safety and rescue items (such as helmets, protective clothing, and metal cutters), ambulance equipment (such as stretchers, splints, blankets, extrication and immobilization devices), and communication devices (radio transmitters and mobile telephones) which are described elsewhere. The minimum amount of diagnostic and therapeutic equipment should include a defibrillator with electrocardiograph monitor (or a separate monitor), pulse oximeter, non-invasive blood pressure monitor, suction aspirator, mechanical ventilator and the all equipment necessary to safely perform any procedure recommended in the advanced cardiac (ACLS or ALS) and trauma (ATLS or EMST) life support protocols that may be appropriate in the prehospital scenario. Equipment used in out-of-hospital environments must be water resistant and be able to withstand the ingress of dust, sand and salt spray. It must be rugged and able to survive a drop from at least one metre on to any face, side or corner, without affecting function, accuracy or reliability.

Helicopter secondary retrieval and transfer missions

In principle, the types of helicopter equipment are no different from equipment fitted to and carried in fixed wing aircraft. However, there is an emphasis on minimizing size and weight because of the smaller cabin space and carrying capability of most helicopter air ambulances compared with fixed wing air ambulances. Every aeromedical organization will equip its aircraft and aeromedical personnel according to the likely mission and requirements of the cases being transported. There are many advisory papers which set out minimum standards of equipment, some endorsed by national authorities, and others by esteemed medical establishments. One such example is a set of recommendations on minimum acceptable equipment produced by the UK Royal Society of Medicine (RSM) working party on minimum standards in medical helicopter systems (Table 9.3).

Interfacility and repatriation operations

Equipment for secondary and tertiary transfers may range from a minimal resuscitation kit for an uncomplicated postoperative or post-infarct repatriation, to a full intensive care capability for critical care patients. When carrying an extensive array of equipment, it is important that all items provide maximum function at minimum cost, size, and weight. Air ambulance and medical assistance organizations should keep lists of recommended *minimum* equipment for the different categories of patients within their sphere of operations. Further items may be needed, and this can only be decided when full information about the patient has been received prior to setting off on the mission. Particular care in planning may prevent the embarrassment of arriving without an essential item, and the danger of continuing the mission without that item.

Table 9.3   Recommendations of the RSM working party on minimum standards in medical helicopter systems: minimum acceptable equipment

Adult	Neonatal
• positive pressure ventilation	• transport incubator
• pulse oximeter	• temperature monitor
• blood pressure measurement	• neonatal ventilator
• electrocardiograph	• pulse oximeter
• defibrillator	• umbilical artery oxygen monitor
• suction device	• blood pressure measurement
• oxygen supply	• electrocardiograph
• intubation equipment	• suction device
• IV fluid equipment	• oxygen supply
• drugs for resuscitation	• air supply
• drugs for continuing management	• intubation equipment
	• drugs for resuscitation
	• drugs for continuing management

Source: *Journal of the Royal Society of Medicine*, Vol 84, pp 242-244.

Fixed wing critical care retrieval and transfer missions

Critical care retrievals and transfers require considerably more equipment. The list in Table 9.4 is one example. It is a comprehensive list, intending to cover a wide range of situations. Readers will be able to think of some items they would like to add and may see some things on the list which they would gladly omit. The point is that no list is perfect, and every aeromedical organization should have a policy or procedure enabling continuous review of medical kit and equipment contents. At least annual review allows updates and advances in medical care and newly introduced management guidelines and protocols to be introduced and ensures the equipment and matériel are available to enable such procedures.

   Many organizations are working towards integrated loading and patient carriage systems with a stretcher-bridge capable of holding all the necessary equipment and devices for the transfer of a ventilated intensive care patient. Readers who are familiar with such systems will also be aware that none is perfect. The concept of putting all the therapeutic and monitoring devices together on one structure, upon which the patient also lays, is an ideal situation. It might be attainable if variables such as aircraft cabin dimensions, patient size, types of devices and access to the patient could be fixed. Unfortunately, these and other confounders make even the neatest system inadequate in some situations. The Swedish National Air Medevac program (SNAM) has developed arguably the most user-friendly and elegant system, and has proven that they can convert a conventional commercial airliner to take six such intensive care systems and twelve other stretcher units within six hours of notification (Figure 9.2).

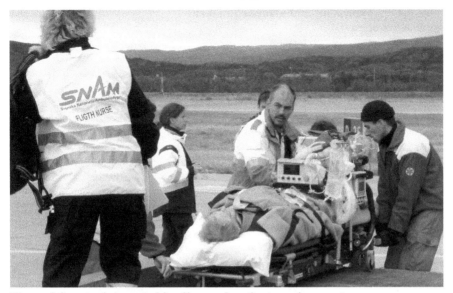

Figure 9.2   An integrated loading and patient carriage system

The flight medical bag

Like all other aspects of aeromedical equipment, the flight medical bag must cover the needs of the individual mission and yet be lightweight and small enough to be easily carried. The bag itself may be a briefcase or holdall, a rucksack ('snatchbag'), or may even be a plastic or metallic case. Ruggedness and durability are important, but weight considerations are paramount since the medical escort may have to carry this bag and other equipment, without assistance, throughout the various stages of the transfer. Another desirable feature is accessibility of the contents. A compartmentalized bag from which equipment can easily be retrieved in the cramped and confined space of an aircraft cabin is a must. It is essential to have a list of the contents of each compartment or pocket, and to be familiar with all the items carried.

In general, it is advisable to avoid carrying too many drugs and medications. Resuscitation drugs (those recommended by the European Resuscitation Council [ERC], American Heart Association [AHA], or other national body) must always be carried. The escort should otherwise try to keep to a small selection of familiar drugs and carry those which are essential to the individual's actual or anticipated requirements during the transfer.

Typical air ambulance equipment

The items listed in Table 9.4 are represented as they would be found in their storage or carrying containers. An alternative would be to list the items alphabetically alongside details of where each item can be found on the aircraft. Extra modules may be added for specialist transfers such as obstetric, paediatric, burns or psychiatric patients.

Table 9.4   Typical air ambulance equipment

Box A (Accessories)

Top	Middle	Base
Labels	IMV Valves x 2	Ventilator
Oxygen Cylinder Spanner	PEEP Valve	Hose and Valve
Digital Thermometer with	APL Valve	Wrights Respirometer
Disposable Covers	Mini-Trach Set	Pressure Cycling
Tubing Clamps x 2	Portex Chest Drain Set	Ventilator Failure Alarm
Mosquito Forceps	Sterile Gloves Sizes 6 ½ & 7 ½	Syringe Driver plus
Drum Cartridge Catheter	Re-Usable Non Re-Breathing	Connecting Tubes
Tongue Depressors	Valve and Plastic Bag	Pressure Infusor Bag
Iodine Tincture BP 25ml x 1		Guide Books
Thermovents x 2		Pall Filter

Box B (Drugs)

Top	First Drawer	Third Drawer
Sharps Box	Needles	Nalbuphine 10mg/ml x10
IV Giving Set x2	21g x8	Naloxone 400mcg/ml x6
Buretrol Giving Set x1	23g x8	Prochlorperazine 12.5mg/1 ml x3
Haemaccel 500ml x2	25g x8	Propofol 200mg/20ml x3
Sodium Chloride 0.9% x2	Tip Caps	Salbutamol 0.25mg/5ml x2
Glucose 5% 500mi x2	String for IV Fluids	Sodium Chloride 0.9% 10ml x7
Glucostix	Safety Pins	Sodium Heparin 2ml x2
Elastoplast Roll		Suxamethonium 100mg/2ml x3
Syringes:	**Second Drawer**	Vecuronium 10mg
20ml x2 10ml x5	Adenosine 3mg/Ml x7	Water for Injection 5ml x5
5ml x5 2ml x5	Adrenaline 1: 1000ml x6	
1ml x2 Insulin x2	Aminophylline 250mg/10ml x2	**Fourth Drawer**
Needles:	Amiodarone 50mg/3ml x6	Glyceryl Trinitrate Spray x1
21g x2 23g x2	Atropine 600mcg/ml x10	Glyceryl Trinitrate Patches x4
25g x2	Calcium Chloride 13.4% 10ml x2	Glucose 50% 50ml x1
Venflons:	Chlorpheniramine 1omg/Ml x2	Salbutamol Inhaler xl
Size 14 x1 Size 17 xl	Diclofenac Sodium 75mg/3ml x2	Salbutamol Solution 20ml x1
Size 18 x1 Size 20 x1	Digoxin 500mcg/2ml x2	Water for Injections 10ml x10
Size 22 x1	Dobutamine 250mg/5ml x1	Disposable Razor x1
Catheter Extension with	Doxapram 20mg/5ml x2	Adrenaline 1 mg/10ml x1
3 way tap x2	Frusemide 20mg/2ml x5	Atropine 1mg/10ml Mini-Jet xl
IV Dressings x2	Glyceryl Trinitrate 25mg/5ml x2	Chlorhexidine Sachets 25ml x2
Scissors	Hydrocortisone 100mg x2	
Gauze Bandage	Isoprenaline 2mg/2ml x2	
Transpore Tape	Labetalol 100mg/20ml x2	
Sterile Gauze Squares	Lidocaine 1 % 1oml x2	
Tourniquet	Lidocaine 2% 5ml x2	
Mediswabs	Metoprolol 5mg/5ml x2	
Ampoule Files	Midazolam 10mg/2ml x10	
Elastoplasts		
Tip Caps		

Box C (General)

Top	Middle	Base
Guedal airway size 1, 2, 3, 4	Laryngoscope handles x 2	Yankauer suction catheter x 1
Sterile stitch scissors	Laryngoscope blade, size 3,4	Suction catheters size 12 fg x 5
Scissors	Gum elastic bougie small x 1	Suction catheters size 14 fg x 5
Disposable scalpel	Gum elastic bougie large x 1	Suction pump adaptors x 1
Spencer wells forceps	Satin slip introducer	Laerdal resuscitation bag
Gauze bandage	Short catheter mount	Non-rebreathing valve
Batteries	Swivel connector	Face masks size 3, 4, 5
Sutures x 2	ET tubes size 5, 6, 7 8, 9	Circular facemask size 2
KY jelly	Nasal airway size 7	Oxygen reservoir bag
Torch	Magill forceps	Disposable nebuliser set x 1
Tissues	Tendon hammer	Oxygen mask with
Transpore tape	Non-sterile gauze squares	tubing (adult) x 1
Sterile gloves for suction	Sterile gloves	Oxygen mask (paediatric) x 1
Stethoscope	Spare laryngoscope bulb x 1	Oxygen tubing x 1
Formulary book	Spare 'o' ring	Oxygen nasal cannulae x 1
Water for injection 20ml x 4	20ml syringes x 2	Pressure regulator with
	Goggles x 2	dual outlet Oxygen
		cylinder spanner x 1
		Oxygen flow meter x 1

Notes on individual items of equipment

Airway and respiratory

Airway Full airway management capability for all age groups includes all equipment for endotracheal intubation, including such aids as bougies, introducers, and airway alternatives such as the laryngeal mask airway (LMA). The equipment, training and ability to perform difficult airway access manoeuvres such as rapid sequence intubation (RSI) and surgical airways are an essential part of any critical care transport system.

Aspirators Although suction pumps (both electrical and mechanical) have improved in recent times, none are as effective as those found in hospital wall systems. Nevertheless effective suctioning is essential for good airway management.

Oxygen supplies Portable oxygen cylinders approved for medical use in aircraft must be separate from aircraft emergency oxygen supplies. In aeromedical organizations cylinders need to be changed more frequently than in a hospital setting. For example, in a hospital it may be reasonable to allow a cylinder to get to as low as a quarter of its full contents before changing it, whereas, in an aircraft, the difficulty with cylinder changes in flight means that they are often changed on the ground if they are below three quarters full. Some air ambulance systems use oxygen concentrators or liquid oxygen containers. This would usually only be when long distance transport is required. The same issues that apply to aircraft oxygen systems apply to medical oxygen systems. Oxygen is classed as dangerous cargo and special arrangements need to be made to carry or use it in flight. Commercial carriers usually supply and fit the oxygen themselves (at a cost, of course). It is essential to know what oxygen supplies you need and to allow a significant margin for error, diversions, delays, and so on. Commonly 50-100% is used as a margin for critical cases.

Likewise, spare cylinders must be available for machines powered by oxygen so that unexpected delays will not erode into the reserves necessary for the patient's respiratory requirements. An alternative to the carriage of bulky and heavy oxygen cylinders is the use of liquid oxygen (LOX) stores. It is now possible to provide flow rates adequate enough to power ventilation equipment, suction devices, and membrane oxygenators without the need for heavy reducing valves and regulators. One litre of LOX stored at -180°C will yield over 800 liters of gaseous oxygen. This expansion rate is almost seven times greater than can be achieved with pressurized gas in conventional cylinders (at 1800 psi). LOX converters are lightweight insulated containers which may contain up to 25 liters of liquid. Insulation is never perfect and, as temperature rises, if oxygen is not being used, more gas is formed and pressure within the container increases. A relief valve will eventually vent this excess but, when calculating oxygen requirements, adjustments must be made to compensate for the fall in oxygen content which starts to occur about ten hours after LOX cylinders are filled.

An alternative method of obtaining high concentrations of oxygen is to generate oxygen on board the aircraft. The best method involves the use of molecular sieves to adsorb nitrogen in compressed air. This effectively enriches the oxygen content as nitrogen is removed. Almost 100 per cent inspired oxygen concentration can be achieved, but flow rates are not sufficient for gas-driven devices. The need for faster flow rates and the danger of compressor failure disrupting the major oxygen supply will always necessitate the carriage of supplemental gaseous or LOX stores.

Compressed air may be used when high oxygen concentrations are not required, for example, to supply incubators during neonatal transfers. Venturi devices can be employed to entrain air for adults requiring intermittent positive pressure ventilation at low or moderate oxygen concentrations, but great care must be made to ensure that the patient's oxygen requirements are being satisfied.

Mechanical ventilators   Many types of mechanical ventilators, with various modes, positive end expiratory pressure (PEEP), continuous positive airway pressure (CPAP) and disconnect alarms, are available for transfers. Simple ones such as the original Drager Oxylog require no power supply at all because the motive forces are supplied by pressure from the oxygen cylinders. This clearly has a great advantage in terms of electrical power usage and risk of power/battery failure. However, the disadvantages include the inadequate alarms and the lack of more complex ventilatory modes, as well as greatly increased gas consumption. Primary missions and a significant number of secondary missions do not usually require complex ventilatory modes. In these cases a patient requiring ventilation can be sedated (and preferably paralysed) and standard Intermittent Positive Pressure Ventilation (IPPV) can be used almost always. The main exception might be severe asthma where the IPPV struggles to provide adequate inflation. Hand (bag-valve-mask) ventilation may then be the only suitable alternative in flight. The safer option may be to remain on scene until the patient's asthma is better controlled. In the tertiary transfer of a patient who may be partially weaned from a ventilator, it may be useful to have other ventilatory modes available. The commonest of these are Pressure Control (PC), Pressure Support (PS), Continuous Positive Airways Pressure (CPAP) and Synchronized Intermittent Mandatory Ventilation (SIMV). The other requisite feature is the ability to provide Positive End Expiratory Pressure (PEEP) with any mode. This can be done in some cases by use of extra circuit valves separate to the ventilator. It seems likely that the use of non-invasive ventilation and in particular mask-CPAP will increase in transport. It can be particularly useful for the cardiac pulmonary oedema patient and, of course, in paediatrics.

Pulse oximetry   These devices have become ubiquitous in acute care medicine and, as such, most medical and nursing personnel understand something about their use. However, it is important to remember that although pulse oximetry provides a valuable estimate of oxyhemoglobin saturation, when used alone it gives no information about the arterial partial pressure of oxygen, nor about the efficiency of pulmonary ventilation. Readers may find it useful to refer back to the oxygen dissociation curve (Chapter 4) to review the relationships between oxygen saturation, partial pressure and altitude. Similarly, it is essential to be aware of the limitations of pulse oximetry, namely that the technique tends to fail or under-read in underperfused patients, that is, in situations of low flow, peripheral cooling and low blood pressure. These are exactly the situations in the field and airborne environment in which we need oximetry to work! Other physiological artefacts, for example, hemaglobinopathies can fool the system. Carboxyhemoglobin and methemoglobin which cause a falsely high reading, and oximetry make no adjustment for patients with anaemia. Physical artefacts also occur. Vibration and strong external ambient light can cause failure or inaccuracy. Oximetry may also be affected by nearby electromagnetic interference sources such as car or aircraft engines. One type of pulse oximeter has also been reported to be adversely affected by ambulance acceleration. Reductions in saturation to as low as 85 per cent were described – this can be worrying unless the medical crew are aware of the phenomenon. Finally, because of the ethical difficulty in calibrating pulse oximeters below 85 per cent, lower readings are derived from mathematical extrapolation and there is clearly a natural tendency towards inaccuracy. Therefore, any value below 80 per cent should be viewed as dangerously low rather than relying on the specific number shown. Pulse oximeters which have ECG gating may be more reliable in low flow states but, in general, they should be considered only in the light of other cardiorespiratory parameters.

Pulse oximetry will work in neonates, but many pediatricians prefer transcutaneous oxygen saturation monitoring in transit.

Capnographs   End-tidal capnography (carbon dioxide [CO_2] measurement) is essential for confirming correct endotracheal tube placement after intubation. A waveform display is necessary. The continuous nature of a waveform provides a valuable assessment of appropriate ongoing ventilation, a visual disconnect alarm, and information about the quality of CO_2 elimination (that is, on the effectiveness of circulation or cardiopulmonary resuscitation, since CO_2 will only be detected if cells are metabolising oxygen and glucose, and circulating blood delivers it to the lungs). Devices with only a numeric display are therefore inadequate for aeromedical use.

CO_2 analysis relies on the absorption of infrared light by CO_2. This occurs in linear proportion to the total amount (or partial pressure) of CO_2 present. However, CO_2 absorption of infrared light is also affected in a non-linear manner by total ambient pressure. At sea level this is not an issue, as many machines are calibrated for a range of +/- 60 mmHg (8.0 kPa). This range of calibration becomes a problem when using these machines in flight and it is useful to check with the manufacturer and also to test a machine at different altitudes before relying on the absolute numbers that they provide. Available hardware is of two main types (mainstream and sidestream) with a third simpler option (colorimetric) available for intubation only:

- *Mainstream*   Older capnographs had cumbersome transducers placed adjacent to the endotracheal tube. These were heavy and hot and susceptible to breakage. Newer models are lighter and more robust.
- *Sidestream*   A fine tube draws expired air out of a side port of the breathing circuit, back to the sensor housed in the main machine. This has the advantage of being simpler, lighter in weight and less liable to damage. The main disadvantage is that the side tube sometimes blocks with condensed moisture.
- *Colorimetric*   These methods are single-use colour change devices used to confirm intubation. They are small disposable devices that fit into the breathing circuit. As gas is drawn through them a colour change occurs to indicate the presence of carbon dioxide. They have no quantitative measurement, but are a cheap, simple and useful aid in confirming intubation.

Blood gas analyser and lab tests   In some settings, particularly for longer transports of complex patients, the ability to perform inflight biochemical tests may be useful. Devices such as the i-STAT analyser can provide blood gas and electrolyte analysis in such a case. Quick hemoglobin estimates can also be useful in some circumstances and a number of simple machines can provide this capability. The i-STAT Portable Clinical Analyser (PCA) is a hand-held device about the size of a palm computer. It is used in conjunction with disposable cartridges for determination of a variety of parameters in whole blood. The analyser stores up to 50 patient records and permits on-screen viewing of test results as well as transmission of records to a data management system using infrared signals. All of the following parameters can be measured or calculated, depending on the type of cartridge used with the PCA:

Blood gases	Biochemistry	Haematology
• pH	• Sodium	• Hematocrit
• PCO_2	• Potassium	• Hemoglobin
• PO_2	• Chloride	• ACT
• Lactate	• Ionized Calcium	
• Bicarbonate	• Glucose	
• Bicarbonate	• Urea Nitrogen	
• Total CO_2	• Creatinine	
• Base Excess		
• O_2 Saturation		
• Anion Gap		

Oxygen supplies   Oxygen cylinders should be checked and replaced regularly. If working in an environment where it is not easy to replenish oxygen from road ambulance crews at a scene, consideration should be given to changing cylinders electively after a case if they are less than ¾ full. This will minimize the risk of running out of oxygen with potentially disastrous results. Spare cylinders must be available – the number depending on the oxygen requirement calculations (usually with a 50-100% reserve). These calculations should also take account of devices powered by oxygen so that unexpected delays will not erode into the reserves necessary for the patient's respiratory requirements. An alternative to the carriage of bulky and heavy oxygen cylinders is the use of liquid oxygen (LOX) stores. It is now possible to provide flow rates adequate enough to power ventilation equipment, suction devices, and membrane oxygenators without the need for heavy reducing valves and regulators. A final word of caution – although space-efficient in the aircraft, the medical crew need to be aware of the availability of decanting sites for replenishment when operating remotely from the home base.

Cardiovascular

Multi-modal monitors   Multi-modal monitors usually display a minimum of ECG, oxygen saturation, invasive and non-invasive pressures, and temperature. They may have channels dedicated to capnography or ventilatory parameters, or spare channels for specific external sources, such as intracranial pressure. Although offering the advantage that modalities are in the one machine, the disadvantage of relying on one device is that if the one and only piece of monitoring hardware fails, the aeromedical escort is left with nothing! For this reason many organizations carry single monitor items as well as a multiparameter device.

Non-invasive pressure monitoring   Non-invasive blood pressure (NIBP) machines are attractive and widely used in the prehospital setting but it is important to be aware of their significant limitations. Although blood pressure can be monitored on multi-modal monitors (such as the Propaq 100 series), stand-alone devices (such as the Dynamap - limb cuff, and Finapres - finger cuff) are also available. These monitoring devices have a tendency to over-read at low blood pressures and under-read at high blood pressures. This can be falsely reassuring. Furthermore, they retain the last blood pressure measurement visible on the screen giving the impression that this is the current blood pressure when in fact it may be nothing of the sort. Finally, the cycle time is usually much longer than for a manual blood pressure and these machines can get into a constant loop of inflation/deflation seeking a 'reading'. However, when invasive pressure is not available and when manual blood pressure cannot be measured (for instance in a high noise or high vibration environment) NIBP may be the only available option. In such cases the significant limitations should be taken into account.

Invasive pressure monitoring   There is no doubt that this is the gold standard for blood pressure monitoring. The advantages include beat to beat real time accuracy (which is important in a dynamic situation), additional information available from the shape of the waveform (and from its response to the ventilatory cycle), and the ability to monitor at a distance. The latter is useful when dealing with trapped patients and in 'shared space' situations. The main disadvantage is that this involves a skilled and invasive procedure. The associated risks are higher than for peripheral intravenous access and it requires an experienced doctor to perform. In untrained hands (and sometimes even for experienced intensivists) it can be time consuming. The increased use of this monitoring modality in all phases of critical care transport is probably one of the most significant changes over the last decades of the 20th century.

Electrocardiography: Cardiac rhythm can be monitored by multi-function devices (such as the Propaq 100 series) or small stand-alone battery powered monitors. Also, many defibrillators have a built in oscilloscope, liquid crystal display (LCD) or similar screen which displays the current waveform. Some machines have the capability of running a rhythm strip, or even a full 12-lead electrocardiogram and, rarely, some patients may require 24 hour ambulatory tape monitoring en route.

Equipment for peripheral and central venous access   Large bore cannulae for peripheral access will be needed and some services also carry central venous cannulae as well. The need for these will depend on the nature of the workload. Primary response teams will also need surgical equipment for access by way of intravenous cut-down techniques.

Intravenous solutions   Simple crystalloid fluids such as Ringer Lactate (compound sodium lactate or Hartmann's solution) can be used in most situations. There is still much controversy about the relative risks of albumin-based solutions but, given the significant weight and volume penalty of carrying fluids, the idea of using colloid solutions which achieve the same volume effect as crystalloids for the carriage of lower volumes of infusate has some potential attraction. The same argument has been made for hyperosmotic crystalloid solutions (but for different reasons). Clinical use of fluids in described in more detail in a number of other modules.

Syringe pumps and infusion pumps Intravenous syringe drivers are smaller, cheaper, and use less power than infusion pumps, and are routinely used on aeromedical flights. Syringe drivers are essential for the administration of vasoactive substances such as inotropes and nitrates, but are also extremely useful for continuous sedation, muscle relaxation, insulin sliding scale and so on. Volume drivers are useful when intravenous volume delivery needs to be accurate, especially with paediatrics.

Pacemakers Therapeutic equipment may be located internal or external to the patient. A rate-responsive cardiac pacemaker may increase its firing rate because of oversensing due to aircraft motion and vibration, or because of interference by electromagnetic fields from security sensors and aircraft avionics. A number of current defibrillators also have an external pacing option which can be used in cases of severe bradycardia. Some services will carry flotation wires for temporary transvenous pacing which can be inserted without the need for fluoroscopy.

Intra-aortic balloon pumps Intra-aortic balloon pumps are becoming progressively smaller and more portable since they were introduced in the 1990s but they tend to be operated by only a select few aeromedical services with experience in the transportation of critically ill cardiac patients. They still suffer from problems with short battery life and the need for external power sources, but inevitably the technology will improve as more and more regional cardiac centres accept acute patients for cardiac investigations and interventional radiology or cardiothoracic surgery.

Defibrillators Defibrillation in flight is considered below. Current evidence indicates biphasic devices give superior results for a given energy level. Implantable defibrillators in patients with recurrent ventricular fibrillation (VF) may operate spuriously in the presence of strong electromagnetic fields and have even been activated by the transmissions of mobile telephones.

Over the years, there has been much debate about the safety to crew and other passengers of defibrillation in flight. Several studies have now categorically proven that defibrillators may be operated quite safely inside aircraft and helicopters. Electricity will always seek the path of least resistance and, unless the patient and his surroundings are wet, this path will be through the patient's chest. Very small current leakage can be detected, but stray electric fields induce no permanent alteration or damage to the function of avionic or navigational equipment in the aircraft.

Early defibrillation is well proven to save lives. American data suggest that sudden cardiac arrest strikes up to 350 000 Americans each year. Most commonly, the victim is in VF and the earlier a direct current (DC) shock is administered, the better the chances of reversion and survival. With every minute after sudden cardiac arrest occurs, the odds of the victim's survival have been estimated as decreasing by seven to ten per cent. The American Heart Association (AHA) estimates that early defibrillation could increase survival rates by 30 per cent or more. Aeromedical organizations where early defibrillation has been introduced have shown even better results. An ongoing study involving defibrillation teams at the Melbourne Cricket Ground during major sporting fixtures has had a remarkable success rate in managing sudden cardiac arrest with success figures well in excess of 50 per cent of total cases.

It is perhaps not surprising that given the enormous number of people who fly on commercial flights, that someone would consider the use of defibrillators in flight in the commercial aviation setting. While the initial use of defibrillators was pioneered by only two airlines (Virgin Atlantic Airways in the UK and QANTAS in Australia) both have reported 'saves' and have proven that defibrillators can be effectively and safely used in the flight environment.

Although safety in flight is an issue often heard, the rules which apply for safe defibrillation on the ground apply equally in flight and, if applied rigorously, should guarantee the safety of the operator and the aircraft. There is still a need to ensure that pads are correctly applied and that the patient is not in contact with personnel or metal. This has been known for many years from the use of defibrillators on mobile road ambulances. In the air ambulance setting, however, it is essential to also warn the aircrew when defibrillation is likely to occur. Since the terrorist atrocities of 9/11 resulted in the locking of flight deck doors, this is usually via the cabin crew (cabin service director [CSD] or purser). Early warning will ensure that any adverse effects on controls and avionic or navigation equipment are recognised and dealt with immediately.

A number of recent studies have shown that semi-Automated External Defibrillators (AEDs) using biphasic waveforms for defibrillation are superior to AEDs that use monophasic waveforms. One study, which involved 115 VF patients, found that defibrillation was achieved with three or fewer shocks in 98 per cent of the patients treated with the biphasic waveform, compared to 67 per cent of those treated with the monophasic waveform. In general, airlines have mostly opted for AEDs without ECG monitoring, since their medical departments agree that the AED must be usable by trained cabin staff. Under these circumstances they feel that an ECG waveform introduces inappropriate (and potentially delaying) decision choices. On the other hand most primary and secondary transfer systems still carry defibrillators in which the ECG waveform can be analysed before manual defibrillation is instigated. Almost all AEDs now use escalating energy biphasic waveforms.

The following extract of a statement made by Dr Jon Jordan, the US Federal Air Surgeon of the Federal Aviation Administration (FAA) on 20 June 2000 concerns the implementation of the Aviation Medical Assistance Act of 1998 and shows the commitment to widespread defibrillator carriage in commercial aircraft.

> With passenger enplanements numbering over 600 million in 1998, nearly double what they were in the early 1980s, and given projections for continued growth in air travel, we anticipate an increase in passengers needing inflight medical assistance. This expectation

is particularly true given the overall aging of the general population in the United States. The most commonly observed serious inflight medical events appear to be cardiac in nature, due to chronic pre-existing conditions or to the sudden onset of previously unknown conditions. The most common form of treatable cardiac event is caused by an abnormal heart rhythm called 'ventricular fibrillation,' (where the heart is still beating, although ineffectively pumping blood). Ventricular fibrillation is treatable with defibrillation, an electric shock that stimulates the heart to resume beating normally. Survival of individuals undergoing ventricular fibrillation can be as high as 90 percent in some circumstances, if defibrillation is provided early during the event.

Cardiac defibrillator technology has progressed to the point that defibrillation similar to that performed in hospitals can, in many cases, be accomplished effectively outside the hospital environment by automated external defibrillators. When activated, AEDs deliver a high-energy electrical pulse to attempt to restore the normal electric heart activity required for normal heart function. At a cost of approximately $3,500 per unit, AEDs are lightweight, compact, virtually maintenance-free, and simple to use. Because these battery-powered systems voice-prompt step-by-step guidance, appropriately trained non-medical personnel may use them fairly confidently to assist in certain cardiac emergencies.

The U.S. Food and Drug Administration regulates the use of AEDs and began approving use of the devices in an aircraft environment in September 1996. Subsequent to this approval, several air carriers voluntarily have begun or have announced plans to carry them on board.

In order to implement the Aviation Medical Assistance Act, in July 1998 the FAA initiated a one-year, inflight, medical event data collection effort in cooperation with the Air Transport Association. Up to 15 different ATA-member airlines, carrying approximately 85 per cent of US domestic airline passengers, contributed some data throughout the year. During July 1, 1998, through June 30, 1999, the data collection revealed there were 188 death or threat-of-death incidents resulting in a total of 108 deaths. It should be noted that 11 of these reported events occurred off the aircraft. AEDs were used to deliver at least one shock in 17 separate events, 14 times on board an aircraft, and three on the ground. From these events, four passengers were reported as having survived. It is believed that the AED use was the event that changed the outcome for those who were reported as having survived. Subsequent to the data collection, further FAA investigation revealed that more passengers, and two flightcrew members, have had similar cardiac events.

Although there are limitations to the use of these data due to variables in the collection process, we concluded that it would be appropriate to propose the use of AEDs on board aircraft because the devices have saved lives. We considered proposing to simply authorize the use of AEDs on board an aircraft, but determined that such an approach would not address issues such as needed emergency medical kit enhancements, maintenance, and safe and appropriate use of the device. Therefore, on May 24 we proposed to require that commercial air carriers operating under part 121 (maximum payload of more than 7,500 pounds) carry at least one AED on board and augment currently required emergency medical kits with additional medications and medical equipment. The rule would also require initial familiarization training for all crewmembers on the location of the AED and its instructions, and the enhancements being added to emergency medical kits. It would also require initial and recurrent training for all flight attendants on AED usage and in CPR [cardiopulmonary resuscitation]. The rule also addresses certain safety concerns about the carriage of AEDs on board aircraft. Currently, lithium batteries power AEDs, which, like many batteries, can be hazardous. Because of concerns over these hazards, the proposed rule would require that carriers meet applicable FAA standards for such batteries and be vigilant about inspecting the device regularly.

In the conclusion of this statement, Dr Jordan summarized the expectations of outcome for passengers who become victims of an unexpected medical emergency in flight. Although this conclusion does not cover the aeromedical transport scenario, it usefully encapsulates the difficulties encountered in the flight environment:

> . . . onboard medical assistance will continue to be discretionary as well as limited and must be regarded as emergency treatment with no unrealistic expectations of favourable outcomes for passengers having medical events in flight. The FAA believes that it is unrealistic to expect crewmembers to achieve the same level of proficiency as emergency medical personnel who perform medical procedures routinely on a daily basis. The availability of these enhancements (equipment and medication) will not eliminate the logistical and medical difficulties experienced in attempting to treat a stricken passenger effectively while in flight. The intent is to provide options for treatment, not to raise expectations in the passenger or medical community regarding the level of care available in flight.

The FAA also examined the need for AEDs at airports. Data on 130 airports indicated that 108 (83 per cent) had defibrillators and 11 (8.5 per cent) had an off-airport response rate of less than six minutes. Thus, 119 airports (91.5 per cent) have the capability to respond adequately to emergency cardiac events. In the light of these results the FAA decided not to propose a rule litigating a requirement for AEDs at airports.

Specific requirements of aeromedical equipment

Electronic monitoring devices are essential to ensure that the patient is continuously and accurately assessed. They need to be easily accessible within the aircraft, legible in both dim lighting and bright sunlight, accurate, and reliable. With few exceptions, the monitoring of physiological trends is usually of more value than point measurements. As a general rule, it is more useful to base assessments on the information combined from monitored variables and clinical acumen, rather than rely on monitor measurements in isolation. This section looks, in detail, at the performance requirements for electronic patient monitoring and life support devices.

Display design

Where numerical displays alone are used, for instance in some pulse oximetry devices, they should be easily readable with large and non-confusable numbers. Waveform and complex mixed displays can also be difficult to read and interpret. Screen displays must be tested in bright sunlight conditions as many of the earlier screens can be 'washed out' and rendered unreadable by bright ambient light. This was a major problem with early model portable defibrillators that made interpreting an ECG rhythm from the screen almost impossible in some conditions. Design should therefore take into account the screen clarity in varying light conditions, with bright reflections, and at varying angles. While cabin lighting may impose glare on monitor screens, special mention must be made of the effect of red cabin lighting during night flight. In fixed wing aircraft with structurally separate passenger cabins, conventional lighting is available and the red light traditionally used to illuminate the flightdeck poses no problems to the medical team. However, in helicopters and smaller fixed wing aircraft, this red light (required by the aircrew to help maintain night vision) may permeate the entire cabin. Red light has been demonstrated to impair the ability of medical personnel to assess patients for cyanosis, interpret colorimetric end tidal CO_2 indicators, and read emergency medication labels. Difficulty may also be encountered with some monitor screens.

Alarms

Whatever systems are used, medical personnel must be familiar with the alarms on the equipment and devices in their charge. Switching off visual systems can lead to disaster, and visual scanning techniques may need to be improved. However, long-term scanning and concentration on multiple monitoring devices is extremely fatiguing, and alertness (that is, the time to respond to an alarm) may be impaired. In theory, audible 'attention-getters' are better than visual alarms, since the medical escort's attention may be focused elsewhere. However, aircraft noise limits the reliability of audible alarms which are often impossible to hear in the flight environment. To be effective in a noisy environment (in the aircraft, helicopter or at the roadside), alarms should therefore have a visual component, especially peripheral vision 'attention getters' such as colour changes and flashing displays. Future systems may incorporate alarms within the aircraft intercom system so that medical attendants can receive auditory information by the same means with which they communicate with other crew. However, this will require specific 'medical-crew-only' wiring so that the pilot is screened from these additional distractions. The possibility of remote vibrating alarms with a tactile connection to the aeromedical escort is also a possible future development.

Size and weight

Equipment must be compact and as light as possible. It must not take up too much room in the aircraft cabin and should have minimal or negligible effects on the aircraft's payload and centre of gravity limitations. Most of the equipment will need to be portable so that it can be carried easily to the patient, and brought back with the patient to the aircraft.

Durability

Equipment must be robust and of rugged design. It must be able to withstand the general rough handling which is inevitable in an out-of-hospital environment to the extent that continuing accurate and reliable working is ensured even after a drop from carrying height on to any face or edge of the equipment. Clearly, every item must be able to function accurately and reliably in appropriate ranges of temperature, humidity, vibration and ambient pressure. The latter causes gas volumes to expand as pressure decreases (Boyle's Law). Equipment susceptible to gaseous expansion include:

- pressure bags
- chest drainage bags
- nasogastric tubes and other closed drains
- endotracheal and tracheostomy tube cuffs
- catheter balloons
- sphygmomanometer cuffs
- pneumatic antishock garment
- air splints
- glass IV fluid bottles
- IV administration sets
- capnography
- mechanical ventilators
- nebulisers
- gas flow generated devices.

Power supplies

Adequate battery endurance and the ability for batteries to be changed readily by teams in transit and also to be capable of being charged from aircraft power sources (DC or AC [alternating current] according to circumstances). Acceptable battery endurance will depend on the missions undertaken but, when treating trapped patients, for example, this time may be hours longer than flight times.

Whenever possible, electrical items should be compatible with aircraft power systems. Clearly this requires advance notice of the precise aircraft type to be used for the mission, and knowledge of its supply system. Although most large passenger carrying aircraft operate a 110 volt AC system, others use 12 volts DC. Most helicopters and light aircraft use a 28 volt DC supply although, again, some operate a 12 volt system. Inverters (which convert the aircraft electrical supply to 110-240 volts AC) are needed for equipment which is not purpose-built or modified for use on aircraft, unless it is capable of independent battery operation. In addition, the aircraft must have the capacity to generate enough electrical power to support the simultaneous operation of all onboard equipment (both medical and operational). Any item which leaves the aircraft with the patient must have an independent power supply and, since battery life is influenced by charge state and temperature, measures must be taken to ensure that adequate power is available for the duration of the entire mission, with sufficient reserves for unexpected delays and diversions. Spare charged batteries must always be readily accessible.

Servicing and care of equipment

Daily maintenance and checking

Ideally, all equipment and medical matériel should be thoroughly checked before and after each mission. Although this need not be by the inflight medical team, they are the crew which take ultimate responsibility for the adequacy of their equipment. The value of checking equipment at the start of each shift is:

- It enables identification of faults and missing items prior to this becoming an issue of critical concern.
- It enables familiarity with the equipment and its exact location, even if not being used on a day-to-day basis.

It is also essential that equipment is checked and replenished after each mission. This is not always done by the off-going crew, especially after a tiring long haul mission. However, consumables used must be replaced, and fouled or infected items must be washed and disinfected or sterilized before being returned to the medical store room. Items may be needed urgently for the following mission, and the next team must be spared the task of replenishing and cleaning equipment before departure. As missions may literally be back-to-back, sufficient stores should be available to manage a number of missions with minimal chance to restock. Emergency restocking available from the patient drop off point will potentially significantly improve crew availability. At a regular time, usually once per week, back-up packs and main packs can be rotated, to maintain their date viability. Disaster response equipment should similarly be rotated.

Battery charge on devices can be more easily maintained at a base during down time than to have the devices aboard an aircraft which will require auxiliary power to be delivered for such purposes. In principle, though, batteries should be on trickle charge whenever the equipment is not in use.

Major maintenance

All electrical, electronic, pneumatic, and mechanical items must be properly maintained under a servicing schedule in accordance with the manufacturer's recommendations and which takes account of the rigors imposed by the aeromedical environment.

Stowage

Finally, all equipment must be safely fitted or stowed, not just in the aircraft or helicopter, but also in vehicles used during ground transfers. American FAA regulations (FAR 25.561) on the stowage and fitting of equipment in aircraft state that all items must be able to withstand deceleration forces of up to 9.0 G in the forward direction (-Gx) and 4.5 G in the downward direction (+Gz). Despite restraint, equipment must remain accessible, but should not be in danger of falling on the patient, crew, or other passengers, and should not obstruct emergency exits or hinder the flight crew in their duties.

Standardization

Clearance for safety of the aircraft

Organizations which fly dedicated air ambulances often have permanent, fixed equipment in situ. This equipment may prove hazardous in terms of spurious and stray electromagnetic fields (which may interfere with radio communications and navigation avionics) and may present a loose object risk during impact or emergency landings. Although the International Civil Aviation Organization (ICAO) does not specifically regulate aeromedical flights or the medical equipment carried on them, in most countries, the carriage of fixed medical equipment for the purpose of monitoring or treating patients in flight is considered to constitute a modification to the aircraft. As such, it must be approved by the relevant national aviation authority. Both the UK CAA and the American FAA have agreed with aeromedical operators that medical equipment on board UK and US registered aircraft can be carried on a 'demonstrated no hazard' basis. Approval implies that no hazard to the aircraft or its passengers has been shown.

Each major item is therefore checked, tested, and approved for use by the relevant national aviation authority. In the UK, for example, all fixed equipment onboard civilian aircraft must be approved by the Civil Aviation Authority (CAA), whereas the Royal Air Force checks and approves airborne equipment for the military. In the USA, a similar situation exists, with FAA being the approving authority for civilian aeromedical equipment. Both the US Air Force and the US Army conduct research and authorize airborne equipment for military use. The USA, UK and other NATO countries contribute to an international working group who collect and pool data on equipment and aircraft types so that individual member countries do not repeat the lengthy and expensive testing process unnecessarily. In principle, rarely used equipment must also be approved before flight, although it is understood that some items may be required at short notice and a common sense attitude must prevail. Close liaison between medical and flight crews should ensure safe operation.

Clearance for safety of the patient

The aviation authority clearance procedures ignore the needs of medical equipment to be unaffected by aircraft systems. As both aviation and medical technology advance, and more emphasis is placed on electronic and computerised monitoring, the likelihood of potential electromagnetic interference increases. To prevent adverse effects of equipment on patients, international standards have been established. Examples:

Description	Standard
Basic aspects of the safety philosophy of electrical equipment used in medical practice	IEC 513
Medical electrical equipment	IEC 601
Medical suction equipment - Electrically powered suction equipment safety requirements	ISO 10079/1
Environmental conditions and test procedures for airborne equipment	RTCA DO 160C
European medical devices directive	93/42/EEC

Regulations for the approval and monitoring of medical devices were introduced throughout the European Community in 1995. All medical devices (except those which are custom made and those used for clinical investigation) must now carry a 'CE' marking before they can be marketed or used within the European Community. The CE mark indicates that the device has been *'designed and manufactured in such a way that, when used under the conditions, and for the purposes intended, it will not compromise the clinical condition or safety of the patient, or compromise the health and safety of the user'*. For certain high risk items of equipment, conformity with these requirements must be based on clinical data, in much the same way that drugs and medications are currently evaluated. Manufacturers are required by law to report serious incidents which will then be investigated and any necessary action taken (such as the issue of a hazard notice).

Although the impact of these regulations has yet to hit the aeromedical industry, many professional committees have attempted self-standardisation, and regulation specifically of ambulance equipment has begun. The CEN (Commission Européenne de Normalization) has embarked on the task of standardizing land ambulance equipment throughout Europe, but has deferred addressing the complexities of air ambulance equipment because of the difficulty caused by the wide variety of aircraft types and missions.

The standards applied to determine whether or not each piece of equipment is suitable vary widely. An indication of the extent of this problem is shown but the following excerpt taken from a *United States Federal Air Surgeons bulletin* commenting on a wide-ranging meeting specifically looking at areas where research or standardization was needed in both rotary wing and fixed wing aeromedical evacuation.

STANDARDIZATION OF MEDICAL EQUIPMENT was the highest priority recommendation from both air ambulance groups. State and federal guidance is minimal and state guidance varies. Much of the state guidance is a carryover from that established for ground ambulances. Approximately 40 of the 50 states have air ambulance regulations, but only about one-third of those dictate equipment.

Workshop participants prescribed basic requirements for equipment used in an air ambulance setting:

- Basic diagnostic items must be present
- Equipment is appropriate to the specific patients and to the duration of the flight
- Equipment has visible alarms
- Equipment is rugged, durable, and securable
- Equipment is of suitable size, power, and backup power for both flight and patient transfer

Medical equipment must not cause electromagnetic interference (EMI) with aircraft equipment, and vice versa. Verification of equipment utility must also be achieved, but is presently unstandardised; there are various entities and programs, i.e., manufacturer, provider, military, and FAA programs.

An appreciation of how equipment testing is conducted was gained by reviewing the Army's medical equipment test program. This is based on Military Standards KL-STD 810-E for environmental testing and MIL-STD 461-D and 462-D for electromagnetic issues. Equipment is tested at 15 000 ft for one hour. Various temperature exposures, including +159°F for one hour and -114°F for six hours, are part of the stress tests. During vibration testing, equipment is tested in each axis for one hour utilizing the vibration profile of helicopter seats. Conditions for humidity testing are 95 per cent Relative Humidity (RH) for four hours at 86°F. The equipment is also tested for radiated emissions, radiated susceptibility, conducted emissions, and conducted susceptibility. Such an extensive program permitted testing of only about a dozen items of equipment per year.

Although related, an equipment test program in the Air Force selects slightly differing limits. Altitude testing takes equipment to 10 000 ft at 5000 ft per minute. A rapid decompression to 40 000 ft is also included. Temperature tests range from +140°F to -400°F for six hours. The humidity tests (at 94 per cent RH and +85°F for four hours) are similar. The vibration challenge is distributed over a two-day period. Fifteen-minute tests are repeated five times, with frequency rates ranging from 5 to 500 Hertz, and displacements from 0.01 to 0.5 inch. Periodic summaries of USAF tests (typically every five years) are available from Brooks Air Force Base.

The report was also insistent on the parallel need for helicopter interior design and equipment placement. In particular:

- Oxygen equipment security
- Placement of hazardous objects within the strike zone of occupants
- Crashworthiness of all systems

Conclusions

The miniaturisation of equipment, so necessary to produce compact equipment, has been made possible because of digital technology and improved microelectronics. In addition, the evolution of display screens using such techniques as liquid crystals and gas plasma, whilst more expensive than cathode ray tubes, are flat and less bulky. There are many other exciting technologies awaiting miniaturisation and application to the aviation environment. It is only a matter of time before further refinement and development makes them available for aeromedical use. However, this anticipation should be tempered by the knowledge that special circumstances dictate special precautions. Equipment must be tested in the flight environment, not just in the laboratory, but also by trialling it in the air ambulance. Once approved for flight, aeromedical crews must be fluid in their knowledge and understanding of the medical devices and monitors which they use. There will likely be no technician to help if a problem occurs mid-flight! Finally, emphasis must be made on the necessity to check and recheck all items of medical material and all devices that are likely to be needed for each patient, and to clean, sterilize, restock and remove medical waste materials at the end of each mission.

References

Bristow, A. et al. (1991) 'Medical helicopter systems – recommended minimum standards for patient management', *J Roy Soc Med.* **84**,:242-4.

Burillo-Putze, G., Herranz, I. et al. (2002) 'Transcranial oximetry as a new monitoring method for HEMS (Helicopter EMS)', *Air Med J.* **21**(1):13-6.

Dedrick, D.K., et al. (1989) 'Defibrillation safety in emergency helicopter transport', *Ann Emerg Med.* **18**(1):69-71.

Department of Transportation, Federal Aviation Administration (1986) 'Emergency medical equipment requirement', in *Federal Register*, **51**:1218-23.

Eljaiek, L.F., (1993) 'Biomedical equipment selection for air medical transport', in Rodenberg, H. and I.J. Blumen (eds.) *Air Medical Physician's Handbook*, AMPA: Salt Lake City.

Fromm, R.E., Campbell, E. and P. Schlieter (1995) 'Inadequacy of visual alarms in helicopter air medical transport', *Aviat Space Environ Med.* **66**:784-6.

Gilbert, B.K. et al. (1999) 'NASA/DARPA Advanced communications technology satellite project for evaluation of telemedicine outreach using next-generation communications satellite technology', Mayo Foundation Participation, *Mayo Clin Proc.* **74**:753-7.

Harding, R.M. and F.J. Mills (1993) 'Medical emergencies in the air', in Harding and Mills, *Aviation Medicine* (3rd Ed.). BMJ: London.

Hatlestad, D.C., Van Horn, J., (2002) 'Air transport of the IABP patient. Intra-Aortic Balloon Pump', *Air Med J.* **21**(5): 42-8.

Heegaard, W., Plummer, D., Dries, D., Frascone, R.J., Pippert, G., Steel, D. and J. Clinton (2004) 'Ultrasound for the air medical clinician', *Air Med J.* **23**(2):20-3.

Hylton, P. (1995) 'What's in a Mark – CE Marking for Medical Devices', *Internat J Intens Care.* **2**(3):98.

Icenogle, T.B., Smith, R.G., Nelson, R., Machamer, W. and B. Davis (1988) 'Long distance transport of cardiac patients in extremis: the mobile intensive care (MOBI) concept', *Aviat Space Environ Med.* **59**(6):571-4.

Jeffries, N.J. and A. Bristow (1991) 'Long distance inter-hospital transfers', *Internat J Intens Care* **1**(5):197-204.

Kobayashi, A. and Y. Miyamoto (2000) 'Inflight cerebral oxygen status: continuous monitoring by near-infrared spectroscopy', *Aviat Space Environ Med.* **71**(2):177-181.

Mallard, D. et al. (1999) 'Testing of the AVL OPTI 1 portable blood gas analyzer during inflight conditions', *Aviat Space Environ Med.***70**(4):346-7.

Martin, S. et al. (1999) 'Use of the laryngeal mask airway in air transport when intubation fails', *J Trauma Inf Crit Care*;**47**(2):352-7.

Martin, T.E. (1993) 'Transportation of patients by air', in Harding and Mills, *Aviation Medicine* (3rd Ed.). BMJ: London.

Martin, T.E. (2000) 'Fatal delay', *Air Ambulance* Sep:4-9.

Mitchell, G.W. and J.E. Adams (1989) 'A Survey of U.S. Army aeromedical equipment', *Aviat Space Environ Med.* **60**:807-810.

Nagappan, R. et al. (2000) 'Patient care bridge – mobile ICU for transit care of the critically ill', *Anaesthesia and Intensive Care.* **28**(6):684-6.

Potapov, E.V., Merkle, F., Guttel, A., Pasic, M., Caleb, M., Kopitz, M. and R. Hetzer (2004) 'Transcontinental transport of a patient with an AbioMed BVS 5000 BVAD', *Ann Thorac Surg.* **77**(4):1428-30.

Price, D. P. et al. (2000) 'Trauma ultrasound feasibility during the helicopter transport', *Air Med J.* **19**(4):144-6.

Randolph, V. et al. (2000) 'Laboratories on the move: blood gas analysis', *Laboratory Medicine* **31**(1):45-8.

Schedler, O., Kalske, P. and H. Handschak (2004) 'Bedside blood gas analysis in airborne rescue operations', *Air Med J.* **23**(2):36-9.

Shaw, E. et al. (2000) 'The application of the Landstuhl frame for air evacuation of patients with femur fractures', *Milit Med.* **165**:521-3.

Spencer, I. (1994) 'A generic specification for special purpose aeromedical equipment, in Aerospace Medical Panel Symposium' *Recent Issues and Advances in Aeromedical Evacuation (MEDEVAC)* , NATO, AGARD: Neuilly-sur-Seine.

PART IV
Clinical Considerations

Chapter 10

Indications for Aeromedical Transport

General considerations

Patients transported by aeromedical services may be any age – adults, elderly, children, and neonates. They usually have an acute medical or surgical problem, and may be flown on an interhospital, international repatriation or direct from the scene of illness or injury. The determination of the patient's need to fly is crucial to the effective operation of any aeromedical system.

In general, aeromedical transport should be reserved for those patients in whom the time required to transport the patient to definitive care by ground ambulance is considered excessive, or where access to care most appropriate for the patient is not available in the local area. It should be restricted to those patients in whom a delay in transport might reasonably be expected to result in adverse consequences or when deterioration might be expected to occur during a long ground journey. Aeromedical transport is also indicated in those situations where the personnel or equipment needs of the patient cannot be met by local transport agencies but may be accomplished by an aeromedical transport service. External factors such as aircraft readiness, weather conditions, costs, and access to appropriate commercial carriers will also affect triage for transport. Suggestions for appropriate use of aeromedical transport services can only be guidelines, and an individual decision on necessity is required prior to every mission.

It may be easier to list those situations where patient transport by an aeromedical service is contraindicated. Patients who are terminally ill with no correctable medical problems, patients who have requested no resuscitative efforts, and patients in cardiopulmonary arrest without return of spontaneous circulation should be excluded. Patients likely to die en route should not be transported if they are already in a medical facility with access to adequate resuscitation equipment. Patients in active labor are rarely transported, especially if cervical dilatation has occurred. The close confines of the aircraft cabin make it a poor location for emergency childbirth. Patients prone to psychotic or violent behavior must not be transported unless appropriate steps (which may include physical or pharmacological restraints) have been instituted. Prisoners of law enforcement agencies should not be transported where there is a potential for violence. The possession of weapons by prisoners or guards carries with it a propensity for use against the crew. Patients whose condition may overwhelm the equipment or personnel resources of the aeromedical program should also not be flown.

Trauma patients

Acute trauma is no respecter of time. Minutes may make the difference between life and death. The injured patient should be transported by the most experienced team available, in the shortest time possible, to a definitive care setting. Any seriously injured patient, or one who has the potential for serious complications, should ideally be treated in a known trauma facility (*trauma center*). Table 10.1 summarizes the factors that suggest a patient might benefit from scene triage and direct transfer to a trauma center. Any of these patients are potential candidates for air transport. Interfacility triage criteria are addressed in Table 10.2.

Table 10.1   Guidelines for the use of aeromedical transport in trauma patients

- Motor vehicle/pedestrian collision at > 10 mph (16 kph)
- Death of another occupant in the same vehicle
- Falls of more than 15 feet (5 m)
- Patient ejected from vehicle during crash
- Motorcycle rider thrown from vehicle at > 20 mph (32 kph)
- Extrication time > 20 minutes
- Acute penetrating injuries of the head, neck, chest, abdomen, or pelvis
- Trauma Score of 12 or less
- Revised Trauma Score of 10 or less
- Glasgow Coma Scale of less than 8
- Intubated patients
- Systolic blood pressure (SBP) < 90 mmHg after initial resuscitation
- Multiple trauma in the pediatric patient

Table 10.2   Interhospital triage criteria

• CNS injury	• Penetrating injury or depressed skull fracture
	• Open injury with or without cerebrospinal fluid leak
	• Glasgow Coma Score (GCS) < 13
	• Deterioration of GCS
	• Lateralizing signs
	• Cord injury
• Chest	• Wide mediastinum
	• Major chest wall injury
	• Cardiac injury
	• Patients who may require protracted ventilation
• Pelvis	• Unstable pelvic ring disruption

- Multi-system injury
  - Pelvic ring disruption with shock and evidence of continuing hemorrhage
  - Open pelvic injury
  - Severe face injury with head injury
  - Chest injury with head injury
  - Abdominal or pelvic injury with head injury
  - Burns with associated injuries
  - Multiple fractures
- High energy impact
  - Car crash or pedestrian injury > 25 mph (40 kph)
  - Rearward displacement of front of car > 20 in (0.5 m)
  - Ejection of car occupant or rollover
  - Death of occupant in same car
- Late sequelae
  - Need for continuing transfusions
  - Mechanical ventilation required
  - Sepsis
  - Single or multi-system failure
  - Major tissue necrosis
- Co-morbid factors
  - Age < 5 or > 55 years
  - Known cardiorespiratory or metabolic diseases

Source: *The American College of Surgeons Committee on Trauma Resources for Optimal Care of the Injured Patient*, 1993.

Non-trauma patients

Patients with non-traumatic illnesses may suffer from any of a variety of medical, or surgical conditions, and may require the input of specialist teams (for example, obstetric, pediatric, or neonatal) to optimize care during transport. The majority will be conducted between hospitals and other health care facilities by road ambulance, but, on occasions, geography, weather, or the lack of local health care may dictate that transfer from the scene of illness by air is more appropriate. Tables 10.3a to 10.3d give summaries of atraumatic patients who may be considered for interfacility transport by air.

Table 10.3a Guidelines for the use of aeromedical transport in non-trauma medical and surgical patients

- Intubated patients
- Patients requiring 100% oxygen, continuous positive airway pressure (CPAP), or positive end expiratory pressure (PEEP)
- Intensive care unit (ICU) to ICU transport where ground transport time may exceed one hour

- Cardiac patients requiring acute intervention (for example, thrombolysis, angioplasty)
- Patients requiring a temporary pacemaker
- Patients < 48 hours after cardiac arrest
- Cerebral edema or congestive heart failure (CHF) requiring active diuresis
- Hypothermia requiring active therapy
- Glasgow Coma Scale < 8
- Patients with indwelling arterial lines, Swan-Ganz catheters, or intracranial pressure monitors
- Decompression sickness (dysbarism)
- Patients with suspected acute aortic aneurysm
- Patients on intra-aortic balloon pumps (IABP)
- Patients with systolic blood pressure (SBP) < 90 mmHg with signs of decreased tissue perfusion or > 200 mmHg with end organ complications
- Acute arterial pH < 7.20 despite therapy
- Patients needing vasoactive medications to maintain adequate SBP
- Patients requiring urgent transport for organ salvage
- Patients requiring urgent cardiothoracic, vascular, or neurosurgical procedure unavailable at the referring institution

Source: Blumen, I.J. and R.S. Gordon, 'Taking to the skies', *Emergency* 1989; 21(11):32-8.

Table 10.3b   Guidelines for the use of aeromedical transport in non-trauma pediatric patients

- Acute dysrhythmias or cardiac failure
- Acute renal failure
- Patients in whom a central line was required for resuscitation
- Cerebral edema or CHF requiring active diuresis
- Complicated overdose or poisoned patients
- ICU to ICU transport where ground transport time may exceed one hour
- SBP < 60 mmHg in a neonate; < 65 mmHg in a one year old; < 70 mmHg in a one to five year old; < 80 in a five to 12 year old
- Patients needing vasoactive medications to maintain adequate SBP
- Patients whose respiratory rate is < 10 or > 60 breaths per minute
- Acute arterial pH < 7.20
- Intubated patients
- Patients requiring 100% O_2, CPAP, or PEEP
- Patients with Reye's syndrome
- Patients with meningitis
- Near drowning patients
- Patients in status epilepticus
- Glasgow Coma Scale < 8

- Hypothermia requiring active therapy
- Non-trauma patients with urgent problems requiring cardiothoracic, neurosurgical, or pediatric surgical care unavailable at the referring institution

Source: Blumen, I.J. and R.S. Gordon, 'Taking to the skies', *Emergency* 1989; 21(11):32-8.

Table 10.3c   Guidelines for the use of aeromedical transport in non-trauma neonatal patients

- Infants requiring mechanical ventilation, CPAP, or PEEP
- Complicated premature infants of gestational age < 30 weeks
- Complicated infants weighing < 1200 grams
- Infants requiring > 60% supplemental oxygen
- Neonates with pneumothorax and thoracostomy tube in place
- Inter-neonatal intensive care unit (NICU) transport where ground transport time may exceed one hour
- Cardiac or respiratory arrest within 24 hours of the flight request
- Infants with temperature instability
- Neonates requiring vasoactive medications or repeated volume challenges to maintain an adequate blood pressure
- Neonates with seizure activity, CHF, or disseminated intravascular coagulation
- Neonatal surgical emergencies (including congenital heart defects, necrotizing enterocolitis, diaphragmatic hernias, abdominal wall defects, intussusception, and volvulus)

Source: Blumen, I.J. and R.S. Gordon, 'Taking to the skies', *Emergency* 1989; 21(11):32-8.

Table 10.3d   Guidelines for the use of aeromedical transport in non-trauma patients in whom aeromedical transport is not indicated

- Terminally ill patients not suffering from an acute correctable medical problem
- 'Do not resuscitate' patients
- Patients in full arrest at the referring institution who cannot be stabilized with a perfusing circulation prior to transport

Source: Blumen, I.J. and R.S. Gordon, 'Taking to the skies', *Emergency* 1989; 21(11):32-8.

Utilization review

All aeromedical transport systems must establish utilization audit procedures that include both prospective screening and retrospective review of all assignments. Prospective procedures may be as simple as mandating that all requests for prehospital flights originate from appropriate EMS personnel. For interfacility missions, a flight physician or crew member might screen all calls. Because of the difficulty of gathering 'secondhand' information and time constraints, preflight screening should always favor the patient.

Retrospective review procedures must create feedback loops with an aim to make future utilization of the aircraft more appropriate. The first step in creating such a system is to identify a set of accepted guidelines for use as a reviewing tool (one such set of guidelines is the Association of Airmedical Services [AAMS]) position paper on the appropriate use of air medical transport). The second step is to apply the guidelines to each mission and have the crew fill out a questionnaire after every flight. Finally, the data is reviewed to determine positive or negative overall trends. Conclusions based on this information may then be used to modify the decision-making process that may have resulted in inappropriate use of transport resources. Examples of subjective and objective utilization review criteria are given in Tables 10.4 and 10.5.

Table 10.4   Outcome indicators for appropriate aeromedical transport

- Patient required urgent medical or surgical intervention during transport not available locally
- Patient transport required a complexity of care or logistical considerations which exceeded local capability or conditions
- Patient required urgent medical or surgical intervention on arrival at the receiving facility
- Patient's predicted mortality was 25% or greater
- Cardiac arrest before, during, or shortly after transport
- Patient not admitted, or discharged within 24 hours of referral

Source: Fromm, R.E. 'Indications for Air Medical Transport', in Blumen, I.J. and H. Rodenberg (eds), *Air Medical Physician's Handbook.*

A recent paper by Silbergleit et al. (2003) examined severity scoring and mortality data to identify trends in acuity and mortality over a 15-year period in one aeromedical system in the USA. APACHE-II scores at the time of transport and hospital mortality data were correlated. Both severity of illness and mortality appear to have increased over the study period, probably in response to changes in the health care system. The strong correlation between APACHE-II performed at the time of transport and mortality validates this technique and offers an outcome-based measure of performance that may allow clinical audit and comparisons between aeromedical systems.

Table 10.5   Injury and illness scoring for appropriate aeromedical transport

- Trauma Score (TS) < 13
- Glasgow Coma Score (GCS) < 13
- Injury Severity Score (ISS) > 15
- Rapid Acute Physiology Score (RAPS) > 4
- APACHE II Score > 15

Source: Fromm, R.E.,'Indications for Air Medical Transport', in Blumen, I.J. and H. Rodenberg (eds), *Air Medical Physician's Handbook*.

Airlines and air ambulances

A resource often overlooked in discussions of aeromedical transport is that offered by commercial airlines around the world. In reality, these airlines perform the majority of 'medical transportation', often bringing patients with known chronic disease or disability to their destinations with no medical assistance requested or required.

When a call for assistance with patient transport is received by an airline, the medical director will often base his initial decision on whether the patient may fly unattended. If it is decided that medical assistance will be required, he may request the aid of colleagues in the aeromedical transport industry to assist with care of the patient, or defer the case for transport by a dedicated air ambulance. While the ability of each commercial carrier to transport the ill and injured varies, nearly all will attempt to make some accommodation for patients who do not inconvenience or pose safety risks to other passengers. This is especially true of national flag carriers, who often feel a special obligation to assist in the repatriation of citizens of the sponsoring nation. While each airline may differ in its capabilities to mobilize airline resources to the aid of the patient, they will certainly allow medical crew to carry their own medical equipment, but only with assurance that it will not interfere with vital aircraft functions. There may also be issues of the carriage of scalpels, scissors and other sharp implements since the increased security measures following the terrorist atrocities of 9/11. Also, the downturn in worldwide air travel that followed the same event caused long-lasting financial hardship for some airlines which have responded with cutbacks in services which affect patient transport. One such example is the carriage of stretcher patients. Although many airlines have never catered for non-ambulant patients, others, such as British Airways, decided in 2005 that the expense of such altruism could no longer be borne. Press releases told of the huge costs of delays and diversions caused by these patients and some airlines instigated immediate bans on stretchers. The knock-on effects have been significant. Many patients now require dedicated air ambulance transfers. This has increased the costs of transport and travel by smaller aircraft considerably increases the complexity of long haul missions which may require several refueling stops to complete the journey. It is also worrying that some patients may be inappropriately re-categorized as ambulant so that they can still fly by commercial carrier. However, at the same time, a few airlines (such as Virgin Atlantic) have purchased completely flat beds for their upper class cabin. Although not designed for very ill passengers, they can be used for low care patients.

Some carriers are able to supply additional oxygen stores for patient use, as well as specific meal services and airport transportation resources (wheelchairs and patient assistance units to aid patient ingress and egress from aircraft).

Those patients who are referred directly to an air ambulance service (or indirectly from an airline) must be subject to careful analysis. The simple fact that the patient contacts an air ambulance service does not mean that he requires transport by dedicated air ambulance. In many cases, it may be easier, more cost-effective, and pose no additional risk to the patient to be transported with a medical escort on a scheduled carrier. The ethical air ambulance provider will try to guard the patient's best interests at all times. While medical concerns are always primary, financial circumstances may be strongly considered if less expensive transport can be expected to have no detrimental effect on patient outcome.

There are few absolute contraindications to the carriage of patients on commercial aircraft. One of these is the unlikelihood of surviving the flight. Though many patients in the last stages of illness wish to travel by air to visit places of importance to them, such travel ought to be discouraged. The logistic problems surrounding death in flight are considerable.

The presence of a highly infectious, virulent contagious disease is also a strong contraindication to commercial flight. As the aircraft cabin is a small, encapsulated, closed space, the chances of passing on illness through droplet spread or casual contact with another passenger is magnified. In these patients, flight represents a disservice to fellow passengers. Immobility, whether from casting of an extremity or chronic disability or debilitation, is a further problem. Not only are these patients at risk of venous stasis and thrombosis, but their immobility prevents active participation in emergency procedures should evacuation of the aircraft be required. It may even delay the evacuation of others.

While it is impossible to state categorically that an ill patient may fly unescorted, a list of conditions which strongly advocate for flight in the minimal company of a medical escort are noted in Tables 10.6a and 10.6b.

Table 10.6a   Absolute contraindications to unescorted air travel

- Unlikelihood of surviving flight
- Active contagious disease
- Immobility

Source: Fromm, R.E. 'Indications for Air Medical Transport', in Blumen, I.J. and H. Rodenberg (eds), *Air Medical Physician's Handbook*.

Table 10.6b   Relative contraindications to unescorted air travel

Cardiopulmonary
- Recent myocardial infarction (until normal activity resumed)
- Uncontrolled hypertension
- Severe congestive heart failure
- Symptomatic valvular disease
- Uncontrolled dysrhythmias
- Hypoxia on room air
- Severe restrictive lung disease
- Pulmonary cysts, bullous emphysema
- Pneumothorax; recent cardiothoracic surgery
- Cystic fibrosis

Neurologic and psychiatric
- Recent cerebrovascular accident
- Uncontrolled epilepsy
- Recent skull fracture
- Brain tumors (primary or metastatic)
- Violent behavior, claustrophobia, or fear of flying

Maxillo-facial, ophthalmic, ear, nose, and throat
- Recent ophthalmologic surgery
- Sinusitis, otitis
- Recent facial or mandibular fracture

Miscellaneous
- Pregnancy: after 36 weeks gestation
- Neonates in first 24–48 hours of life
- Unstable premature infants
- Sickle cell disease
- Uncontrolled diabetes mellitus
- Recent casting of an extremity
- Diverticulitis, peptic ulcer disease, recent gastrointestinal (GI) bleed
- Recent abdominal surgery
- Diving within 24 hours before flight

Source: Fromm, R.E. 'Indications for Air Medical Transport'. in Blumen, I.J. and H.Rodenberg (eds), *Air Medical Physician's Handbook*.

References

Association of Air Medical Services (1990) *Position Paper on the Appropriate Use of Emergency Air Medical Services*, Association of Air Medical Services: Pasadena, California.

Benson, N.J., Alson R.L., Norton E.G. et al. (1993) 'Air medical transport utilization in North Carolina', *Prehosp Disast Med.* **8**:133-7.

Biewener, A. et al. (2004) 'Impact of helicopter transport and hospital level on mortality of polytrauma patients', *J Trauma Injury Infect Crit Care.* **56**(1):94-8.

Bledsoe, B.E. (2003) 'Air medical helicopters save lives and are cost-effective', *Emerg Med Services.* **32**(8):88-90.

Boyd, C.R., Corse K.M. and R.C. Campbell (1989) 'Emergency interhospital transport of the major trauma patient: air versus ground', *J Trauma.* **29**:789-94.

Falcone, R.E. (1994) 'Indications for air medical transport: practical applications', in Blumen, I.J. and H. Rodenberg (eds), *Air Medical Physician's Handbook*, AMPA: Salt Lake City.

Gabram, S.G.A., Stohler S., Sargent R.K., et al. (1989) 'Interhospital audit criteria for helicopter emergency medical services', *Connecticut Med.* **55**:387-92.

Lerner, E.B., et al. (2003) 'Is total out-of-hospital time a significant predictor of trauma patient mortality?', *Acad Emerg Med.* **10**(9):949-54.

Rhee, K.J. and R. J. O'Malley (1994) 'Indications for air medical transport: general concepts', in Blumen, I.J. and H. Rodenberg (eds), *Air Medical Physician's Handbook*, AMPA: Salt Lake City.

Rosenberg, B.L. et al. (2003) 'Aeromedical service: how does it actually contribute to the mission?', *J Trauma Injury Infect Crit Care.* **54**(4):681-8.

Silbergleit, R. et al. (2003) 'Long-term air medical services system performance using APACHE-II and mortality benchmarking', *Prehosp Emerg Care.* **7**(2):195-8.

Thomas, S.H. (2004) 'Helicopter emergency medical services transport outcomes literature: annotated review of articles published 2000-2003', *Prehosp Emerg Care.* **8**(3):322-33.

Chapter 11

Clinical Considerations in Transport of the Ill and Injured

Introduction

A knowledge and understanding of the physical, physiological and psychological constraints imposed by travel and the flight environment will allow anticipation and prevention of any problems that may otherwise occur during the transfer. As air pressure declines with increasing altitude, less oxygen is available for cellular metabolism and gases trapped within body cavities will expand. Passenger carrying aircraft maintain a cabin pressure which rarely exceeds 6000 ft (1800 m). Although healthy passengers will feel no ill effects, there is a significant decline in alveolar partial pressure of oxygen, from 13.7 kPa (103 mmHg) at sea level to about 10 kPa (75 mmHg) at 6000 ft (1800 m). With ascent from sea level to the same altitude, gas volumes in body cavities will expand by over 25 per cent. There may also be problems with motion sickness, vibration, noise, cold or humidity, not to mention the psychological terror felt by some who can imagine nothing worse than being locked in a flying metal tube!

Aeromedical transport encompasses an entire array of medical conditions and operational situations. These range from the transfer of a medically fit but elderly and frail patient on a scheduled flight to the primary transfer of a patient with multiple injuries from the roadside to the receiving hospital. Although some aspects of assessment and care are universal, there is a clear difference in approach between the transfer of a critically ill patient during a primary or secondary transfer and the planned transfer of a stable patient to a medical facility near to home, or a quaternary transfer to the patient's home address.

The initial approach to the severely ill or injured patient should follow the traditional ABCD assessment taught in all advanced life support courses. This is the sequential appraisal and management of the airway (A), breathing (B), circulatory status (C), and an assessment of neurological dysfunction (D). This assessment and management must proceed in an orderly fashion, with airway concerns taking priority over breathing, breathing over circulation, and circulatory status over isolated neurological impairment. The ABCD plan is not only key to initial patient assessment, but provides a template for the care of patients when inflight problems or complications arise. By consistently examining all patients using this system, life threatening problems can be anticipated and dealt with at the earliest opportunity.

Only after these initial priorities have been secured is it sensible to examine the whole patient to exclude other problems.

Critically ill and injured patients are often difficult to manage on conventional passenger aircraft, and airline medical authorities may refuse medical clearance for some types of patients. These aircraft are not designed to carry the medical equipment needed to effectively care for such patients and, despite screening, it is almost impossible to maintain privacy from the inquisitive eyes of other passengers. Whenever possible, small, dedicated air ambulances should be used to transport those in need of intensive therapy who might otherwise be refused carriage by the airlines (Figure 11.1).

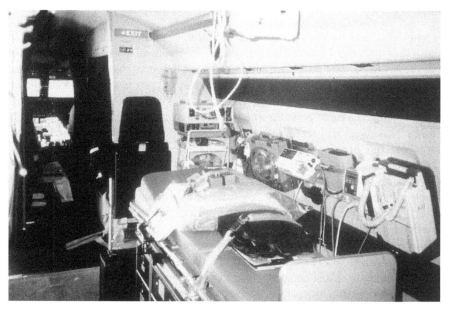

Figure 11.1 Dedicated air ambulance. Note the space restrictions and difficulty with stowage and access to equipment

When distances are short, piston or turboprop aircraft are used. These aircraft are often unpressurized, and great care must be taken to ensure that the patient's requirements for inflight oxygen are adequately met. Over greater distances, faster jets may be used. These aircraft are inevitably pressurized due to the altitude of their normal operations. The final decision on aircraft type best suited to any individual medical transfer is a fine balance based on speed, range, cabin size, internal fit, and cost.

This chapter is written with the intention of providing a summary of the major conditions which may pose problems during aeromedical transport. The focus is on anticipation and management of difficulties before and during flight but any discussion of the indications and contraindications for flight can only be relative.

There are few clinical reasons for refusal of aeromedical transportation, and none are absolute. To a large extent, aeromedical services exist to transport patients whose condition would make them ineligible for flight by normal airline. Many suitable texts are available for those who require more clinical information on individual conditions.

Airway considerations

An obstructed airway is life threatening but easily managed if recognized early. Any patient who is obtunded and unable to maintain patency of the upper airway is at serious risk of obstruction, especially during movement and transport. Such patients should have the airway cleared and secured prior to flight. In addition to those with obvious airway obstruction, any patient who is unable (or likely to become unable) to protect his own airway against the possibility of aspiration after regurgitation should have a cuffed endotracheal or tracheostomy tube inserted prior to departure. Once inserted, the tube must be checked to ensure correct placement and secured against accidental dislodgment. Patients who suggest the need for intubation prior to leaving the scene or referring facility include those who are obtunded (head injury, medical coma, or sedated), require artificial ventilation, have obvious upper respiratory tract obstruction (maxillofacial injuries or epiglottitis), and whose airway is likely to become compromised in the immediate future (respiratory tract burns). These patients are best escorted by someone skilled in the practice of intubation and ventilation, such as an anesthesiologist, intensivist or, in some countries, respiratory therapist or nurse anesthetist. To replace a malpositioned tube is difficult enough in the protected environment of a hospital; it is even more so in the back of a moving ambulance or in the cabin of an aircraft moving in three dimensions simultaneously.

Tracheostomy tubes must be changed before flight. Humidified oxygen administered via a stoma mask will overcome the low humidity of the artificial cabin atmosphere and help prevent dry mucous plugs. Further problems may be avoided by frequent, careful, aseptic suction of the airway. There is controversy over the inflation of cuffs on tracheostomy and endotracheal tubes. Some argue that they should be filled with sterile water, since air is subject to expansion with the lowered ambient pressure as altitude increases. Cuff volume expansion is likely to increase pressure on the tracheal wall and may result in necrosis if pressures are of sufficient intensity and duration. If the medical escort recognizes this potential problem and releases some of the air in the cuff on ascent but subsequently forgets to reinflate it on descent, an air leak will occur, oxygenation may be impaired, and the airway will no longer be protected. Antagonists to this argument state that the problem is unlikely to occur with modern high volume, low pressure cuffs, and that a pressure limiting pilot balloon will prevent over-inflation at altitude. This is true, but it can not prevent an air leak on descent when air has already been spilled out of the cuff. Like most aeromedical dogma, there is simply no evidence base upon which to guide good practice.

Care of the cervical spine is an integral part of airway management. All patients who are the victims of trauma, regardless of the mechanism of injury or the presence or absence of neurological deficit, should be considered to have an unstable cervical spine injury until clinically and radiogically disproven. All trauma patients should be fully immobilized with a hard cervical collar and head restraint applied (Figure 11.2). Immobilization is essential whilst lifting and loading the patient but restrained patients are at risk of aspiration after emesis, and of pressure sores at points of prolonged contact. Patients with suspected cervical spine injury who require endotracheal intubation may be intubated orally or nasally as long as the integrity of the cervical spine is maintained by immobilization and manual in-line stabilization. The operator should take care to avoid flexion, extension, and rotation of the head and neck.

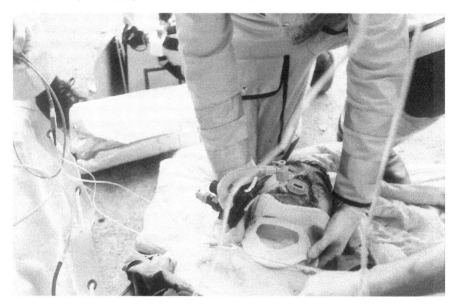

Figure 11.2   Immobilization of the head and neck in suspected cervical spine injury

Respiratory considerations

Patients with problems of oxygenation or pulmonary function at ground level will likely exhibit increased difficulty at altitude. Such patients must be identified well before departure so that adequate oxygen supplements, mechanical ventilation, or other special requirements can be met. A decision on the required aircraft cabin pressure must be made early in flight planning, and the aircraft operator duly informed. Oxygen calculations should always include at least 50 per cent reserve in case of delays or diversions and, if large volumes of oxygen are required, an extra refueling stop may be necessary to collect or replenish cylinders. Such decisions require advance communications and planning with airline and airport authorities.

Whatever the disease process, if oxygen is required at ground level, the requirement for oxygen at altitude can be calculated using the FiO_2 required to maintain an alveolar partial pressure of oxygen (PaO_2) of 13.3 kPa (100 mmHg) as measured at the originating hospital. Even if a patient does not appear to require oxygen at ground level, there may be enough respiratory impairment to reduce PaO_2 to such an extent that the patient is, from a respiratory point of view, already equivalent to being at altitude. With a knowledge of expected PaO_2 at various altitudes, it is simple to estimate the effects of a 'further' 6000 ft (1800 m) on oxygen tension. It should be remembered, however, that these figures refer to normal respiratory physiology, and that the 'ground' altitude should be calculated above sea level. Patients requiring more than 40 per cent oxygen at ground level are likely to need positive pressure ventilation when cabin pressure exceeds 4000 ft (1200 m). Clearly, care should be taken with the use of 100 per cent oxygen in patients who rely on hypoxic drive for respiratory stimulus (as in chronic obstructive pulmonary disease). However, although ventilation may be reduced when oxygen in high concentration is given, most of the deterioration in such patients occurs as a result of adverse ventilation/ perfusion inequalities consequent upon the increased oxygen concentration.

Arterial oxygen tension (PaO_2) at altitude may also be predicted in normocapnic patients through the use of the equation:

$$PaO_2 \text{ (at altitude)} = 22.8 - 2.74 \text{ (x)} + 0.68 \text{ (y)}$$

where (x) is the anticipated altitude in thousands of feet above sea level and (y) is the patient's sea level PaO_2. This equation has been found to be most accurate when used two hours before flight. Varying oxygen concentrations can be administered in patients who are being tested using the equation. Supplemental oxygen will increase the sea level PaO_2 and increase the PaO_2 at altitude accordingly.

Whatever method is used to screen pulmonary patients for flight, PaO_2 at sea level should be at least 9.3 kPa (70 mmHg). This will yield a PaO_2 at cruise altitude of 6.7 to 7.3 kPa (50 to 55 mmHg), and should preserve oxygen hemoglobin saturation at or above 90 per cent in the absence of other confounding pathology. Pulmonary function laboratories may be able to perform specific altitude challenge tests, where the patient breathes in a gas mixture which simulates that at altitude. These tests can be especially helpful in evaluating the patient with chronic hypercapnia. The British Thoracic Society provides an excellent summary of such hypoxic challenge testing as well as the assessment of the fitness of respiratory patients for air travel (www. brit-thoracic.org.uk).

Once the flow rate required to maintain an adequate FiO_2 and PaO_2 is known, oxygen carriage requirements can be determined. If the volume of the oxygen cylinder and the pressure within it is known, then the amount of gas emanating from the cylinder at sea level can be calculated according to Boyle's Law:

$$(V_1) (P_1) = (V_2) (P_2)$$

Where V_1 = volume of usable gas
         V_2 = volume of cylinder
         P_1 = ambient pressure at 1 atmosphere ($\approx$ 100 kPa at sea level)
         P_2 = pressure of gas in cylinder

Example - To calculate volume of usable gas:

2 liter (V_2) oxygen cylinder under 13 000 kPa (P_2) at 100 kPa SL ambient pressure (P_1) of pressure will yield:

$$(V_1) = (P_2) \times (V_2) \div (P_1) \text{ that is:}$$
$$(V_1) = (2000 \times 13\ 000) \div 100 = 260\ 000 = 260 \text{ liters}$$

Because P_1 is nearer 101.3 kPa, a little less than 260 liters of usable gas will be available at sea level. If oxygen is administered to a patient at a rate of 5 liters per minute, the cylinder in the example above will provide about 50 minutes of oxygen flow.

Pneumothorax, whether spontaneous, iatrogenic, or caused by disease or trauma, will be exacerbated by the effects of gaseous expansion if not properly drained. Although surgical emphysema may worsen alarmingly, it is the potential for impairment of gaseous exchange and life threatening tension pneumothorax which is of most concern. If a thoracostomy drain has been recently removed, a suitable delay should elapse before flight is considered, and only then with radiographic evidence of a fully expanded lung. If in doubt, it is better to keep the drain in place during the transfer, since an open, draining air leak is preferable to a closed, expanding lesion. Those who are to be transported with a chest drain in situ should have a preflight chest Xray to ensure that the tube is well sited and draining correctly, and to demonstrate the absence of significant residual pneumothoraces. Chest tubes should be fitted with a functioning Heimlich valve or a valved drainage bag. Fluid draining from the chest may demonstrate faster flow at altitude if the pleural cavity contains free air.

Placement of chest tubes in the field or transport setting is controversial. A correctly placed chest tube can release trapped air and fluid from within the pleural cavity, promote lung re-expansion, and reduce ventilation/perfusion mismatching. However, it may also release any tamponade effect that the mass of blood and air has on internal chest bleeding, and aeromedical personnel may have difficulty keeping pace with ongoing fluid losses from within the chest. Some would argue that while a hemothorax, unless massive, is generally not life threatening in isolation, tension pneumothorax is. Therefore, efforts should concentrate on diagnosing the presence of tension pneumothorax and treating it appropriately with needle thoracostomy, usually in the midclavicular line of the second intercostal space.

Some thought should be given to the likelihood of other injury in patients with a pneumothorax. Trauma patients also suffer underlying pulmonary contusions which may impair gaseous exchange. There may also be myocardial contusions which predispose the patient to cardiac dysrhythmias and abnormalities of heart wall motion. Patients with significant flail chest are best transported with the support of intermittent positive pressure or jet ventilation.

Any condition which increases the basal metabolic rate will also increase oxygen demand. Supplemental oxygen must be provided for thyrotoxic patients and those with pyrexia, recent exposure to extremes of temperature, and significant burn injuries (including those who have suffered major internal damage from electrical burns).

The best way to measure oxygen sufficiency is by evaluation of arterial blood gases. A reasonably accurate assessment of oxygen saturation can be achieved with pulse oximetry methods, but the problems and limitations of this method are discussed in Chapter 9. Clinical acumen is the key. In addition to altered respiratory parameters, the hypoxic patient is likely to exhibit confusion, tachycardia, and cyanosis.

Although pulmonary disease affecting gas exchange may exist in isolation, it often accompanies disease affecting other organs. Patients with isolated pulmonary disease (such as an otherwise fit patient with a respiratory tract infection) usually tolerate moderate short duration hypoxia without significant sequelae. Patients with no pulmonary disease but organs at risk of hypoxia, such as a recent cerebrovascular accident (CVA), will be no more hypoxic at altitude than the escorting doctor or nurse. However, a patient with a combination of pulmonary or other disease which affects gas exchange and 'organs at risk' will often suffer severe effects of hypoxia at altitude. All patients with respiratory disease must therefore be assessed for evidence of ischemia in other organs.

Cardiovascular considerations

The cardiac patient is at risk from the reduction of PaO_2 which occurs within the aircraft cabin, but may also be affected by fear of flight, the stress of travel, time zone changes, gastric distention, and confinement in the aircraft cabin. Many are smokers, and it has been estimated that the carboxyhemoglobin level of a heavy smoker impairs oxygen carriage to such an extent that he may be considered to have a 2000 ft (610 m) disadvantage at sea level. Any known impairment of cardiac reserve will require transportation in a pressurized aircraft with careful planning before departure. All such patients, and in particular those with symptoms of myocardial ischemia or a diagnosis of myocardial contusion, will require inflight oxygen supplementation and close monitoring by the flight medical team.

For the purposes of planning transport by air, it is helpful to divide patients who have had a myocardial infarct into two groups – those whose recovery has been so far, free of complications, and those who have experienced any of the signs or symptoms listed in Table 11.1.

Table 11.1   Significant complications of myocardial infarction

- Chest pain persisting beyond 48 hours
- Rhythm disturbances or heart failure beyond the first 24 hours
- Ejection fraction of less than 50%
- Residual ischemia as assessed by
    - resting or exercise ECG
    - angiography
    - radio-isotope scanning
- If it is a second or subsequent infarct

Although there is no clear supporting medical evidence, it is often stated that those who have suffered a myocardial infarction should not be transported by air until after at least one week of complication-free recovery. Like all such rules, much depends on the facilities at the patient's location, the capabilities of the transferring aircraft, and the skills of the inflight team. It may be necessary to transfer a patient earlier, especially if he is in a remote place or at a location which cannot offer specialty cardiac care. Indeed, it might be argued that the whole point of transporting cardiac patients is to transfer them early in the course of their illness so that maximum benefit can be derived from specialist care. If early transportation is required, thought should be given to the logistics of the assignment and to the provision of resuscitation equipment and skills in an aircraft large enough for cardiopulmonary resuscitation (CPR) to be performed well.

A review of over 100 patients with acute myocardial infarction (AMI) transported by one aeromedical service revealed that 12 per cent suffered complications en route requiring treatment, but no patients died during flight. In another study of 150 patients with AMI, none suffered a major complication or death during transport even though 55 received thrombolytic therapy en route. The growth of regional cardiac imaging and interventional radiology facilities has seen a marked increase in the secondary transfer of patients with ischemic heart disease. Of 250 patients with AMI transported for cardiac catheterization and coronary angioplasty, 50 patients suffered complications. Transient hypotension, third degree atrioventricular block, and ventricular tachycardia were the most common inflight problems, but no patients died during transport. The overall evidence suggests that major inflight events are infrequent and can be managed effectively while aloft. Although at first it seems that these complications are not specific to the flight environment, another study compared patients with AMI or unstable angina transported by air and by road. Although patients transported by air were no more ill than those who were carried in ground vehicles, serious untoward events were significantly more likely in the aeromedical group.

In the prehospital environment, it seems clear that aeromedical transport provides no survival advantage to the patient in cardiopulmonary arrest unless spontaneous circulation has been restored prior to helicopter arrival. The benefits of air transport of patients with evolving AMI are unclear but early results suggest there is little difference when compared with those transported by road ambulance. However, the weight of evidence does not yet support a specific conclusion. The safety and efficacy of aeromedical care for patients with other cardiac conditions is poorly defined.

Care should be taken in the preflight assessment of any post-infarct patient in an effort to detect residual ischemia which may take the form of dysrhythmias, cardiac failure, and/or pain. Examination of the patient and review of the latest electrocardiogram, chest Xray, biochemistry, and hematology results will allow anticipation of potential problems and treatment of such complications as anemia and electrolyte imbalances or other precipitants of dangerous instability before departure. Preflight sedation may be required as prophylaxis against airport and flight stresses. In addition to their anxiolytic and cardiopreservative effects, beta blockers are no longer contraindicated in the presence of cardiac failure, but may exacerbate asthma and bradydysrhythmias. Long haul patients may benefit from a hypnotic agent to facilitate sleep, but not at the expense of respiratory drive. As with cardiac care on the ground, the aims of management should be to prevent myocardial hypoxemia and metabolic acidosis, to promote cardiac contractility, prevent cardiac failure, and to treat pain and anxiety.

Any deleterious changes in cardiac rhythm at altitude may be due to hypoxia, and supplemental oxygen should be immediately administered or increased. Although much has been written about the use of defibrillators in aircraft, there is no evidence that aircraft or occupant safety is at risk. However, because of the possibility of stray electric fields affecting aircraft avionics, it is mandatory to warn the flight crew before defibrillation or synchronized cardioversion is performed. The overall treatment of dysrhythmias is no different to that which would occur at ground level, and should follow guidelines established by the European Resuscitation Council, American Heart Association, or other current principles of practice. Exacerbation of angina or the presence of new chest pain may be relieved by supplemental oxygen alone, but may also be due to the psychological stresses of flight and respond to mild sedation in addition to conventional treatments.

A significant decrease in myocardial perfusion, as may occur with altitude-induced hypoxemia, is likely to result in an element of congestive heart failure. This may be heralded by increasing pulse and respiratory rates in the presence of distended neck veins. The noisy cabin environment may render pulmonary auscultation for rales and rhonchi virtually useless. However, audible wheezes without a previous history should alert the inflight team to the possible presence of left ventricular failure, as should expectoration of frothy, blood-stained sputum and the presence of pulsus alternans. As at ground level, initial treatment should be the administration of 100 per cent oxygen. Drug therapy may include the use of nitrates, opiates, and diuretics. For the supine patient, every effort must be made to place him in an upright posture. This is not always possible on some stretcher types, and extra pillows or rolled blankets should be used. All patients at risk of cardiopulmonary complications should have a patent intravenous cannula in place before departure. Urinary catheterization may be required in view of the difficulties of using and emptying bedpans and bottles and of moving seriously ill patients to onboard lavatories.

As the cardiac and pulmonary systems are interlinked, the American College of Chest Physicians (ACCP) developed a list of altitude limitations for cardiorespiratory disease. The reference is rather old now, and the recommendations are broad. In some respects they may appear completely irrelevant because it is unlikely that a modern established aeromedical organization would consider transferring any cardiorespiratory patient without supplemental oxygen. But, is that necessarily the case throughout the world and in all situations? As this chapter is written, two of the biggest natural disasters in recorded history have recently taken place – the Indian Ocean tsunami and the earthquakes in Kashmir and Pakistan. Both disasters resulted in tens of thousands of deaths and thousands of injured survivors. These were exceptional and terrible experiences, but any scale of disaster will inevitably result in the use of ad hoc ill-equipped general purpose aircraft and helicopters for casualty evacuation purposes. Victims of such events are likely then to be emplaned without the luxury of inflight supplemental oxygen. Table 11.2 notes the ACCP criteria, and can be helpful in recognizing safe altitude limits in specific patient populations, and aid in the prediction of the need for supplemental oxygen perhaps when resources are scarce.

Pacemaker oversensing can occur in the presence of extraneous electromagnetic fields and stray currents. Such conditions are highly likely in the aircraft and as a result of airport security devices. The possibility of lead movement and dislodgment always exists. While little can be done for internal pacemaker problems in the transport setting, failure of external pacemakers should dictate that leads be checked before an attempt to regain capture is made by increasing the pacing output and the use of inotropic agents. Supplemental oxygen must be given, and dysrhythmias treated appropriately.

The efficient carriage of oxygen by blood depends on the quantity and quality of hemoglobin in the circulation (see Chapter 4). Since pulse oximetry can be misleading, a knowledge of the most recent Hb level is mandatory for proper interpretation. Although increases in cardiac output and ventilation can compensate for some reduction in hemoglobin, these mechanisms may themselves be subject to the adverse effects of hypoxia. For instance, myocardial ischemia will be exacerbated by anemia, and poor cardiac reserve will minimize the compensatory capability of increasing cardiac output. Compensatory effects are more efficient with chronic anemia, but a small degree of acute blood loss may also be beneficial. The most efficient hematocrit is 35 per cent. This level represents the maximum oxygen carrying capacity of blood. Ideally, all patients for aeromedical transport should have a stable hematocrit of at least 35 per cent and a minimal hemoglobin level of 7.5 g/dl. Although effective safe altitudes for various levels of Hb can be calculated from a graph of altitude equivalents (Figure 11.3), patients with a Hb level lower than 7.5 g/dl will require continuous oxygen support throughout the flight and possibly preflight or even inflight transfusion.

Table 11.2   Altitude restrictions for patients with cardiopulmonary disease without supplemental oxygen

Altitude limit	Patient condition
10 000 feet	Suspected or mildly symptomatic cardiopulmonary disease
8000 feet	More than mildly symptomatic cardiopulmonary disease
	Marked ventilatory restriction
6000 feet	Myocardial infarction (> 8 weeks)
	Angina pectoris
	Sickle cell anemia
	Cyanosis (regardless of etiology)
	Cor pulmonale
	Respiratory acidosis
4000 feet	Severe cardiac disease with cyanosis or recent decompensation
	Patients with two of the following:
	• Cyanosis
	• Cor pulmonale
	• Respiratory acidosis
	Congestive heart failure,
	Myocardial infarction (< 8 weeks)
2000 feet	Concurrent cyanosis
	Cor pulmonale
	Respiratory acidosis

Source: The American College of Chest Physicians, Committee on Physiologic Therapy, Section on Aviation Medicine. *Air Travel in Cardiorespiratory Disease*. Dis Chest 1960; 37:579-88.

When oxygen carrying capacity is impaired, whether by derangement of the Hb molecule or by gaseous competition, supplemental oxygen will be required. Sickle cell anemia is a specific problem. Sickling crises may be provoked by hypoxia and circulatory stasis exacerbated by enforced immobility during flight. Patients particularly at risk are those with Hb C disease and sickle cell beta thalassemia. Sickle cell trait does not appear to cause problems. If air travel cannot be avoided, cabin pressure should be as high as possible, supplemental oxygen should be administered throughout the journey, and patients should be encouraged to increase their intake of non-alcoholic fluids.

Finally, postoperative cardiac patients are often much fitter than they might have been before operation. As long as the patient is stable, asymptomatic, and free of trapped pleural or mediastinal air, there is no specific contraindication to flight.

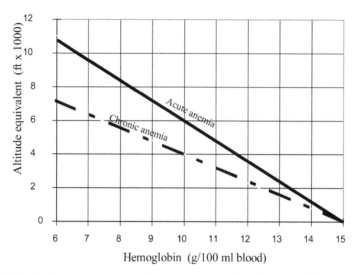

Figure 11.3   Altitude equivalents for various levels of hemoglobin

Neurologic and neurosurgical considerations

The major considerations for any patient suffering neurological illness or injury are to prevent secondary damage by cerebral hypoxia and the effects of cerebral compression, whether due to increasing intracranial pressure or the effects of lowered ambient pressure on gases trapped within the cranial vault or ventricular system. A Glasgow Coma Score (GCS) should be recorded and documented in the preflight notes, along with the date and time of the examination. Although the GCS is essentially a qualitative score, the assignment of numbers adds a degree of objectivity, especially when the same observer records consecutive scores. A decrease in the score of two or more points constitutes a neurological deterioration likely to require acute intervention. A decrease of more than three points is highly suggestive of serious deterioration and constitutes a neurosurgical emergency.

In many countries, neurosurgical and other trauma services are organized on a regional basis. As a result, patients with serious head injuries are often transferred between hospitals by air. Several studies in the UK have provided evidence that the transfer phase is potentially hazardous, often poorly managed, and patients subsequently deteriorate en route. All this can be avoided if adequate preparation and clinical excellence are applied in practice. Nothing can be done to minimize primary brain damage which is inflicted at the time of the injury, but the main causes of secondary brain damage – cardiovascular instability, hypoxia, and hypercarbia – are all preventable.

Safe transfer of patients with head injuries requires an effective and communicative partnership between the referring hospital, the neurosurgical unit and the transport agencies. It is important to agree local guidelines between the referring hospitals and the neurosurgical unit in advance. Knowing which patients should be referred, when a transfer should be made, and the essential preparations and arrangements for the journey prevents unnecessary delay and delivers the patient to definitive specialist care more promptly. However, guidelines do not replace clinical judgment, although they do provide a safe framework within which judgment can be exercised.

The issue of prompt delivery to a specialist center requires a little more discussion. We all know that seriously ill or injured patients tolerate transport, by air or ground, badly, so the issue becomes do we 'stay and play' rather than 'scoop and run'? Remembering rule number one – transfer decisions are always made on an individual basis – the severity of an intracranial bleed in a closed head injury is important in patients who have yet to undergo definitive surgery. If there is evidence of an expanding lesion or a continuing bleed, the hematoma needs to be evacuated immediately. Put another way, in this neurosurgical emergency, the issue is how soon can I get this patient to a surgeon who has the skill to evacuate this hematoma, rather than how soon can I transfer this patient to the neurosurgical center. The two might be the same thing, but all general surgeons should be able to drill a burr hole to deal with the initial emergency, and this skill may be considerably nearer than the neurosurgical centre. An alternative approach is to move the skilled surgeon to the patient who is too unstable to be transported.

Once the mass lesion is dealt with, the intracranial pressure (ICP) is under control, and the patient is stabilized with appropriate monitoring, then the transfer can be undertaken with less haste, and hence less risk. These decisions should be made conjointly between the accepting and transferring teams, if possible with computerized tomography (CT) evidence to guide decision making.

The Neuroanaesthesia Association of Great Britain and Ireland has published guidelines for the transfer of head injured patients, and states that these patients must be accompanied by an anesthesiologist or other doctor with suitable training, skills and experience if the patient is intubated, undergoing therapy to reduce ICP, receiving cardiovascular support, or has a deteriorating GCS. Some neurosurgical centers operate a retrieval service whereupon the retrieving team is dispatched to the patient and undertake their management and stabilization prior to the transfer. When distances are long, it is usually more expedient for the transfer team to be drawn from local staff. They must then rely on advice provided by the neurosurgical center on specialist management such as the use of mannitol or anticonvulsants. Although sedation, analgesia and muscle relaxation will help to decrease an elevated ICP, other measures may well be needed in patients waiting for definitive neurosurgery. Mannitol may be administered to decrease ICP by initiating a diuresis, and if ICP is proven to be high and unmanageable, barbiturates, such as thiopentone (*Pentothal*) may be prescribed to further lower ICP and cerebral oxygen demand. But the question must always be asked – is there a hematoma which needs evacuating before this patient can be transported?

Whoever undertakes the initial management, meticulous resuscitation and stabilization before transfer are the key to avoiding complications during the journey.

The fundamental requirement is to ensure satisfactory and stable tissue perfusion and oxygen delivery and, in doing so, appropriate respiratory support must be established. Intubating conditions in an aircraft, helicopter or road ambulance are far from ideal, and even the remotest possibility of later development of a compromised airway or respiratory failure merits endotracheal intubation prior to departure. Only in exceptional circumstances should a patient with a significantly altered conscious level not be sedated, intubated and ventilated. Table 11.3 gives the currently accepted indications for the intubation of head injury patients.

Further supportive care is essential to minimize the risk of secondary brain injury. Intravenous fluids should be given to maintain or restore satisfactory peripheral perfusion, blood pressure and urine output. The circulating volume should be normal or supra-normal before transfer, preferably with a haematocrit over 30%. A central venous catheter may be useful to optimise filling pressures and for the administration of drugs and fluids during the transfer. A patient persistently hypotensive despite resuscitation must not be transported until all possible causes of the hypotension have been identified and the patient stabilized. Correction of major hemorrhage takes precedence over transfer. It is important that these measures are not omitted in an attempt to speed transfer of the patient, as resultant complications may be impossible to deal with once the journey has commenced. Although there is no strong supporting evidence, it is obvious that brain metabolism (and hence oxygen consumption) should be minimized. It may be that future research will show a convincing place for active cooling but, until then, patients should at least not be allowed to become hyperthermic or pyrexial, and crystalloids containing glucose (dextrose) should initially be avoided.

During the transfer, management will be focused upon maintaining oxygenation and adequate blood pressure, and preventing dangerous elevations in ICP. Monitoring ECG, invasive blood pressure, SpO_2 (venous oxygen saturation) and $ETCO_2$ (end-tidal carbon dioxide) and the administration of drugs and other infusions should be continued. A patient who has been physiologically stabilized before departure is more likely to remain so for the duration of the transfer. This does not abrogate the requirement for constant vigilance and prompt action to deal with complications if they arise. However, the need to perform any procedure during the transfer probably indicates inadequate preparation for the transfer and should be avoided if at all possible. There is a universal truism which states that 'the best type of transfer is the one where you don't have to do anything to the patient'.

Patients with a known head injury but who do not meet the criteria for intubation will need an intravenous cannula inserted for the prophylactic or therapeutic management of nausea, vomiting, and seizures. Since the conscious head injured patient is more prone to nausea and motion sickness, an antiemetic may be recommended to prevent the elevated intracranial pressure (ICP) that accompanies vomiting and retching. Most antiemetics affect alertness, potentially making the GCS unreliable.

Table 11.3   Indications for intubation and ventilation after head injury

Immediately:

*   Coma – GCS 8 or less
    *   – not obeying commands
    *   – not speaking
    *   – not eye opening
*   Loss of protective laryngeal reflexes
*   Ventilatory insufficiency as judged by blood gas analysis
    *   – hypoxaemia (PaO_2 < 9 kPa on air or < 13 kPa on oxygen)
    *   – hypercarbia ($PaCO_2$ > 6 kPa)
*   Spontaneous hyperventilation causing $PaCO_2$ < 3.5 kPa
*   Respiratory dysrhythmia

Before the start of the journey:

*   Significantly deteriorating conscious level, even if not in coma
*   Bilateral fractured mandible
*   Copious bleeding into the mouth (for example, from skull base fracture)
*   Seizures
*   An intubated patient must be ventilated with sedation, muscle relaxation and analgesia
*   Aim for
    *   – PaO_2 > 13kPa
    *   – $PaCO_2$ 4.0 - 4.5 kPa

Source: Modified from Gentleman et al. *BMJ* 1993; 307: 547-552.

Many aspects of the aviation environment can predispose patients to seizure activity (for example, hypoxia, psychological stress, and excitement). Any patient at risk may be sedated during the journey, but the GCS will again be affected. Known epileptic patients may require premedication prior to departure. This prophylaxis may be achieved by either an increase in their normal anticonvulsant therapy (previously prescribed anticonvulsants may be given within one hour of aircraft departure regardless of the time of the last dose) or with diazepam at least one hour before flight. All patients known to be at significant risk of having seizures should travel as stretcher patients and any epileptiform activity that does occur must be stopped, to prevent further cerebral damage. Convulsions occurring during flight should be treated in the same way as they would be on the ground. Recommended management includes: diazepam (as *Diazemuls*), midazolam, or phenytoin. A convulsing patient must have a secure and patent airway, be given 100 per cent oxygen, kept warm, and prevented from self-harm. Paraldehyde should never be used, as adverse reactions to preservatives within the medication are common, and spillage can be corrosive to aircraft materials.

Since air in the cranium will expand at altitude, any patient who has had a craniotomy should generally not fly before the seventh postoperative day unless the aircraft is pressurized to the altitude of the site where the operation was performed. Similar care should be taken for those who have recently suffered a penetrating head injury, or have had cerebrospinal fluid (CSF) leakage from the ears or nose suggesting a basilar skull fracture. If a CSF leak is present at ground level, it will drain slightly faster at altitude. With the advent of high tech imaging techniques, air encephalograms and ventriculograms are virtually unheard of, but if they have been done, the same concerns apply.

Medical escorts should be aware that patients with significant head trauma are likely to have suffered associated cervical injury, especially if chest trauma has also occurred. Fractures of the clavicle and the first or second ribs are closely associated with cervical spine injury. In the presence of such a history, suitable protection of the cervical spine is essential even if a fracture or subluxation has not been diagnosed. Up to 15 per cent of cervical fractures are missed on initial Xrays.

Facial injuries may also complicate head trauma, and may compromise airway patency. Open reduction and fixation (ORIF) is the commonest method of repair to facial fractures, but any patient who has had external fixation of the jaws must have either a quick release device fitted to the apparatus or have wire or band cutters easily accessible, preferably affixed to his person for the duration of both ground and air phases of the transfer. Prior to the start of the journey, patients with mandibular immobilization may benefit from a suitable antiemetic by intramuscular or intravenous injection, and the placement of a nasogastric tube through which the stomach can be aspirated or drained. Patients with unstable midface fractures awaiting definitive correction are likely to require intubation and packing of the posterior pharynx to prevent secondary hemorrhage. The deranged anatomy and inflammation of a severely injured face may disrupt the sinuses and their drainage, causing subcutaneous emphysema and sinus pain which will worsen with altitude. All patients with severe facial injuries should be considered to have a basilar skull fracture until proven otherwise.

The clinical features of a cerebrovascular accident (CVA) are likely to be exacerbated by hypoxia, and continuous supplemental oxygen will be required for all patients during transport. For those with proven CVA, transfer is recommended after ten days, as long as deterioration or complications have not occurred. Hard and fast rules cannot be enforced, since much of the transport decision relies on the facilities of the referring hospital, the condition of the patient, and the capabilities of the inflight team. When CVA patients are transferred early, supplemental oxygen must be administered throughout the flight to maintain, or exceed, the ground level oxygenation status. In addition consideration should be given to the use of stretchers, especially if the patient is incontinent.

Elderly patients who have not suffered a stroke but are transferred for other reasons may become confused at altitude. Many elderly people have considerable cerebral arteriosclerosis, yet not severe enough to prevent normal functioning at ground level. However, at the lower ambient pressures of flight, some areas of the brain (the so called *lethal corners* at the far reaches of the arterial tree) may become ischemic and will infarct if this exposure to hypoxia is prolonged.

Patients with closed head injury or tumor may be carried safely by air, as long as cerebral metabolism and oxygenation are ensured and vigilant observation is maintained for sudden elevations in ICP.

Acute subarachnoid hemorrhage (SAH), from whatever cause, can be difficult to manage, but a ruptured aneurysm is the cause in 75 per cent of patients, and the risk of rebleeding is significant. Informed clinical decisions can best be made after CT angiography, but these techniques may not be available in some referring hospitals. Depending on the cause and severity of the bleed, the initial issue which needs resolution is where is the nearest and best place for this patient to be treated. In the case of a long haul repatriation, it may be that transfer to a nearer neurosurgical center with appropriate expertise in interventional radiology and surgical clipping may be a more appropriate option than a long and risky flight back home. A recent grading system from the World Federation of Neurosurgeons (Table 11.4) provides a validated prognostic index which correlates well with final outcome. Discussions between the referring hospital, neurosurgical center and the aeromedical team should carefully examine the risks and benefits of patient transfer.

Table 11.4   World Federation of Neurosurgeons (WFN) grading for SAH

GCS	Motor deficit	WFN grade
15	absent	I
14-13	absent	II
14-13	present	III
12-7	present or absent	IV
6-3	present or absent	V

However, because of the risk of rebleeding and cerebral ischemia and infarction between days 3 and 14, longstanding published recommended times for patient transfer after the acute event are either during the first 48 hours or after two weeks have elapsed. Figure 11.4 gives a graphical representation of the risk of rebleeding after aneurysmal SAH, and it shows that the risk does not plateau until about 30 days after the initial event. If, for example, a patient survives the first 40 days after a bleed, there is still approximately an 18 per cent chance of a rebleed in the remaining four to five months. From a medical insurance point of view, the risk of a rebleed remains about five per cent for at least ten years, and the risk of death from a rebleed is more than twice that of the initial bleed. About a quarter of patients develop clinical evidence of ischemia/infarction, and, in turn, a quarter of these will die as a result. Other complications include hydrocephalus, expanding intracerebral hematoma, pulmonary edema, epilepsy, cardiac and dysrhythmias.

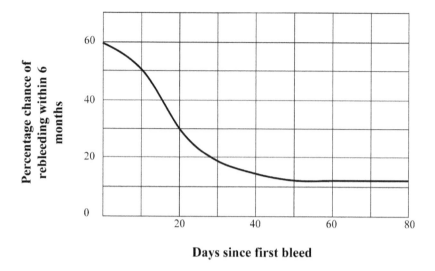

Days since first bleed

Figure 11.4   Risk of rebleeding after an aneurysmal SAH

Orthopedic considerations

Plaster of Paris or fiberglass casts may contain air pockets which may expand during flight and apply pressure to the underlying skin and disrupt the structural integrity of the cast. Although air within the soft padding under a cast will normally vent without restriction, if soft tissue swelling interrupts the escape of this air at the top or bottom of the cast then tissue ischemia and further swelling will result. Compressive effects from the expansion of soft tissues at subatmospheric pressures may also occur. There is some research evidence that the compartment pressure in an uninjured limb which is encased in plaster and taken to altitude may increase to a sufficient extent to cause a true compartment syndrome. Bivalving the cast down to the layer of the skin cover may eliminate these risks. Splitting the cast will also allow easy access to wounds should they require attention during the flight. If this is not possible, serious wounds (especially those involving vascular structures) may require the cutting of an appropriate window in the cast to allow access for observation and/or treatment. Exchanging full circular casts for backslab splints before transport may be preferred. All internal drains should be subject to negative pressure or free drainage.

Due to the confined cabin space and the effects of acceleration, all forms of traction should use closed systems, such as springs or cords under tension. Free-hanging weights are not to be used. External fixators must be checked for security prior to departure, and care should be taken in the movement of patients (and people around the patient) to avoid jarring the metalwork. Military antishock trousers (MAST, also known as pneumatic antishock garment, or PASG) may be used to stabilize pelvic and lower extremity fractures. They may be used in prehospital flights and short duration interhospital transfers. The MAST suit is inflated by air and, when used for the purposes of immobilization, it is crucial to maintain stability of the pelvis and long bones of the lower extremity without causing vascular obstruction to the legs. It is essential on flights of long duration to deflate the suit, one compartment at a time in rotation.

Any patient with multiple long bone fractures who suddenly appears hypoxic with dyspnea and confusion may have suffered a fat embolism. This event is especially likely if the presentation includes convulsions, pyrexia, and a petechial rash. Life threatening emboli may lodge in the lungs or the brain. Initial treatment should include administration of high concentrations of inspired oxygen and management of any ensuing shock.

Patients with hand injuries requiring elevation are likely to require extra occupant space (such as a business class seat) and some form of suspension for the sling. It may be more appropriate to consider carriage as a stretcher patient. Those who have undergone arthroscopic examination of any joint will be fit to fly 48 hours after surgery, as long as the postoperative period has been uneventful. Many patients with injuries are young and otherwise fit. Provided that adequate early treatment has been concluded, a small delay may significantly improve both the comfort and safety of the transfer.

Patients with multiple trauma

Two major studies from the United States describe the impact of aeromedical transport on the mortality of trauma patients. In the first, 150 victims of blunt trauma treated at the scene of injury and transported by ground were compared with another 150 blunt trauma victims transported by air. Patients transported by aeromedical services exhibited a 52 per cent reduction in mortality when compared with controls. A second survey of primary responses by helicopters revealed that, in over 1200 victims of blunt trauma, a 21 per cent reduction in actual versus expected mortality was observed when these patients were compared with controls.

Work from the United Kingdom provides mixed messages. One suggests that in rural settings, total patient transport time does not differ between ground services which transport patients to the closest hospital facilities and a helicopter service which transported patients to the regional tertiary referral center. No outcome criteria were reviewed. A review of helicopter EMS operations in London revealed no overall improvement of survival in patients transported by air versus ground, although those more severely injured patients did exhibit a survival advantage if transported by air. Studies form both sides of the Atlantic must be interpreted in the context of viewing the air transport service as part of a trauma system, and not as an isolated unit unto itself.

Other studies have tried to quantify the effect of aeromedical transport on patients with traumatic cardiopulmonary arrest. In general, trauma victims in cardiac arrest showed no survival advantage from aeromedical transport unless vital signs were noted by EMS personnel. Studies reviewing on-scene thoracotomies performed by physician flight crew also revealed no benefits from this intervention.

Gastrointestinal considerations

The main considerations in patients with abdominal hollow viscus disease or injury are gaseous expansion and hemorrhage. The normal volume of intraluminal gas in an adult is between 100 and 400 ml, formed predominantly by fermentation and swallowed air. Although normally able to vent, any passenger may experience moderate discomfort after ascent to altitude. Problems may occur after flatulent foods or with intestinal obstruction, infection, ileus and after gas is introduced into the peritoneal cavity at laparotomy or laparoscopy.

Preferably, patients who have had laparotomy or repair of the gastrointestinal tract should not be transported by air until the seventh postoperative day, since volume expansion may weaken or disrupt sutures. Similarly, expansion of intraluminal gas may cause secondary hemorrhage in healing wounds and peptic ulceration. A decision to transport the patient earlier should be made in conjunction with the referring surgeon, and then only if there is no evidence of ileus or gross abdominal distention and no risk of wound dehiscence. Patients who require urgent transport despite these conditions may require placement of an orogastric, nasogastric, or rectal tube prior to flight. Cabin altitude should be maintained as close to sea level as possible. Patients who have undergone laparoscopic examination will be fit to fly 48 hours after surgery, assuming an uneventful postoperative period.

Gas in colostomy and ileostomy bags at ground level will also expand with altitude, and removing the bag in flight can lead to fecal overflow. Stoma outputs of gas and fecal material will likely increase as gas expands in the intestinal tract. Changing the bag before departure and venting before removal may prevent problems in transit. All patients requiring nasogastric suction, or who have any other form of enterostomy tube, should have appropriate drainage into a collecting bag during the flight.

Any patient susceptible to motion sickness, or in whom vomiting would cause considerable medical problems, should be given a preflight antiemetic. Those complaining of nausea en route should be similarly treated, although antiemetics may be ineffective once nausea has occurred.

Endocrine considerations

Endocrine problems which deserve special consideration during air medical transport center on those conditions where time factors are important for symptomatology or therapy. Diabetic patients may require feeding, insulin administration, and assessment of serum glucose levels at specific intervals. Similarly, patients on supplemental corticosteroids may require their medications to be administered at specific intervals in order to avoid precipitating an adrenal crisis. The prevention of many inflight problems related to endocrine disorders lies in maintaining the patient on the local (overseas) time, irrespective of the number of time zones crossed in flight. Gradual adjustment of medications and routines to home local time should occur under supervision at the accepting hospital.

Ophthalmic considerations

Traditional aeromedical wisdom holds that those patients who have suffered penetrating eye injury or who have been subject to surgery where an air bubble remains in the eye should fly only when the aircraft cabin altitude can be maintained at sea level or otherwise at least a week after surgery. In theory, expansion of gas bubbles within the eye may precipitate acute glaucoma. Recent studies, however, have failed to demonstrate any appreciable effect of the expansion of gas within the eye, presumably because the gas bubble floats within the liquid non-compressible vitreous humor. However, there has been one account of temporary blindness in a patient with air in the globe. This resolved completely when the cabin altitude was reduced.

Finally, vibration, acceleration, and gaseous expansion may cause increased leakage of vitreous fluids in patients with unsealed penetrating injury to the globe.

Infectious diseases

Infectious diseases are important, not only when considering the patient, but they also have implications for the aeromedical team, flight crew, other passengers, aircraft, and equipment onboard. The majority of these patients will need transport in a dedicated air ambulance. Even if the condition is not critical, the possibility of spreading infection and the often unpleasant sights and smells of infectious diseases cause most airlines to be reluctant to accept these passengers.

The nature of the illness dictates the level of precautions to be taken in the care of the patient. Clearly, patients with tuberculosis require appropriate respiratory precautions, while those with the acquired immune deficiency syndrome (AIDS) or hepatitis need thorough care and disposal of blood, body fluids, and contaminated medical materials. While the use of barriers such as gowns, gloves, and goggles may seem intimidating and uncaring, safe practice dictates the use of these universal precautions in the unknown or undiagnosed patient. Inflight personnel may also desire, or be required, to take prophylactic medications to counter exposure to infectious disease. Examples include the use of rifampicin for prevention of meningococcal meningitis and the chronic use of antimalarial agents. Flight team policy should dictate vaccinations necessary prior to flight duty, and should also specify methods of cleaning and disinfecting of equipment, uniforms, and aircraft structures. The development of individual program policies is best dictated by the inflight team and medical director working in conjunction with specialists in infectious disease and infection control. The World Health Organization (WHO) is a fundamental source of information (see International Health Regulations, Chapter 19), and have recently produced revised guidelines on 'Tuberculosis and air travel'.

Psychiatric and psychological considerations

Any frankly psychotic patient, those with active hallucinations, or patients experiencing withdrawal symptoms should be sedated before flight and should ideally travel as a stretcher patient if considered to be a danger to himself or others. Location within the cabin is also important. It is unwise to place the violent or suicidal patient next to an emergency exit or near to emergency equipment such as flares and axes. Appropriate manpower and restraints should be available in the event that patient control be lost. Other patients who may react adversely to air travel should be identified by the flight team and considered for mild sedation prior to flight. Special concern should be given to those patients who have been involved in any form of recent transport accident, regardless of their apparent willingness to fly.

The psychological aspects of aeromedical transport on the patient must be recognized and addressed. Patients may have unfounded fears relating to the aircraft, crew, equipment, receiving facility, or simply the idea of air travel. Family and friends may have similar concerns. It is incumbent upon aeromedical personnel to answer all questions as best they can, and be prepared at all times to provide for the psychological as well as the clinical wellbeing of the patient.

General considerations

Other than for emergency evacuation direct from the location of injury or to a center for definitive medical or surgical care, all patients should have stable vital signs, be adequately hydrated and have no active hemorrhage. Any patient in pain must be given analgesia suitable for the mode and duration of the journey, preferably before departure from the point of injury or evacuating hospital.

With the exceptions described above, movement of most postoperative patients can be arranged for 24 hours after surgery, although for a long duration transfer a longer delay is prudent. Patients who have undergone minor surgery may be transferred after 12 hours. Finally, a full and comprehensive aeromedical summary, completed by the inflight medical escort or team, must be completed and attached to the notes of all patients.

Conclusions

The decision to evacuate any patient by air must be made with the best interests of the patient in mind. A clear understanding of the stresses of flight is essential, and decisions must take into account the latest information on flight times, delays, flight duration, stopovers and the level of medical care available at each stage in the transfer.

Every effort must be made to minimize the clinical workload for the inflight teams. Unnecessary dressing changes, poorly sited IV cannulae and missed medications or meals are examples of procedures which will detract from the care which can be given to the more seriously injured patients.

Finally, a concise but thorough handover is required at each stage of the evacuation 'chain'. Any patient whose condition, or its treatment, may give rise to an aeromedical problem should be identified early, so that adequate supervision and appropriate treatment can be given prior to, or during, the journey.

References

A group of neurosurgeons (1984) 'Guidelines for the initial management after head injury in adults', *Brit Med J.* **288**:983-985.

American College of Surgeons Committee on Trauma (2005) *ATLS Course Manual 7th Ed.* American College of Surgeons: Chicago.

Baxt, W.G. and P. Moody (1983) 'The impact of a rotorcraft aeromedical emergency care service on trauma mortality', *J Am Med Assoc.* **249**:3047-51.

Baxt, W.G. and P. Moody (1987) 'The impact of a physician as part of the aeromedical prehospital team in patients with blunt trauma', *J Am Med Assoc.* **257**:3246-50.

Baxt, W.G., Moody O., Cleveland H.C. et al. (1985) 'Hospital-based rotorcraft aeromedical emergency care services and trauma mortality: a multicenter study', *Ann Emerg Med.* **14**:859-64.

Belinger, R.L., Califf R.M., Mark D.B. et al. (1988) 'Helicopter transport of patients during acute myocardial infarction', *Am J Cardiol.* **61**:719-22.

Gentleman, D. and B. Jennett (1981) 'Hazards of inter-hospital transfer of comatose head-injured patients', *Lancet* **2**: 853-855.

Gentleman, D. (1997) 'Head injury' in Morton, N.S., Murray, M.P. and P. G. M. Wallace, *Stabilization and Transport of the Critically Ill*, Churchill Livingstone: London.

Gentleman, D. et al. (1993) 'Guidelines for resuscitation and transfer of patients with serious head injury', *Brit Med J.* **307**: 547-552.

Glanfield, M. (2001) Predicted oxygen requirement at altitude (card calculator). *www.ccat-training.org.uk*

Jenkinson, J. L., Saunders D A. et al. (1996) *Recommendations for the Transfer of Patients with Acute Head Injuries to Neurosurgical Units*. The Neuroanaesthesia Society of Great Britain and Ireland and The Association of Anaesthetists of Great Britain and Ireland: London.

Kaplan, L., Walsh D. and R. M. Burney (1987) 'Emergency aeromedical transport of patients with acute myocardial infarction', *Ann Emerg Med.* **16**:55-7.

Lindsay, K.W. and I. Bone (2002) *Neurology and Neurosurgery Illustrated*, Churchill Livingstone: London.

Neuroanaesthesia Society of Great Britain and Ireland (1996) *Recommendations for the transfer of patients with acute head injuries to neurosurgical units*. AAGBI: London

Rodenberg, H. (1992) 'Aeromedical transport and inflight medical emergencies', in Rosen, P., Barkin R., Braen R. et al. (eds*)*, *Emergency Medicine: Concepts and Clinical Practice*, (3rd Ed.), Mosby: St. Louis.

Rogers, G., Ruplinger J., Spencer W. et al. (1988) 'Helicopter transport of patients with acute myocardial infarction', *Texas Med.* **84**:35-7.

Staniforth, P. (1994) 'Head injuries – to be transferred or not?' *Injury* **25**: 491-492.

Wright, S.W., Dronen S.C. and T.J. Combs (1989) 'Aeromedical transport of patients with post-traumatic cardiac arrest', *Ann Emerg Med.* **18**:721-6.

Chapter 12

Transport of Patients with Spinal Injuries

Spinal injuries

Normal physiology may be grossly deranged in patients who have suffered spinal cord injury. The exact nature of the dysfunction depends on the level and severity of the damage. Clearly this information will not be available to air ambulance crews in the primary retrieval role, but time spent at the roadside ensuring proper packaging and movement of the patient will be time well spent. If in doubt, all patients with the potential for spinal injury should be treated as such.

On the other hand, aeromedical escorts involved with secondary and tertiary transfers will be expected to have a thorough knowledge and understanding of the injury or condition before departure. This usually requires an in-depth, face-to-face handover between the flight medical team and a senior neurosurgeon (or orthopedic surgeon in some centers), as well as a senior member of the nursing team.

Advanced trauma life support (ATLS) skills and knowledge are essential but the knowledgeable flight team will also take special aeromedical factors into consideration. Like all critically ill patients, spinal patients are particularly susceptible to the hypoxic environment at altitude, gas expansion, G forces, vibration, and variations in temperature. In essence, they have a number of potential issues and complications which, unless managed preemptively, can lead to significant deterioration en route.

Airway and breathing

Paralysis of intercostal muscles and the diaphragm may impair ventilation and lead to hypoxia. In the acutely traumatized patient, accompanying chest injuries are likely to exacerbate the situation. A full preflight pulmonary assessment is essential to ensure that those patients requiring supplemental oxygen or ventilation are identified and appropriately managed. Close monitoring of oxygen saturation is essential, and measurement of end tidal carbon dioxide will help to identify hypoventilation (which will be seen as hypercapnia) in those at risk. Regular suction of the airway and chest physiotherapy may be essential to prevent aspiration in those who are conscious. A cuffed endotracheal or tracheostomy tube will be required in those who are not.

Neurogenic shock

When the sympathetic chain is also injured due to trauma in the high thoracic and cervical spine, vasomotor control becomes unbalanced. The combination of unopposed vagal (parasympathetic) stimulation and loss of vascular tone results in neurogenic shock. This state is pathognomically characterized by hypotension in the presence of bradycardia. Such 'relative' hypovolemia caused by vascular dilation and venous pooling will exacerbate the physiologic effect of any true fluid losses. The differential diagnosis of shock can be difficult in the victim of multiple trauma. As a general rule, hypotension is never due to an isolated head injury and, as hypovolemic and neurogenic shock will both respond to fluid therapy, the differential diagnosis becomes somewhat moot prior to the decision to undertake surgical intervention. Intravenous access is essential and should be in place before the journey is started.

The lack of opposition to vagal influence on the heart produces a bradycardia which may progress to asystole when the vagus is further stimulated by the placement of an oropharyngeal or nasopharyngeal airway, nasogastric tube, or urinary catheter. Atropine, a potent parasympatholytic agent, may be administered prior to all such maneuvers, and the electrocardiogram should be monitored throughout the transfer. Guidelines for the treatment of cardiac arrest should follow those recommended by the European Resuscitation Council (ERC), the American Heart Association (AHA), or other recognized authorities. Priority is given to the rapid restoration of circulating volume and oxygenation.

Thromboembolic complications

The spinally injured patient with circulatory impairment is also at risk of pulmonary embolism, which may result in ventilation/perfusion mismatches, hypoxia, acute right sided heart failure, and pulseless electrical activity (electromechanical dissociation). Whenever possible, patients without other acute traumatic injuries at risk of bleeding should be stabilized on anticoagulant therapy prior to departure. The risk of emboli is greatest during the second and third weeks after injury. Patients who have not been anticoagulated should receive 5000 units of heparin subcutaneous before flight. Mild massage may stimulate sluggish circulation. Elastic stockings should be worn to minimize the risk of deep venous thrombosis.

Thermoregulation

Vasomotor lability and sensory deficits also prevent adequate thermoregulation, and patients may be prone to both hypothermia and heat intolerance. Great care should be taken to ensure that the internal milieu of the aircraft cabin is comfortable for the patient, especially in smaller aircraft which often have poor cabin heating. The patient also requires thermal protection from both heat and cold during the ground phases of the transport.

Skin care

Even when the cord is not transected, significant injury may cause paralysis and impaired sensation. In combination, these may lead to pressure sores, especially in the presence of hypoperfused and hypoxic tissues. Care should be taken to ensure that the patient is lying on a soft, smooth surface, and that no hard objects or intrusions impinge upon the patient's skin. A Spenco blanket, sheepskin, or egg-crate mattress will minimize the potential for injury. Extra diligence is required to treat those areas at particular risk. Soft fluid packs over the heels and ankles or sheepskin booties are helpful, but no substitute for frequent movement of the patient to disperse the load onto other areas.

Primary transfer of spinal patients

In the early transfer of spinal patients to the primary receiving facility, those who are at risk of cervical injury should have the neck and back immobilized on a rigid spine board and supported in the neutral position. This is best done with a hard collar and sand bags, rolled towels, or foam blocks placed on either side of the head. Tape should be placed over the forehead to secure the head to a spinal board or the stretcher upon which the patient is lying. A vacuum mattress-type neck collar may also be used, but care should be taken to ensure that all air is evacuated from the collar, since residual air will expand with altitude, causing the collar to lose its rigidity. Patients whose neck injury has not been formally diagnosed should not have the cervical spine placed under traction. Exacerbation of spinal lesions by distraction injury may be catastrophic.

Secondary and tertiary transfer of spinal patients

Lifting and moving devices

When the journey is likely to exceed two hours, arrangements for the safe turning of the patient must be made. Simple arrangements may include the use of a rigid backboard, cervical collar, and head restraint. The board/patient unit is periodically turned from side to side to relieve pressure areas and help ventilation by recruiting closed alveoli. Although transfer on a spinal board is preferable for prehospital patients being moved to an initial receiving facility, this mode of carriage is uncomfortable in those with residual sensation and may cause pressure sores in patients with sensory loss. Modern spinal boards offer a degree of protection with soft padding, but the problem still occurs with long transfers. A scoop (clamshell) stretcher is useful for safely transferring patients between stretcher types and between stretchers and beds, but should not be used in place of a turning frame or vacuum mattress. Extrication devices (such as the Kendrick and Russell devices), although useful during the release of entrapped patients at complex trauma scenarios, are unsuitable for the secondary or tertiary transfer of such patients.

While most larger aircraft can accommodate a Stryker or Povey frame (Figure 12.1), bulk and weight will necessitate a dedicated lifting device to elevate the frame to the aircraft door. If a turning frame is used, it is recommended that the patient not be turned into the prone position for fear of reducing ventilation by diaphragmatic splinting. Rather, the patient should be alternately rotated 30 degrees to each side of the long axis of the body interspersed with periods lying supine. Most patients on short haul transfers can be transported satisfactorily on a vacuum mattress conformed to the patient's body contours and lined with a sheepskin blanket (Figure 12.2).

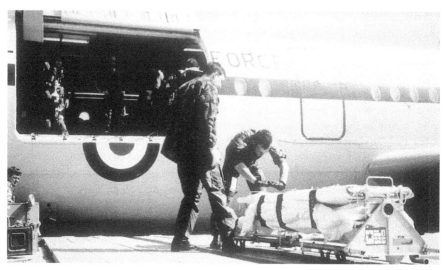

Figure 12.1   Povey turning frame being loaded onto a military VC10 strategic casevac aircraft

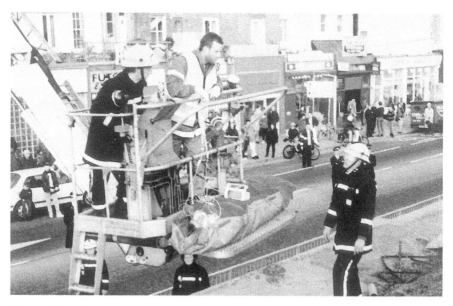

Figure 12.2   Vacuum mattress conforms to the patient's body contours

Cervical traction

A patient whose cervical spine has already been stabilized may well have traction tongs in situ. They are expensive items and the referring hospital may be reluctant to allow them to leave with the patient. This is an example of the importance of good communication between referring hospital and the flight medical crew. Do not rely on the hospital team to think of this problem in advance! Arriving at a distant hospital without the correct equipment is highly embarrassing and an expensive oversight. It is also a great inconvenience to all the health professionals in the various chains of medical care either side of the transfer, and may well result in compromise or deterioration of a patient in urgent need of evacuation.

Crutchfield's and Cone's tongs may be most suitable for use in aircraft. Like any form of skeletal traction, cervical traction must be maintained by a closed system. Free-hanging weights are susceptible to movement in all three axes of flight, and to the effects of increased gravitational forces. During acceleration or turning maneuvers exerting a force of 2G, a one kg mass will weigh two kg and a three kg mass will weigh six kg. The extra 'weight' may result in distraction injury. As a result they should not be used at any stage in the transfer of patients by air.

The chest piece of a halo vest or Minerva jacket system may impede ventilation while aloft, and should be split prior to departure in case of urgent need for removal in flight.

Miscellaneous considerations

It is essential to decompress stomach gas which may splint the diaphragm and impede adequate ventilation and to prevent possible regurgitation and aspiration. A freely draining nasogastric tube should be placed before flight, and metoclopramide (a gastric prokinetic) may be useful to help empty the stomach. Conscious patients are more prone to motion sickness and a more reliable anti-emetic may be offered, such as cyclizine. In the presence of ileus, persistent abdominal distention may be due to the expansion of intestinal gas. This may be relieved by the passage of a flatus tube.

Consideration should also be given to the placement of a urinary catheter for the duration of the transfer. If a catheter is in situ, it may be worthwhile replacing it before departure, since sensory loss will mask a full bladder caused by a blocked tube. Even if the full bladder is detected, catheter replacement in flight can be difficult. A further advantage to an indwelling catheter is the ability to measure hourly urine output as a guide to the adequacy of circulating volume.

Documentation

It is the author's practice to undertake a witnessed neurological examination during the receiving handover of a spinal patient. This is then documented fully, along with the date and time of the examination plus the names of the health professionals present. This may need to be repeated at intervals during the transfer but, at the very least, should be undertaken again at the final destination handover. Deterioration of spinal function is a devastating potential complication of transportation and one which has profound long-term implications for the patient and his family. Excellent clinical and nursing care should be documented so that the discovery of any complications can be chronologically pinpointed (see Chapter 19), thus avoiding the potential for blame shifting at subsequent investigation.

Psychological support

Finally, conscious patients with spinal injuries require reassurance, tact, and psychological support. In doing so, aeromedical personnel should freely talk to patients about why such fastidious precautions are being taken on their behalf. This will help to bond the patient and his carers, and to invoke trust. Similarly, conversations to family members about unconscious and sedated patients should seek to reassure all concerned that the appropriate standard of care is being given even though the patient is in between hospitals. It is worth remembering that most lay people will view the transport phase as a 'treatment vacuum', and may well judge the aeromedical crew against the hospital staff that they have probably come to know quite well. It would not be surprising if they view the transfer as a move from one place of safety to another, with a stressful and dangerous period of uncertainty between the two. A view sometimes shared by our terrestrial medical and nursing colleagues!

However, it is not advisable for the flight medical crew to enter into discussion about the likely outcome of the patient's injuries. All such enquiries should be politely referred to the receiving medical team stating that they are the experts in the next stage of the patient's care and, as such, will soon be in possession of more information. Failure to avoid being drawn into such a discussion may lead to your comments being quoted (or, often, misquoted) at a later stage, especially if the patient, family member, or legal representative are looking for possible blame factors for the patient's condition. As a final guard against unnecessary litigious involvement, it is worthwhile documenting all clinical discussions with the patient and any other significant persons.

References

Baxt, W.G and P.Moody (1983) 'The impact of a rotorcraft aeromedical emergency care service on trauma mortality', *J Am Med Assoc*, **249**:3047-51.

Baxt, W.G., Moody O., Cleveland H.C. et al. (1985) 'Hospital-based rotorcraft aeromedical emergency care services and trauma mortality: a multicenter study', *Ann Emerg Med*, **14**:859-64.

Rodenberg, H. (1992) 'Aeromedical Transport and Inflight Medical Emergencies', in Rosen P., Barkin R. et al. (eds), *Emergency Medicine: Concepts and Clinical Practice*, (3rd Ed.), Mosby: St. Louis.

Bridges, E.J., Schmelz J.O., and S. Mazer (2003) 'Skin interface pressure on the NATO litter', *Milit Med.* **168**(4):280-6.

Hauswald, M. and T. McNally (2001) 'Confusing extrication with immobilization: the inappropriate use of hard spine boards for interhospital transfers', *Air Med J.* **19**(4):126-7.

Hesse, R. and B. Plaisier (2003) 'Gunshot wounds of the cranium or torso: implications for spinal immobilization and airway management', *Air Med J.* **22**(6):21-3.

Chapter 13

Transport of Burns Patients

Burn injuries

Victims of burn trauma pose a challenge to the inflight medical team. Although minor burns (less than 15 per cent of body surface area) should not present physiological problems during flight, patients with burns to cosmetic areas, or when appearance or odor may cause offense to other passengers, may be refused permission to fly on commercial aircraft. Although criteria for referral to tertiary burns centers may differ, the American Burns Association recommended criteria are widely promulgated on the ubiquitous ATLS course (Table 13.1).

Patients with major burns have derangements of normal anatomy and physiology which are likely to be severe. The simplest approach to these patients is to follow the traditional ABCD approach to emergency care.

Airway

Airway obstruction due to laryngeal edema following a respiratory tract burn should be considered in all patients being transferred to a primary receiving center and those being transferred to a burns unit within the first twelve hours of injury. Facial and oropharyngeal burns, carbonaceous sputum, burnt nasal hairs, or a decreased level of consciousness are all indicative of inhalation injury and respiratory tract burn. It is essential to provide a definitive airway (endotracheal intubation, tracheostomy, or cricothyroidotomy) before complete laryngeal obstruction occurs and neck edema distorts anatomic landmarks. Nasal intubation is preferable, since the tube is better tolerated and easier to maintain in position, but naso-tracheal tubes may obstruct sinus ostia and predispose the patient to barosinusitis.

Table 13.1   The American Burns Association criteria for transfer to a specialist burns unit

- Full thickness burn >5% body surface area (BSA) in any age group
- Partial thickness and full thickness burns >10% BSA in age under 10s and over 50s
- Partial thickness and full thickness burns >20% BSA in other age groups
- Inhalation injury
- Burns of:

- face (especially eyes and ears)
- hands and feet
- genitalia and perineum
- overlying major joints
• Electrical burns and lightning injury
• Significant chemical burns
• In the presence of:
  - pre-existing illness or concurrent trauma that might affect mortality or morbidity
  - special social emotional or rehabilitative problems

Breathing

Bronchodilators may be necessary for those with troublesome airway spasm and are best given as nebulized solutions. Continuous monitoring of oxygen saturation is essential for all patients, and intubated burn victims require continuous end tidal carbon dioxide measurement to ensure correct tube placement and adequacy of ventilation. Patients should ideally be nursed in the head-up position, and chest physiotherapy, bronchial lavage, and suction may be necessary to maintain airway patency in the dry atmosphere of the aircraft cabin.

Patients with circumferential full thickness chest burns are likely to suffer respiratory impairment as swelling and scar tissue prevent excursion of the chest wall. Escharotomies may be necessary. This requires incision through the eschar until viable tissue is reached. Although often described as painless because of the loss of sensory nerve endings, there is no guarantee that the scalpel will not reach uninjured tissue. It is therefore kinder to use some analgesia for this procedure.

Patients with less severe inhalation injury may not develop significant signs for several days, but even the patient without respiratory tract burn is at risk of pulmonary dysfunction as part of an overall systemic response to major injury (acute respiratory distress syndrome, ARDS). Severe necrotizing parenchymal damage is frequently seen with large burns and appears to be related to immunosuppression. It is vital that all patients have an evaluation of pulmonary function prior to departure (including arterial blood gases if possible) so that appropriate equipment and facilities can be provided in flight. The treatment of patients with known ARDS should follow the ARDS-net protocol.

Circulation

Although hypovolemia is expected in the early hours after a significant burn injury, the fall in cardiac output may be by as much as 65 per cent. This drop is much greater than would be anticipated as a result of fluid loss alone. The balance is due to sequestration of tissue fluid. This forms edema around and beneath the burn in tissue that has been damaged but not destroyed. Fluid replacement strategy should be based on the requirements calculated by one of the many formula available for the purpose. The Parkland formula (crystalloid-based) is often used in the USA (Table 13.2), whereas the Mount Vernon (albumin-based) regime (Table 13.3) is most often used in the UK. An additional volume of fluid should be considered to compensate for enhanced fluid losses at altitude.

Table 13.2   The ATLS recommended fluid regime for burns

Fluid	Ringer lactate (Hartmann's Solution)
Formula	2-4 ml per kg body weight per 1% BSA burned in 24hr
Regime	Half in first 8 hours after injury, half in the next 16hr
Monitoring	Aim for urine output of 30-50 ml/h in adults and 1.0 ml/kg/h in children under 30kg

Table 13.3   Mount Vernon fluid resuscitation regimen

- Time starts from the time of the burn
- The first 36 hours are divided into six consecutive blocks
  - 4hr, 4hr, 4hr
  - 6hr, 6hr
  - 12hr
- Give 4.5% albumin: 0.5ml x body weight (kg) x % BSA burn
  - over each block of time
- Give blood as necessary to maintain Hb > 10.5 g/dl
- Give 1.5-2.0 ml/kg/hr 5% glucose
- Use this regimen as a guideline and adjust fluid input accordingly
- Start enteral feeding at the earliest opportunity

Fluid management requires central line placement and central venous pressure (CVP) measurement, and a urinary catheter should be inserted so that hourly urine output can also be measured. Urine output is best kept above 1 ml/kg/hour.

Deposition of hemoglobin and myoglobin from necrotic tissues may result in hemoglobinuria. Acute treatment consists mainly of adequate hydration. Forced diuresis may be required, but should be performed only under the direction of the specialist physician. Hemoglobin and hematocrit should be measured, and any necessary steps taken to optimize the hemoglobin (> 10.5 g/dl) or hematocrit (35 per cent) before embarkation.

Electrolyte abnormalities are unusual immediately after burn injury, but hyperkalemia may follow extensive tissue necrosis. Evaluation of serum electrolytes should be reviewed before leaving the referring hospital so that appropriate corrections may be performed. If intubation is required, suxamethonium must be avoided to prevent dysrhythmia-inducing levels of potassium which can cause cardiac arrest.

Electrocardiogram monitoring is therefore essential for all patients throughout the out-of-hospital phase. Abnormalities of acid/base balance will depend on metabolic rate, the adequacy of circulation and oxygenation, and the provision of suitable metabolic substrates. Attempts should be made to correct significant abnormalities before departure.

Limbs

The leathery eschar can threaten patency of blood supply to limbs or digits with circumferential burns, and limb-threatening compartment syndrome may follow rapidly. Full thickness circumferential burns, or those extending over a limb compartment, should be considered for escharotomy before departure from the referring hospital depending on the presence and risk of vascular compromise.

Skin and dressings

When the skin is breached the normal physical barrier against microbial infection is lost. Furthermore, the presence of devitalized tissues is an ideal medium for bacterial culture. The combination of both results in a much decreased resistance to infection. Although the burn is sterile soon after the injury, the gradual fall in immune responses means that infection may inevitably follow. Wounds must be redressed prior to transfer under sterile conditions, since the inside of an aircraft is a less than ideal place for the prevention of contamination. Any seepage of dressings during the journey should be covered with sterile cotton wool and bandages. Plastic hand bags or cling-film dressings should not be disturbed unless absolutely essential. If repatriation necessitates a stopover, arrangements should be made so that the patient can be admitted temporarily to the nearest hospital capable of offering facilities for sterile dressing changes under anesthesia or with suitable analgesia.

Hypercatabolic state and pain

Following extensive burn injuries, metabolic rate and oxygen demand is greater than normal. This results from increased tissue catabolism and to an elevation of catecholamine production. Minimizing stress of any sort will prevent even higher levels of circulating catecholamines. Pain, discomfort, emotional distress, fear, excess movement and vibration, hypoxia, and extremes of temperature should be avoided. Pain control utilizing potent agents is a crucial aspect of burn management. If a sedative is deemed necessary, chlorpromazine is a useful choice. In addition to being a major tranquilizer, it potentiates the analgesic actions of narcotic agents and has antiemetic effects.

Healing itself requires a high metabolic turnover, and unless nutritional requirements are met, catabolism of body stores (predominantly muscle) will occur. This will result in negative nitrogen balance, loss of muscle mass, and impaired wound healing. Calorific and protein requirements for each patient must be calculated and supplied in increased amounts for the duration of the journey.

Thermoregulation

Temperature regulation is also likely to be disturbed. Loss of skin and subcutaneous tissue results in a deficit in body insulation. Loss of body heat is made worse by the evaporation of fluids from the surface of the burn wound. Evaporation will be exacerbated by the dry atmosphere of the pressurized aircraft cabin. Covering the wound at all times to prevent excess fluid loss is key. The use of warming or reflective ('space') blankets may prove useful to maintaining an adequate thermal environment.

References

ARDS Network (2000) 'Ventilation with lower tidal volumes compared with traditional tidal volumes for acute lung injury and acute respiratory distress syndrome', *N Engl J Med.* **22**;1568-78.

Baack, B.R., Smoot, E.C., Kucan, J.O. et al. (1991) 'Helicopter Transport of the Patient with Acute Burns', *J Burn Care & Rehabilitation*, **12**:229-33.

Clarke, J.A. (1982) *A Colour Atlas of Burn Injuries*, Chapman & Hall: London.

Judkins, K.C. (1988) 'Aeromedical Transfer of Burned Patients: A Review with Special Reference to European Civilian Practice', *Burns, including Thermal Injury*, **14**(3):171-179.

Martin, T.E. (1990) 'The Ramstein airshow disaster', *J R Army Med Corps*, **1**(36):19-26.

Pirson, J. and E. Degrave (2003) 'Aeromedical transfer to Belgium of severely burned patients during the initial days following the Volendam fire', *Mil Med.* **168**(5):360-3.

Saffle, J.R., Edelman, L. and S.E. Morris (2004) 'Regional air transport of burn patients: a case for telemedicine?', *J Trauma-Injury Infection & Critical Care* **57**(1):57-64.

Santos, F.X., Sanchez-Gabriel, J., Mayoral, E. and C. Hamann (1995) 'Air evacuation of critically burned patients', *Mil Med.* **160**(11):593-6.

Settle, J.A.D. (1986) *Burns – the first five days*, Smith & Nephew: Romford.

Chapter 14

Transport of the Obstetric Patient

Introduction

In the United States, many hospital-based transport services were first implemented to bring newborn infants to tertiary care. Problems with early transport incubators, as well as increasing recognition that the mother was the ideal incubator, encouraged the development of transport programs to bring the gravid woman to specialized obstetric and neonatal facilities prior to delivery. It was the availability of rapid and safe aeromedical transportation, surmounting the problems of time and distance, which promoted the development of regional perinatal centers to provide care to those mothers and neonates at increased risk of morbidity and mortality. Transport of the high risk gravid patient, with delivery of the newborn at a tertiary care facility, has probably resulted in increased maternal and fetal survival, decreased short and long-term morbidity, and decreased hospitalization costs for infants transported in utero.

The goal of perinatal care systems is the safe and timely transport of the mother, and not neonatal transport. This may necessitate early transport of patients in preterm labor (PTL) or with premature rupture of membranes (PROM) in order to avoid panic transfers when cervical dilation is advanced, and the emergency transport of unstable neonates.

Maternal anatomy and physiology

Pregnancy alters normal female anatomy and physiology, and these changes will affect the care provided during aeromedical transportation. Anatomically, the enlarging uterus becomes vulnerable to traumatic injury. Engorged with blood and lacking vascular tone, it may represent a major source of hemorrhage. More critically, the enlarging uterus can affect cardiovascular and respiratory dynamics. In the supine gravid female, the uterus falls backwards onto the inferior vena cava, causing a partial obstruction and decreasing venous return to the heart. This, in turn, leads to decreased cardiac output and lowers both the systolic and diastolic blood pressure. A slight reflex tachycardia may be seen as the cardiovascular system compensates for this change. The partial obstruction of the inferior vena cava also results in vascular congestion within the lower extremities, increasing the risk of stagnant flow and thrombophlebitis. This is a key factor in aeromedical patients who will be immobile for long periods of time ('economy class syndrome'). The rising uterus also reduces diaphragmatic motion and diminishes tidal volumes. An increase in maternal respiratory rate is a frequent compensation. The uterus also places pressure inferiorly upon the bladder, resulting in increased frequency of micturition. The continuous need to urinate may pose problems for team members escorting immobile patients, especially in small dedicated air ambulances without lavatory facilities.

Physiologically, other major alterations include increases in maternal intravascular volume and enhanced renal excretion of drugs. As a result of these changes, signs and symptoms of shock will not be apparent until blood loss reaches 2000-2500 ml, and dosages of medications excreted by the kidneys may need to be increased.

Fetal heart tones and cardiotocography provide unique measures of maternal and fetal wellbeing. While the latter technique requires special equipment and skilled interpretation, the presence and rate of fetal heart sounds can, and should, be monitored in all gravid patients. The fetal heart may first be heard with Doppler sound amplification devices at 10-12 weeks of gestation, and with the fetoscope or ordinary stethoscope at 20 weeks. However, the latter are useless in the noisy aircraft cabin environment, and a Doppler probe is essential during the transfer.

Flight team composition

Maternal transfers should be flown under the medical direction of an obstetrician or other doctor who has expertise in the management of high risk pregnancy and also of aviation physiology. The decision to perform the actual transfer should be made by the entire transport team, based on their collective experience and training. Consultation with referring and accepting obstetricians is crucial.

Obstetric flight nurses and midwives have extensive experience in caring for high risk patients in tertiary obstetric referral centers. Their specialist clinical judgment allows them to undertake more demanding maternal transports, such as patients with advanced cervical dilation, heavy vaginal bleeding, or eclampsia. Cross-trained general adult or pediatric flight crew can safely perform many transfers, but time, distance, and knowledge may limit the types of transports these crew members may accept. If there is the possibility of precipitous delivery en route, a neonatal flight nurse or pediatrician should accompany the team. Obstetricians are not usually required in the actual flight crew, especially when experienced maternal transport personnel operate under strong on and off-line medical control.

The obstetric trained flight physician or nurse must have an excellent working knowledge of maternal physiology and the processes of both normal and accelerated labor. Experience with tocolytic drugs is essential, and fetal assessment skill using cardiotocographic monitors and Doppler instruments is also required. In addition, critical care skills are crucial, as bleeding problems and hypertensive crises may comprise up to a quarter of all maternal transfers.

Transport issues

Maternal transport may seem to be unduly complicated by the physiological alterations of pregnancy and the need to care for two patients rather than one. However, awareness of the principles of emergency care (the ABCs of resuscitation), coupled with knowledge of the anatomical and physiological changes in pregnancy, and the effects of flight on the materno-fetal unit, should enable aeromedical escorts to anticipate and avoid or manage any inflight problems that may occur.

Air transport of the gravid female is usually safe for both mother and fetus. At a cabin altitude of up to 7500 ft (2315 m), maternal inspired oxygen concentration is adequate to meet the metabolic demands of both mother and fetus. Any fetus at risk should enjoy maternal hyperoxemia in flight. In a review of over 350 maternal helicopter transports, no deliveries occurred in flight, although nine flights were aborted due to the abrupt acceleration of labor. Nearly 90 additional patients were transported by fixed wing aircraft. Only one delivered en route, and she had exhibited no signs of labor prior to flight. Premature labor and third trimester vaginal bleeding were the major reasons for transfer in both groups.

Another retrospective review of 80 long distance fixed wing obstetric air transports for the two years up to July 2002 confirms the expected finding that aeromedical transfer is safe. The most significant inflight complication was nausea and vomiting, present in 80 per cent of cases. On a more serious note, increased contractions occurred in 8.8 per cent, but there was no control group to ascertain if this is an unexpectedly high number. Since an increase in frequency and strength of contractions is a normal consequence of labor, this 'complication' may simply reflect a normal physiological event. Of the other reported complications, hypertension occurred in 1.3 per cent of cases, hypotension in 1.3 per cent, and decreased maternal respiratory drive in 1.3 per cent.

Specific disorders

Vaginal bleeding

Vaginal bleeding in the gravid female can be due to a number of causes, including intrauterine infection, spontaneous abortion, or hormonal etiologies. These causes of bleeding tend to predominate in early pregnancy. The vast majority of patients transported for vaginal bleeding, however, will be in their third trimester. Life threatening causes of vaginal bleeding in this group of patients includes placenta previa, abruption, and postpartum hemorrhage. In all cases, maintenance of adequate circulating volume with infusions of crystalloid, colloid, and/or blood is the key to management. There is also a growing evidence base for the use of Factor VII.

Patients suffering from postpartum hemorrhage may respond to oxytocin infusion, intended to contract the atonic uterus and decrease flow from any retained placental fragments. Uterine massage and nipple stimulation (manually or while breast feeding) may further stimulate uterine contraction.

Patients with known bleeding disorders may benefit from the administration of fresh frozen plasma, platelets, or specific coagulation factors as required.

Patients with placenta previa may have placental tissue overlying the cervical os which can be damaged during vaginal examination and cervical checks. Vaginal examination is absolutely contraindicated in these individuals.

Premature rupture of membranes

Premature rupture of membranes is more attention-getting than injurious. However, it may signal the need for the medical team to prepare to manage preterm labor or anticipate precipitous delivery. In addition, the breach in fetal intrauterine isolation may predispose the mother and fetus to intrauterine infection and endometritis. Avoidance of excessive emotion and careful attention to perineal sterility and hygiene is crucial. The prophylactic or therapeutic administration of a penicillin or cephalosporin agent active against skin, vaginal, and anaerobic flora may be indicated.

Preterm labor

Preterm labor may occur at any time during the maternal transport, and is often the primary reason for the flight. In general, a fetus is at maximum risk if delivered outside the hospital at less than 34 weeks of gestational age. Preterm labor may be managed with intravenous administration of magnesium sulfate in accordance with the instructions of the obstetrician. Some authorities advise the prophylactic administration of magnesium sulfate in any gravid patient being transported by air.

Precipitous delivery

Delivery of the fetus cannot always be predicted. The best management scheme for the flight crew is preparation. Advance plans should be made with regard to patient positioning, methods of management of fetal presentations, and familiarity with, and accessibility to, neonatal resuscitation equipment.

Pre-eclampsia and eclampsia

Pre-eclampsia (more formally known as pregnancy induced hypertension, or PIH) is a pathological state of pregnancy characterized predominantly by hypertension and proteinuria. Left untreated, PIH can lead to eclampsia, which is the presence of the above findings coupled with generalized tonic-clonic seizure activity.

Seizure prophylaxis in these patients centers on the administration of magnesium sulfate; the acute treatment of seizures should follow traditional patterns of the use of benzodiazepines, phenytoin, and barbiturates. The use of these drugs should be tempered with the knowledge that the use of phenytoin in early pregnancy is associated with fetal malformations, and the use of benzodiazepines and barbiturates, with maternal and fetal respiratory depressions.

The hypertension itself can be acutely treated with oral or intravenous hydralazine. The use of nitrates should be avoided due to the risk of induced methemoglobinemia and maternal-fetal hypoxia. Eclampsia may be present up to several weeks post partum, and should be considered in the differential diagnosis of new onset seizures in all women.

Amniotic fluid emboli

Emboli from within the amniotic sac may migrate throughout the bloodstream, resulting in cerebrovascular accident or pulmonary embolism. Amniotic fluid emboli are also a major cause of perinatal disseminated intravascular coagulation. Care is supportive, with special attention paid to respiratory and neurologic status, but the flight medical crew must be aware that the 'normal' hypoxia experienced in the hypobaric cabin atmosphere will be exacerbated by further, detrimental, disruption to oxygen carriage.

References

Elliot, J.P., O'Keeffe, D.F. and R.K. Freeman (1982) 'Helicopter transportation of patients with obstetric emergencies in an urban area', *Am J Obst & Gyne*, **143**:157-62.

Elliott, J.P., Foley, M.R., Young, L., Balazs, K.T. and L. Meiner (1996) 'Air transport of obstetric critical care patients to tertiary centers', *J Reprod Med.* **41**(3):171-4.

Elliott, J.P., Sipp, T.L. and K.T. Balazs (1992) 'Maternal transport of patients with advanced cervical dilatation – to fly or not to fly?', *Obstetrics & Gynecology*, **79**:380-2.

Jones, A.E., Summers, R.L., Deschamp, C. and R. L. Galli (2001) 'A national survey of the air medical transport of high-risk obstetric patients', *Air Med J.* **20**(2):17-20.

Low, R.B., Martin, D. and C. Brown (1988) 'Emergency air transport of pregnant patients: the national experience', *J Emerg Med.* **6**(1):41-8.

O'Brien, D.J., Hooker, E.A., Hignite, J. and E. Maughan (2004) 'Long-distance fixed-wing transport of obstetrical patients', *South Med J.* **97**(9):816-8.

Parer, J.T. (1982) 'Effects of hypoxia on the mother and fetus with emphasis on maternal air transport', *Am J Obstet Gyne.* **15**;142(8):957-61.

Van Hook, J.W., Leicht, T.G., Van Hook, C.L., Dick, P.L., Hankins, G.D. and C. J. Harvey (1998) 'Aeromedical transfer of preterm labor patients', *Tex Med.* **94**(11):88-90.

Chapter 15

Transport of Neonatal and Pediatric Patients

The child as a special patient

A child's response to illness and injury is often different to that of an adult, and appropriate management requires specialist pediatric knowledge and a new set of skills. This is well known to pediatric intensive care units, many of whom have their own retrieval transport teams.

The range of children's weights and sizes, and their physical differences, may have a significant influence on transfer requirements both in logistical considerations and in terms of preparation of equipment and medications. Neonates (babies within the first month of life) are commonly transported to and from specialist units. Whilst sharing some of the problems of older children, they have their own special pathologies and needs, even further removed from the problems of adults. Many of these babies are critically ill and it is usual for a suitably trained neonatal pediatrician and neonatal nurse to accompany them. In most centers the transportation of the newborn is considered a specialty in its own right.

Prehospital versus interhospital transportation

The same principles and logistics apply for children as for adults, but there are a number of unique problems in prehospital pediatric management:

- There are fewer professionals skilled in prehospital pediatric medical management.
- Comprehensive pediatric equipment may not be readily available.
- Children can deteriorate faster than adults, for example, respiratory obstruction may occur more rapidly because of the small diameter of the airways.

A 'scoop and run' policy may therefore be appropriate at an earlier stage in the sick child, although adequate oxygenation before leaving the scene is still essential. If this is not possible, immediate and rapid transportation to definitive care is mandatory.

Secondary and tertiary transportation

During secondary and tertiary (interhospital) transfer, as with adults, the child's condition should be optimized before moving, although undue delay should be avoided once the decision has been made. The concept of 'an intensive care bed on the move' indicates the quality of care expected from a good pediatric intensive care transport system. With all transfers, the details of the patient must be discussed between the referring and receiving medical teams at senior level. Full details of the history, current therapy and planned management should be discussed before departure.

Efficacy and safety of pediatric transport

Published data describing the demographics of pediatric and neonatal aeromedical transport is scarce. The experience of one American flight program notes that, of over 700 pediatric patients transported by either fixed or rotor wing aircraft, 32 per cent suffered from neurologic disease, 19 per cent were victims of trauma, and 19 per cent were ill from non-neurologic infectious disease. Only one per cent of all patients required major resuscitative measures en route. A review of over 600 patients transported by another pediatric service revealed that 25 per cent were victims of trauma, 24 per cent of neurologic disease, and 20 per cent suffered respiratory failure or infection.

As rare as these demographic studies are, clear evidence of the efficacy of air versus ground transport of pediatric patients is virtually non-existent. The benefits of rapid transport of critically ill or injured pediatric patients by skilled crews to specialist facilities seems intuitively logical but, given the current medicolegal climate and the impossibility of performing a truly controlled study on the out-of-hospital environment, little progress in the literature may be expected in the very near future.

Understanding the differences

A knowledge of the major differences in anatomy and physiology is essential for the medical flight team, and the most critical of these can best be summarized according to the familiar principles of advanced life support, that is, in terms of the airway, respiration and circulation.

Airway

Under six months of age, the tongue and tonsils are relatively large in comparison with the oropharynx. This impairs visualization of the larynx during endotracheal intubation, and also ensures that infants are obligate nose breathers. Any compromise or obstruction to the nasal passages may cause respiratory distress. In addition, since the trachea is soft and the cartilaginous rings not yet fully formed, extension of the neck can cause kinking of the tubular structure with subsequent obstruction. Often all that is needed is a slight adjustment to the position of the head on the neck. The correct position for maintaining the airway in a child is to have a small support under the child's shoulders (*sniffing the morning air* position), since the relatively large occiput tends to cause flexion of the neck.

The larynx is slightly more cephalad in a child than in an adult, also causing more difficulty in viewing the cords during intubation. If intubation is required, it should be remembered that the trachea grows to only 7 cm by 18 months of age and it is easy to intubate the right main bronchus, and that tubes correctly positioned at the carina are easily displaced by movement of the patient. The narrowest point of the airway in children under 8 years of age is at the cricoid cartilage below the cords (as opposed to the cords themselves in older patients), obviating the need for a cuffed tube. A useful rule of thumb for choosing the correct endotracheal tube size in young children (internal diameter in mm) is to divide the age by 4, then add 4.

Respiration

The lower airways are small, and even a minimal decrease in the already small bronchiolar diameters can result in large reductions in cross-sectional area with subsequent respiratory impairment. Furthermore, tidal volume is much more dependent on the proper functioning of the diaphragm in children than in adults, and gastric or abdominal distention can have a marked effect on chest expansion. In addition to the types of respiratory considerations already discussed, some children or infants may have problems of lung compliance (with poor gaseous transfer and also increased work of breathing) and mismatching of ventilation and pulmonary perfusion caused by shunting of blood between the right and left sides of the heart. Children also have a relatively high basal metabolic rate (almost double that of an adult), and the onset of respiratory impairment due to any cause rapidly results in hypoxemia. A full assessment of cardiopulmonary function is therefore essential for all severely ill and injured children prior to transportation. Oxyhemoglobin saturation, electrocardiogram monitoring and capnography may be necessary in flight.

There are many aeromedical implications of these differences in airway and pulmonary anatomy. As infants have limited mobility and even more limited communication, vigilance must be paid to patient position to avoid respiratory impairment. The presence of gas in the stomach or intestinal tract will expand with altitude and may restrict diaphragmatic motion and further compromise respiratory status. Placement of an orogastric or nasogastric tube may be required. Children with congenital pulmonary anomalies may be at risk of spontaneous pneumothorax, and those with cyanotic heart disease may exhibit precipitous falls in oxyhemoglobin saturation during transport at altitude. Low humidity in aircraft cabins may increase airway responsiveness and promote bronchospasm, while the increased thickness of pulmonary secretions may cause mucous plugging, atelectasis, and hypoxia because of mismatches in pulmonary ventilation and perfusion. The latter problem is of special concern in patients with cystic fibrosis and congenital bronchiectasis. Hypoxia at altitude will also worsen pulmonary hypertension, which will cause particular difficulties in patients with right sided cardiac failure from septal or valvular abnormalities. As infants have an increased body surface area to body mass ratio and have less developed thermoregulatory mechanisms, temperature control may also be a problem.

If a respiratory emergency does occur, it may not be easy to make a definite diagnosis. If the airway is patent, warm humidified oxygen should be administered in the highest possible concentration. Caution should be used in giving high concentrations of oxygen to children with chronic respiratory insufficiency (chronic hypercapnia), such as those with advanced cystic fibrosis and those with bronchopulmonary dysplasia. Even very ill children may not tolerate an oxygen mask. If all else fails, nasal cannulae may provide up to 52 per cent FiO_2. However, to provide this concentration requires a flow rate of eight liters per minute, which is highly irritating to the nasal and pharyngeal mucosa.

If, despite a patent airway and the administration of humidified oxygen, ventilation is clearly inadequate, the child's breathing should be assisted by the use of a bag-valve-mask (BVM) system or, in an emergency, by mouth-to-mouth, mouth-to-nose, or mouth-to-pocket mask ventilation. In the absence of specific pediatric equipment, it is possible to use an adult BVM device as long as gentle positive pressure ventilations are used to assist the child's own efforts. Uncoordinated ventilations in a breathing child will cause coughing, retching and gastric distention. A useful rule of thumb in estimating the effective depth of ventilation is to ensure the child's chest rises enough to resemble the normal excursion of a deep breath for the child's size. Pediatric rebreathing bags have pop-off valves indicating when positive airway pressure has exceeded critical limits.

The child who remains apneic will inevitably require mechanical ventilation. Tidal volumes can be estimated at 10-15 ml/kg; minute volumes (tidal volume x respiratory rate) should approximate 100 ml per kg/min. The maximum normal respiratory rate in infants is 40/min. It is 30/min in toddlers and 20/min in older children. Mechanical ventilation should only be undertaken by those experienced in pediatric endotracheal tube placement and ventilatory management.

Circulation

The recognition of shock can be extremely difficult in children, not only because of the wide variation in normal ranges of physiological parameters (Table 15.1) and the problems of palpation of pulses and detection of blood pressure, but also because of relatively large physiological reserve allowing prolonged compensation and maintenance of apparently normal parameters until significant hypovolemia has occurred. Tachycardia is an early sign, but it can also be caused by fear, pain and other stressors. Repeated evaluation is essential and, for those especially at risk, hourly urinary output should be measured. The inflight team should be aware of the rapidity by which a seemingly well child can deteriorate, and it would be wise to secure intravenous access in those at risk before leaving the referring hospital or scene of injury (Figure 15.1). In flight, the best means of emergency access is via an interosseous needle, placed in either the distal femur or proximal tibia, avoiding the growth plates and not distal to a fracture. Crystalloids, colloids and drugs can be infused by this route, although they are best administered using a syringe under pressure.

About a quarter of the child's circulating volume can be lost before obvious clinical shock is seen. As soon as shock is diagnosed, the child should be given a bolus of warmed crystalloid solution. The bolus should be a quarter of the normal circulating volume[1] stat, that is, 20 ml/kg. Failure to improve is an ominous sign which necessitates a further bolus of crystalloid or, if available, 10 ml/kg of type specific blood. Surgical opinion is urgent.

Table 15.1   The wide variation in normal ranges of physiological parameters in children

	Heart rate (per min)	Mean blood pressure (mm Hg)	Respiratory rate (per min)
Under 18 months	160	80	40
18 months to adolescence	120	90	30
Adolescence	100	100	20

Source: American College of Surgeons (2005), *Advanced Trauma Life Support Manual* (7th Ed.): ACS, Chicago.

Drugs and equipment

The wide range of ages and sizes of children can cause confusion in deciding upon appropriate drug doses and in selecting equipment for use. Aircraft participating in primary responses must stock a complete range of pediatric equipment. For those flight services which can plan in advance to transport a single known patient, a much narrower range of equipment need be carried. Help can be provided by the use of a Pediatric Vade Mecum, Broselow Pediatric Emergency Tape© (Vital Signs Inc) and the British Medical Journal Paediatric Resuscitation Chart (Figure 15.2). 'Drug doses', published by the Intensive Care Unit of the Royal Children's Hospital in Victoria, Australia, is another excellent source of information.

The Broselow Pediatric Emergency Tape utilizes the association between a child's age, height, and weight to identify the correct drug dosages and equipment sizes for pediatric emergency procedures. Each age/size group is color coded. For

---

1   A child's normal circulating volume is about 80 ml per kg body weight.

simplicity, many who frequently manage pediatric emergencies keep equipment and drugs of the correct size and dose in appropriately colored bags or boxes which correlate to the Broselow Tape.

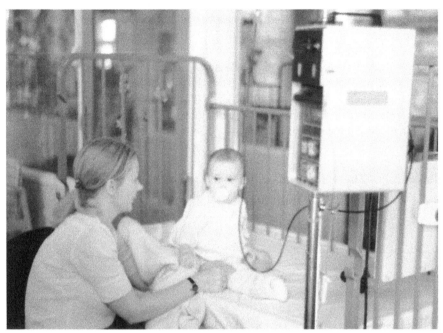

Figure 15.1 Intravenous access is often necessary before leaving the referring hospital or scene of injury

Gaseous expansion

Gaseous expansion at altitude can cause problems other than the effects on diaphragmatic contractility. Although both potential and actual gas filled cavities are smaller in children, the effects of expansion are relatively greater. Otic barotrauma is frequently seen in children under six because catarrhal syndrome (the common cold) obstructs small eustachian tubes when only mildly inflamed. Interestingly, however, children with serous otitis do not experience undue difficulties during flight. This is probably because the obstructed middle ear is filled with non-compressible fluid rather than air.

Any gas producing illness (such as necrotizing enterocolitis) or endoscopic procedure where gas is infiltrated may herald gastrointestinal problems when cabin pressure is low. Children are naturally prone to motion sickness, and air in the stomach and intestinal tract may worsen nausea with expansion at altitude. Fizzy drinks immediately before or during flight should be avoided.

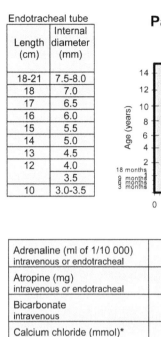

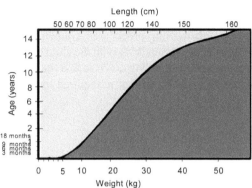

Endotracheal tube	
Length (cm)	Internal diameter (mm)
18-21	7.5-8.0
18	7.0
17	6.5
16	6.0
15	5.5
14	5.0
13	4.5
12	4.0
	3.5
10	3.0-3.5

Adrenaline (ml of 1/10 000) intravenous or endotracheal	0.5	1	2	3	4	5
Atropine (mg) intravenous or endotracheal	0.1	0.2	0.4	0.6	0.6	0.6
Bicarbonate intravenous	5	10	20	30	40	50
Calcium chloride (mmol)* intravenous	1	2	4	6	8	10
Diazepam intravenous per rectum	1.25 2.5	2.5 5	5 10	7.5 -	10 -	10 -
Glucose (ml of 50%) intravenous	10	20	40	60	80	100
Lignocaine (mg) intravenous or endotracheal	5	10	20	30	40	50
Salbutamol (μg) intravenous	25	50	100	150	200	250
Initial DC defibrillation (J)	10	20	40	60	80	100
Initial fluid infusion in hypovlaemic shock (ml)	50	100	200	300	400	500

* One millilitre calcium chloride 1 mmol/ml ≡ 1.5 ml calcium chloride 10% ≡ 4.5 ml calcium gluconate 10%

Figure 15.2   BMJ Paediatric Resuscitation Chart
Source: Oakley P.A. (1988) *Br Med J 297*, 1 October.

Child psychology

Although a child is easier to physically load and manipulate aboard aircraft and does not take up as much space as an adult, he may be fractious or excitable and may need special arrangements such as feeding, diapering, and entertainment.

Children are naturally more emotionally labile and dependent than adults. Fear and anxiety will elevate heart rate, blood pressure, and intracranial pressure, and crying will increase oxygen demand and may exacerbate hypoxia. A child may feel vulnerable in the strange environment of the airport and aircraft, especially if ill or injured and in the company of strangers. Often a familiar toy or blanket can ease anxiety, but it is unwise to bribe children with snacks or toys before subjecting them to painful or embarrassing procedures. Gaining trust with the help of cooperative parents is key. Time spent talking with the child to encourage acceptance, and simple considerations such as bending down so that the patient is not intimidated by figures towering above, may be all that is required to ensure cooperation throughout the journey.

Parents

It is important not only to obtain parental consent for all aspects of treatment and transfer, but also to use parents as a trusted buffer between medical team and patient whenever possible. It is therefore extremely helpful if a parent or, occasionally, another trusted adult, accompanies the transfer team, and it is generally preferable to keep parent and child in contact for as much of the flight as possible. Parents should be regarded as an integral third party of the child/doctor relationship and must be kept constantly informed of all interactions and developments en route. However, the parent will also be anxious and concerned, so the inflight team must keep the parent informed of all procedures necessary for the safe conduct of the transfer and must avoid being drawn into discussions on the recent past management of the child or the potential prognosis. Parents watch carefully and pay great attention to what is said about their child.

Thus, there is great emotional benefit if a parent can accompany a conscious child. However, the desire to carry family members on the flight should always be secondary to the actual needs of the patient and the flight crew and space constraints may make this impractical, particularly if an emergency occurs en route. If parents cannot accompany the child, it is encumbent on the medical team to ensure:

- They have a means of traveling to the receiving unit.
- They have clear directions to the receiving unit and the ward.
- They are instructed that, under no circumstances, should they attempt to follow an ambulance that is using blue lights and sirens.
- If they cannot go to the receiving unit themselves, they understand clearly where the child is to be admitted. They should have the telephone number of the new hospital and ward.

Neonatal transport

Many of the principles of pediatric transfers are applicable to neonates but there are some important differences. It is usual for a pediatrician or neonatologist trained in neonatal transport to transfer the baby along with a neonatal intensive care nurse.

These babies most commonly require transfer to a specialist unit for the reasons outlined in Table 15.2.

Table 15.2   Indications for neonatal transfer

- Complications of prematurity
- Complications of delivery, for example, birth asphyxia and meconium aspiration
- For urgent surgery, for example,
  - Diaphragmatic hernias
  - Tracheo-esophageal fistula
  - Gastroschisis
  - Necrotising enterocolitis
- Congenital heart disease
  - May involve the use of alprostadil to keep the ductus arteriosus open
  - Alprostadil can cause apnoea and these babies must be sedated, intubated and ventilated prior to transfer
  - Oxygen concentrations should be tailored to the individual needs of the patient because of the effect oxygen has on the adult/foetal circulation balance
- Other medical congenital or acquired problems, for example,
  - Hydrops foetalis
  - Renal failure

In all cases, the management of the baby before and during transfer must be discussed in detail with the receiving unit (preferably consultant to consultant). Treatment which needs to be initiated prior to and during transport may be complex and specific to the disorder.

Neonatal physiology

An understanding of neonatal physiology is key to understanding many of the unique problems affecting this subset of patients, as well as their aeromedical implications.

Before birth, oxygenated blood flows to the fetus from the placenta through the umbilical vein. This vein empties into the inferior vena cava, which in turn channels this blood into the right atrium and ventricle. In the fetus, pulmonary vascular resistance is high, and this high pressure is transmitted back to the right side of the heart. While some blood is pumped into the pulmonary system, most flows through the foramen ovale, a one way flap valve in the atrial septum, into the left atrium. There it is mixed with blood coming form the lungs and pumped to the body by the left ventricle through the aorta.

The aorta is joined to the left pulmonary artery just distal to the heart. This juncture is known as the ductus arteriosus, and allows for the passage of oxygenated blood into the pulmonary parenchyma in order to nourish the developing lungs. Once used by peripheral body tissues, blood collects in the umbilical arteries and is carried away from the body to the placenta for gaseous and metabolic exchange.

Fetal haemoglobin (HbF) has a greater affinity for oxygen than its adult counterpart, hence, a lower PO_2 is required to bind a given amount of oxygen, i.e. oxygen is bound more avidly, but results in less liberation in the tissues. The lower PO_2 in an aircraft cabin therefore facilitates oxygen delivery to the baby, but hinders its release into the baby's tissues. In other words, HbF and altitude both shift the oxygen dissociation curve to the left (see Chapter 4). The practical implications are not well established, but common sense dictates that a pressurized cabin is essential and the lowest possible cabin altitude is ideal.

At birth, a major physiological change occurs as a result of the sudden increase in arterial PO_2 associated with pulmonary ventilation. Increased levels of oxygen in the blood cause vasodilatation of the pulmonary vascular bed, lowering pulmonary vascular pressure while relatively elevating systemic vascular resistance. As a result, the pressure balance in the heart shifts, and the left side of the heart now becomes the high pressure channel. Higher pressures on the left side of the heart effectively close the flap valve of the foramen ovale. The increased arterial PO_2 causes narrowing and closure of the ductus arteriosus over the following few days, effectively isolating the pulmonary and systemic circulations and producing normal adult pattern blood oxygenation and flow patterns. Exposure of the newborn to altitude and the rigors of flight may result in hypoxia that may assist in maintaining the patency of the ductus arteriosus, but also promote increased pulmonary vascular resistance and pulmonary hypertension in an attempt to recreate fetal circulatory patterns.

Much of the initial therapy of neonatal disorders, especially those involving cardiac anomalies, is dedicated to maintaining the abnormal fetal physiology until definitive care can be provided. In patients with obstruction or impedance to pulmonary flow resulting in congenital cyanotic heart disease, preservation of the patency of the ductus arteriosus may be the only noninvasive method by which blood can traverse the gap between the systemic and pulmonary circulations.

Specific neonatal disorders

Hypothermia

A key aspect of neonatal care is the maintenance of an optimal thermal environment. Cold or heat stress consumes calories and oxygen at rates which readily exceed the capabilities of the compromised newborn. Frequent monitoring of the temperature of the neonate and of his or her environment is crucial. A normal axillary temperature does not assure that the thermal environment is appropriate. Adult patients can maintain their body temperature within a normal range for some period of time in adversely high or low environmental temperatures. Unlike the adult, however, the neonate is severely limited in his capability to compensate.

Heat loss occurs through evaporation, radiation, convection, and conduction. Within the confines of the warm, closed transport incubator, heat loss by convection and conduction are minimal. Because of the neonate's large body surface area and rapid respiratory rate, significant heat loss occurs by radiation and evaporation. In addition, evaporative heat losses from the administration of dry medical gases contribute to the thermal imbalance. Each time the incubator is opened, time is required to re-establish a stable environment.

Respiratory distress

Numerous conditions may cause increased work of breathing and elevated oxygen requirements. The lungs of premature infants may be deficient of surfactant, resulting in the diffuse atelectasis of hyaline membrane disease. The use of prenatal betamethasone and/or postnatal installation of surfactant has diminished the severity of this disorder. In full-term and post-term infants, the aspiration of meconium prior to or at birth can result in focal areas of atelectasis, air trapping, and persistent pulmonary hypertension of the newborn with right to left shunting through the foramen ovale or ductus arteriosus.

It is imperative that the transport team understand the complications of neonatal hypoxia and how respiratory status is affected by altitude. Compromised neonates are highly susceptible to the effects of Boyle's and Dalton's Laws. The transport team must be prepared to identify and manage the occurrence of hypoxemia or pneumothorax.

Diaphragmatic hernia

This congenital defect occurs in 1 in 2200 live births. The presence of abdominal organs in the thorax may severely affect lung growth and development. A high incidence of pulmonary hypoplasia combined with persistent pulmonary hypertension of the newborn may result in pneumothoraces, especially following resuscitative efforts. It is essential that the gastrointestinal tract remain decompressed and the pneumothorax be evacuated. The impact of expanding gases trapped in the thorax or intestine can be lessened by maintenance of patency and suction on the chest and or gastric tubes. Fortunately, many neonates afflicted with diaphragmatic hernia are being identified by antenatal ultrasound. The best method of transfer is the materno-fetal unit, that is, when the baby is transferred in utero to be delivered at a tertiary center.

Intestinal obstruction

Some forms of intestinal obstruction can be diagnosed prenatally with subsequent maternal-fetal transfer; others present after birth, with marked abdominal distention. Gaseous distention may cause elevation of the diaphragm. Respiratory status may be severely compromised, as the neonate's tidal volume is primarily dictated by diaphragmatic excursion. Gastric decompression and elective intubation for transport should be considered.

Omphalocele and gastroschisis

This abdominal wall defect results in exposure of the gastrointestinal tract exterior to the patient. Significant heat and fluid can be lost from the exposed gut by evaporation. Altitude effects upon gas volumes may compromise circulation to trapped segments. Early placement of an orogastric tube to suction may minimize the accumulation of intraluminal air. These children require strict attention to both temperature control and cardiovascular support.

Cyanotic congenital heart disease

Acute non-surgical therapy for most forms of cyanotic heart disease are dependent upon maintenance of patency of the ductus arteriosus and control of pulmonary blood flow. Prostaglandin E is helpful to maintain ductal patency but has significant side effects, including hypoventilation, apnea, and hyperthermia.

Proper ventilation technique to control the arterial partial pressures of oxygen and carbon dioxide and ensure optimal acid-base balance is critical. Management of the patient during transport should be discussed in advance with the pediatric cardiovascular team to determine the optimal plan for care.

Neonatal intensive care unit (NICU) equipment

Sophisticated neonatal retrieval services generally have something much more akin to an 'intensive care unit on a trolley' providing some or all of the equipment listed in Table 15.3.

Neonatal intensive care trolleys are extremely heavy to lift and thought must be given to loading before the ambulance arrives. In an emergency a slope up to the back of the vehicle may suffice if a hydraulic system is not available but only if used with great care. A final word of warning – some aircraft doors are too narrow, or the angles inside too tight to accommodate these cumbersome incubators. It is important to ensure that any aircraft to be used to transport an incubator is suitable for the purpose.

Table 15.3   Typical neonatal transfer equipment

- Incubator with thermostatically controlled heat source (Figure 15.3)
- Ventilator (of a quality which may be found in a neonatal intensive care unit) with humidifier
- Oxygen and air compressor with oxygen blender
- Suction aspirator
- Syringe pumps as required
- Monitoring equipment:
  - ECG
  - Inspired oxygen monitor
  - Pulse oximeter
  - Transcutaneous oxygen and carbon dioxide
  - Noninvasive/invasive blood pressure monitoring
  - Peripheral/core temperature
- Comprehensive battery and mains power system.
- Drawers containing all necessary equipment for emergencies including:
  - Chest drains
  - Umbilical venous catheters
  - Endotracheal tubes
  - Resuscitation drugs

In some countries, dedicated ambulances are equipped specifically for carrying these systems and the retrieval staff. These vehicles may have additional features such as a resuscitaire for emergency procedures that may occur en route. Occasional equipment such as extra corporeal membrane oxygenation may also be available as part of an extremely specialized retrieval service. Nitric oxide therapy during transport has also been described.

Team composition and training

Pediatric and neonatal team members may include doctors, nurses, respiratory therapists (in the USA), and paramedics. A diverse pool of transport personnel allows for teams to be designed to meet specific patient needs. The impact of different team configurations on patient outcome has not been studied in the neonatal population, although one Canadian study suggests that appropriately trained and experienced paramedics can perform well as pediatric flight team members. Each program must evaluate the needs of its region and its own service capability in determining optimal crew configuration. The team composition for specific patient types must be decided before transport requests are received. Roles and responsibilities of team members should be well defined, yet remain flexible enough to meet unexpected patient care contingencies.

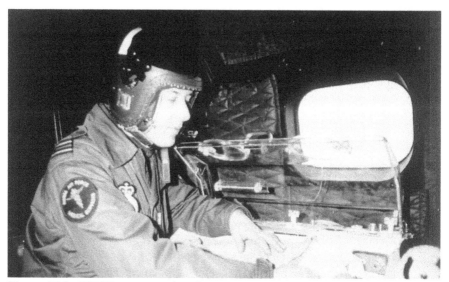

Figure 15.3   NICU transport incubator

All transport team personnel should have a sound knowledge of pediatric and neonatal resuscitation, stabilization for transport, and frequently encountered diseases. Well organized content can be found in education programs offered by the American Heart Association, the American Academy of Pediatrics, and the American College of Emergency Physicians. Advanced skill training should be considered based upon team composition and program's transport mission.

References

Advanced Life Support Group (1999) *Prehospital paediatric life support*, BMJ Publishing Group: London.

Atkins, D.L. and R.E. Kerber (1994) 'Paediatric defibrillation: current flow is improved by using 'adult' electrode paddles', *Pediatrics*, 94(1); 90-3.

Barry, I.W. and C. Ralston (1994) 'Adverse events occurring during interhospital transfer of the critically ill', *Arch Dis Child*, **71**: 8-11.

Bergman, K.A., Geven, W.B. and A. Molendijk (2002) 'Referral and transportation for neonatal extracorporeal membrane oxygenation', *Eur J Emerg Med.* **9**(3):233-7.

Biswas, A.K., Thompson S.L. and M.R. Mutert (2002) 'Air medical transport of a pediatric patient with a pulmonary artery catheter and inhaled nitric oxide', *Air Med J.* **21**(5):10-1.

Black, R.E., Mayer T., Walker M.L. et al. (1982) 'Air transport of pediatric emergency cases', *New Eng J Med.* **307**:1465-8.

Bowers, W.R. and P. L. Wyrick (2003) 'Extracorporeal life support: a transcontinental transport experience', *Air Med J.* **22**(2):8-11.

Brink, L.W., Neuman, B. and J. Wynn (1993) 'Air transport', *Pediatr Clin North Am.* **40**:439-50.

Chameides, L. and M.F. Hazinski (eds), (1994) *Textbook of Pediatric Advanced Life Support*, American Academy of Pediatrics and American Heart Association, Dallas.

Cornish, J.D., Carter, J.M., Gerstmann, D.R. and D. M. Null (1991) 'Extracorporeal membrane oxygenation as a means of stabilizing and transporting high risk neonates', *ASAIO Trans.* **37**(4):564-8.

Cunningham, M.D. and F.R. Smith (1973) 'Stabilization and transport of severely ill infants', *Pediatr Clin North Am.* **20**: 359-366.

Dobrin, R.S., Block S., Gilman J.I. and T.A. Massaro (1980) 'The development of a paediatric emergency transport system', *Pediatr Clin North Am.* **27** 633-646.

Doyle, E. et al. (1992) 'Transport of the critically ill child', *Br J Hosp Med.* **48**: 314.

Eckstein, M., Jantos, T., Kelly N. and A. Cardillo (2002) 'Helicopter transport of pediatric trauma patients in an urban emergency medical services system: a critical analysis', *J Trauma.* **53**(2):340-4.

Grubbs, T.C. and N. L. Kraft (2002) 'Neonatal transport issues with prostaglandin E1 infusions', *Air Med J.* **21**(3):8-12.

Harris, B., Orr R. and E. Boles (1975) 'Aeromedical transportation for infants and children', *J Pediatr Surg*, **10**:719-24.

Holleran, R.S. (2003) 'Transporting the family by air', *Pediatric Emerg Care.* **19**(3):211-4.

Jesse, N.M., Drury, L. and M.D.Weiss (2004) 'Transporting neonates with nitric oxide: the 5-year ShandsCair experience', *Air Med J.* **23**(1):17-19.

Lavelle, J. (1996) 'Transport case 1: a time to fly? A dilemma in pediatric transport', *Pediatr Emerg Care*, **12**(2):122-5.

Letts, M., McCaffrey M., Pang E. and F. Lalonde (1999) 'An analysis of an air-ambulance program for children', *J Pediatr Orthop.* **19**(2):240-6.

Macnab, A.J. (1991) 'Optimal escort for interhospital transport of paediatric emergencies', *J Trauma.* **31**: 205-9.

McKay, S., Cruickshanks J. and C. H. Skeoch C (2003) 'Transporting neonates safely', *J Neonat Nurs.* **9**(1):Step by Step Guide.

Martin, T.E. (2005) 'The oxygen dissociation curve', in: *Principles and practice of trauma nursing.* London:, Elsevier.

Martin, T.E. (2001) *Handbook of patient transportation*, London: Greenwich Medical.

Mayer, T.A. and M.L. Walker (1984) 'Severity of illness and injury in pediatric air transport', *Ann Emerg Med,* **13**:108-11.

Morse, T.S. (1969) 'Transportation of critically ill or injured children', *Pediatr Clin North Am.* **16**: 565-571.

Orf, J., Thomas, S.H., Ahmed, W., Wiebe, L., Chamberlin, P., Wedel, S.K., and C. Houck (2000) 'Appropriateness of endotracheal tube size and insertion depth in children undergoing air medical transport', *Pediatr Emerg Care.* **16**(5):321-7.

Paediatric Intensive Care Society (1996) *Standards for paediatric intensive care*, Saldatore: Bishops Stortford.

Robb, H.M., Hallworth, D., Skeoch, C.H. and C. Levy (1992) 'An audit of a paediatric intensive care transfer unit', *Br J Intens Care*. **2**: 37-9.

Robertson, D.N. (1999) 'A mother's care: Do we include the family when the situation is critical?', *J Emerg Nurs*. **25**(3):206-7.

Samuels, M.P. (2004) 'The effects of flight and altitude', *Arch Dis Childhood*. **89**(5):448-55.

Shann, F. (2003) *Drug doses (12th Ed.)*, Pub: Intensive Care Unit, Royal Children's Hospital,Victoria, Australia,

Smith, D.F. and A. Hackel (1983) 'Selection criteria for paediatric critical care transport teams', *Crit Care Med*. **11**: 10-12.

Task Force on Interhospital Transport, American Academy of Pediatrics (1993) 'Guidelines for air and ground transport of neonatal and pediatric patients', *Am Acad Pediatr*, Elk Grove: Illinois.

Tortella, B.J., Sambol, J., Lavery, R.F., Cudihy, K. and G. Nadzam (1996) 'A comparison of pediatric and adult trauma patients transported by helicopter and ground EMS: managed-care considerations', *Air Med J*. **15**(1):24-8.

Wynn, R. (1994) 'Air medical transport of the neonate', in Blumen, I. J. and H. Rodenberg (eds), *Air Medical Physician's Handbook*, AMPA: Salt Lake City.

Chapter 16

Critical Care Transfers and Retrievals

Introduction

The frequency of interhospital transfers of patients is increasing, mostly due to the increasing complexity of healthcare with concentration of skills into specialized centers and the relative lack of intensive care bed availability. This chapter focuses on the transport of high dependency and intensive care patients and, although the principles of safe transport between intensive care units are no different to those discussed in previous chapters, critical care patients offer the most difficult challenges and require immense planning, preparation, skill, knowledge and teamwork to achieve success.

The aim of transfer is to improve the quality of care provided to the patient. The safe surroundings in the ambulance must attempt to mirror the attention provided in an intensive care unit (ICU), but the transfer should at least do no harm. Even this aim is not always possible. Table 16.1 gives some facts about inter-ICU transports in the UK.

Table 16.1   Inter-ICU transfers in the UK

- Over 10 000 intensive care patients are transferred annually in the UK
- Most hospitals transfer fewer than 20, too few to allow medical and nursing personnel to gain expertise
- 90% of patients are accompanied by staff from the referring hospital
- Recommendations from the UK Intensive Care Society and the Association of Anaesthetists of Great Britain state that retrieval teams from the accepting hospital should conduct the transfer

Hazards of transportation

Critically ill patients have deranged physiology and require organ support and invasive monitoring. They tolerate movement, changes in temperature and vibration poorly, and complications are not uncommon. Audits suggest that 15 per cent of patients arrive at the destination hospital with detrimental hypoxia or hypotension, and 10 per cent have injuries that were undetected before transfer. Complications en route may be less frequent if senior anesthesiologists accompany the patients, or if fewer personnel in specialist teams are allowed to gather experience. Once in the aircraft, supervision and advice are difficult to obtain.

Organization

Most critical care authorities now advise that a retrieval service (where the patient is collected by a team from the accepting hospital) is preferable to a transfer team (from the referring hospital or an independent air ambulance provider). A regional approach, in which designated centers accept specific subspecialty patients, allows a more rational approach to the establishment of retrieval teams but, at the very least, each hospital should have:

- designated consultant(s) responsible for transfers ;
- guidelines for referral and for the transfer itself;
- equipment specifically prepared and packed;
- personnel nominated to check, replenish, clean and recharge equipment;
- nominated medical and nursing transfer personnel;
- training for transfer personnel;
- good communication within and between hospitals;
- proper routines for referral between hospitals;
- regular audit.

Initial communication

Poor initial communication is a frequent occurrence to which there is no easy solution. The details of the patient to be transferred must be discussed between the referring and receiving medical teams at senior (preferably consultant) level. The escorting medical team must raise any valid concerns at the outset and should never assume that decisions already taken to transfer are the correct ones. Clear answers are needed to the following questions:

- Why is transfer occurring now?
- Is the medical risk acceptable?

The aim is to gather as much information as possible. This must include history, previous treatment and operations, current care and treatment requirements and future management plan. Modern information and communication technology enables real-time discussion and data transfer by telephone, telemetry or via the Internet, so distance (even international) is no longer a problem.

Transfer decisions

The timing of transfer for certain groups of patients is critical. Guidelines have been published to help the decision-making process, for example, in head injury patients, but for others it is more difficult. For instance, in patients with multiple organ failure, the balance of risk and benefit needs to be carefully considered before the decision on whether and how to send or retrieve the patient is made.

The choice of transport mode depends on:

- urgency
- mobilization time
- distance
- weather
- traffic conditions
- cost.

Table 16.2   The advantages and disadvantages of different modes of transport

Mode	Advantages	Disadvantages
• Road ambulance	• Low cost • Rapid mobilization • Less weather dependency • Easier patient monitoring	• Slow over long distances • Dependent on traffic conditions
• Helicopter air ambulance	• Recommended for journeys over 50 miles • Fast and (possibly) direct	• Slow to mobilize • Requires ground ambulances at either end if no dedicated hospital landing sites • Noisy • Vibration • Small cabin • Often only available during daylight • Expensive

• Fixed wing air ambulance	• Recommended for journeys over 150 miles
	• Compared to a helicopter:
	  – faster
	  – more space
	  – less noise and vibration
	  – less weather dependent
	  – less costly
	  – 24-hour service
		• Slow to mobilize
		• Requires ground ambulances at either end
		• Distance to nearest airport may be great

The advantages and disadvantages of different modes of transport are highlighted in Table 16.2. All vehicles, whether they are road or air ambulances, must have:

- trolley access and fixing systems;
- sufficient space for two or three medical attendants;
- lighting and temperature control within the cabin;
- adequate gases and electricity supply;
- storage space for drugs and equipment;
- good means of communications.

Equipment

General equipment issues are discussed in detail in Chapter 9, but some extra notes are important when considering intensive care patients.

Electrical equipment

It is important to know a machine's expected battery life and ensure it is fully charged. Most monitors have a three to six-hour published life. This is notoriously inaccurate. A shortened life occurs with age of battery and increased electrical demands, such as frequent noninvasive blood pressure cuff cycling or constant use of backlight. Spare batteries are essential.

Multi-function units

Compact multi-function monitors are available from several leading manufacturers (for example, Hewlett Packard, Datex, and Protocol). They are convenient and greatly improve patient safety but expensive (up to £12 000 or US$20 000 per unit). An acceptable device should be capable of monitoring continuous ECG, pulse oximetry, two pressure waveforms, noninvasive blood pressure, capnography and temperature. The ability to produce a strip-chart printout is also useful. It should have a clear display readable in a variety of lighting conditions. Although full colour is best, an orange/black display gives good clarity but grey liquid crystal displays are difficult to read in bright light.

Ventilators

Gas-powered fluid-logic ventilators are ideal (for example, Draeger Oxylog first series, Pneupac, Ventipac). They are small, lightweight, reliable and robust and need no electrical supply. Inspiratory and expiratory times are set, together with a flow rate. There is usually a choice between ventilation on 100 per cent oxygen, or 'air-mix' (approximately 40 per cent). More sophisticated models are usually electrically powered and have a synchronized intermittent mandatory ventilation (SIMV) mode, airway pressure alarms and positive end expiratory pressure (PEEP). Most current models are able to provide pressure support, and some have other complex ventilatory modes such as bitlevel peak airway pressure (BPAP). Lowes and Sharley (2005), have recently completed a survey and comparison of the following models:

- Breas PV403
- Pulmonetic LTV1000
- Newport HT50
- Uni-Vent 754
- Puritan Bennet LP10

Although humidification must be provided via a heat/moisture exchange (HME) filter, most of these ventilators are suitable for children (over the age of 18 months) and adults with a variety of lung pathology and are able to generate a peak inspiratory pressure of 60-80 cmH$_2$O.

Oxygen

Ventilator oxygen consumption depends on inspired oxygen fraction and minute volume. A 10 l.min^{-1} estimate is a useful starting point. A size E (640 l) oxygen cylinder will last approximately one hour, the larger size F (1360 l) approximately 2¼ hours. Oxygen failure or supply exhaustion when transporting patients with increased oxygen demand is catastrophic. Carriage of approximately twice the total calculated oxygen requirement is recommended.

   Novel solutions to the perennial problem of carrying oxygen cylinders have been tried. LOX (liquid oxygen) has been used by the USAF medevac service with some success, although it is considered to be dangerous air cargo by all airlines and carriers. On board oxygen generators (OBOGs) still suffer from the problem of low flow rate, but linking several together has been suggested as a viable possibility. Perhaps the single most useful advance is the development of a modified closed circle system in New Zealand (Pacific Air Ambulance) which, when used in conjunction with an electrically powered ventilator, allows a large reduction in oxygen requirements for long flights.

Defibrillator

Traditionally, manual defibrillators (such as Hewlett Packard, Lifepack, and Laerdal) have been said to be preferable to semi-automatic models (AEDs) because the electronic algorithm may, in theory, be confused by vibration artifact. Modern biphasic AEDs are extremely reliable and robust, but the larger manual machines will still be necessary when an external pacing facility is needed.

Syringe drivers

Syringe pumps are essential for accurate drug delivery. The double-syringe types are more compact and convenient than those taking a single syringe, but it is important to ensure that pumps and syringes are compatible.

Doctor's bag

A comprehensive doctor's bag should contain all routine anesthetic and emergency drugs in sufficient quantity for the entire transfer. Several manufacturers make custom-designed emergency bags for the ambulance and mountain rescue services. These are ideal. There should be ample storage space for drugs, together with a variety of compartments for essential airway equipment, cannulae, syringes, intravenous fluid, chest drain sets (with underwater seal kit or Heimlich valve), and sundry items such as gloves, swabs, tape, sharps box, and so on. An inventory of drugs and equipment is essential for checking contents and recording expiry dates.

The medical team

Successful interhospital transfer requires a well coordinated team effort. A full-time hospital consultant in intensive care medicine should be responsible for the service, training of transfer personnel and audit of transfer activities. In addition to the crew of the ambulance, a critically ill patient should be accompanied by a minimum of two attendants:

- doctor, usually an anesthesiologist trained in intensive care with:
  - previous transfer experience
  - at least two years' postgraduate experience
  - a qualification in the specialty;
- assisted by a qualified anesthetic or intensive care nurse, paramedic, or technician familiar with intensive care procedures and equipment.

Final preparation

Stabilization of the patient should follow the principles outlined by the advanced trauma life support (ATLS) and advanced cardiac life support (ACLS) ABC approach and, since hypovolemic patients tolerate movement poorly, circulating volume should be normal or supranormal before departure. Intravenous loading will usually be required to maintain satisfactory blood pressure, perfusion and urine output, but inotrope therapy may also be needed. Particularly unstable patients may need central venous pressure or pulmonary artery pressure monitoring to optimize filling pressures and cardiac output. In addition, monitoring immediately prior to transfer should include ECG and blood gas analysis

Documentation must include a referral letter, radiographs, the clinical notes, and results of all investigations. Any unused cross-matched blood or blood products must accompany the patient. Finally, the consultant and nurse in charge from the receiving intensive care unit (ICU) must be informed of the estimated time of arrival and travel arrangements should be discussed with relatives.

The transfer

If possible, the patient should be positioned to provide maximum access during the transfer. Space at the head end will allow monitoring and management of the airway. All-round access is ideal but not always achievable in road ambulances, and all but impossible in aircraft.

The transfer should be undertaken smoothly and rarely at high speed. The staff/patient ratio during the journey is better than normally expected in the hospital ICU and the aim is to provide the same standard of monitoring, nursing care and medical intervention. The caveat, of course, is that in transit it can be difficult or impossible to undertake major procedures. During the ground phase of the transport, any significant incidents may be best managed after the ambulance has pulled over to the side of the road – a luxury not available in aircraft.

Specialized critical care transfers

Specialized coronary care transport teams have been operating in the USA since the 1980s and, although it is recognized that America has widely differing patient transport needs because of vast distances between hospitals, it is likely that an ever increasing number of schemes will operate out of the UK, Europe and Australia in the future. Recent advances in intraortic balloon counterpulsation (IABC) technology have made transport of selected patients safer. Accepted indications for transfer of a patient on an IABC pump are given in Table 16.3. Similarly, even though the RAF pioneered the international aeromedical transfer of renal dialysis patients in the 1960s, civilian practice has not followed. However, new hemofiltration technology may prove small and robust enough to be useful for long journey times.

Table 16.3   Indications for IABC transport

- Accelerating angina (transport to a cardiac facility for bypass surgery)
- Ischemic or idiopathic cardiomyopathy when cardiac transplantation is an option
- Emergency repair of structural defects, such as mitral valve defect
- Hemodynamic instability during a cardiac catheterization
- Need for advanced pharmacological therapy necessitating transfer to a tertiary care facility
- IAB pump-dependent patient has exhausted the resources of the referring facility

References

A group of neurosurgeons (1984) 'Guidelines for the initial management after head injury in adults', *Brit Med J.* **288**:983-985.

Association of Anaesthetists of Great Britain and Ireland (2000) *Recommendations for standards of monitoring during anaesthesia and recovery*, AAGBI: London.

Donelly, J.A. and G.H. McGinn (1997) 'Equipment for the transfer of the critically ill', Morton N.S.et al. (eds), in: *Stabilization and Transport of the Critically Ill*, Churchill Livingstone: London.

Fischer, D., Veldman, A., Schafer, V. and M. Diefenbach (2004) 'Bacterial colonization of patients undergoing international air transport: a pro-spective epidemiologic study,' *J Travel Med.* **11**(1):44-8.

Flabouris, A., Schoettker P. and A. Garner (2003) 'ARDS with severe hypoxia – aeromedical transportation during prone ventilation', *Anaesthesia & Intensive Care.* **31**(6):675-8.

Intensive Care Society (1997) *Guidelines for the transport of the critically ill adult.* Intensive Care Society: London.

Lamb, D. (2003) 'The introduction of new critical care equipment into the aeromedical evacuation service of the Royal Air Force', *Intensive & Critical Care Nursing* 19(2):92-102.

Lowes, T. and P. Sharley (2005) 'Oxygen conservation during long distance transport of ventilated patients', *Air Med J.* **24**(4):164-171.

Mertlich, G. and S. J. Quaal (1989) 'Air transport of the patient requiring intra-aortic balloon pumping', *Crit Care Nurs Clin North Am* **1**(3):443.

Neuroanaesthesia Society of Great Britain and Ireland (1996) *Recommendations for the transfer of patients with acute head injuries to neurosurgical units*, AAGBI: London.

Reily, D.J., Tollok, E., Mallitz, K., Hanson, C.W. and B.D. Fuchs (2004) 'Successful aeromedical transport using inhaled prostacyclin for a patient with life-threatening hypoxemia', *Chest* **125**(4):1579-81.

Shirley, P. (2003) 'Prone ventilation and aeromedical transport', *Anaesth Intensive Care* **31**(6):675-8.

Veldman, A., Diefenbach M., Fischer D., Benton A. and R. Bloch (2004) 'Long-distance transport of ventilated patients: advantages and limitations of air medical repatriation on commercial airlines', *Air Med J* **23**(2):24-8.

Wallace, P. G. M and Ridley, S.A. (1999) 'Transport of Critically Ill Patients', in: Singer M. and I. Grant (eds), *ABC of Intensive Care*, BMJ: London.

Chapter 17

Nursing Care in the Air

T. Martin and I. MacLennan

Introduction

Nursing care within the harsh environment of an aircraft cabin is not the sole responsibility of nurses and, although they are the most effective practitioners, a nurse is not always present during the transfer to deliver this type of care. This chapter utilizes a systems-based model to provide an overview of elements of nursing care related specifically to the flight environment, enabling the reader (who may not be a nurse) to identify solutions to some of the more common nursing care problems.

Safety and risk management

The safety of self and patient will always be the most important consideration during any aeromedical transfer. Although not solely the domain of the nurse, when planning a transfer, attention should always be paid to strategies to minimize risk. For instance, these include:

- ensure at least basic airway adjuncts and hand-held suction apparatus are always carried;
- ensure all time-limited equipment and drugs are within date;
- carry appropriate antidotes to drugs (for example, naloxone for opiates);
- carry appropriate medication for the treatment of anaphylaxis if new drugs are likely to be administered;
- ensure all single use items are discarded after a single use, and that all single patient items are discarded after patient hand-over or left with the patient at the receiving facility;
- ensure all electrical equipment has been maintained and checked as per manufacturer's instructions;
- ensure all equipment has been checked for function prior to undertaking a transfer and that spare working batteries are carried;
- secure all invasive equipment, especially during times of maximum movement such as transfer from road vehicle to aircraft;
- check equipment contents for allowable items. Since the atrocities of 9/11 airlines have restricted the carriage of sharp objects and other items in the cabin on commercial flights. There are, however, certain exceptions. Most

airlines will permit the carriage of needles for medical use, but will insist on blunt ended, as opposed to pointed, scissors.

Equipment

As with most aspects of patient care, nursing is heavily reliant on the use of appropriate equipment. The aircraft cabin will not have a store equipped with specialised nursing consumables and supplies, and so anticipation of such needs is vital before undertaking a patient transfer. When planning, it is easy to become fixated on the patient's primary diagnosis and peripheral requirements can sometimes be neglected. A competent practitioner caring for a cardiac patient is likely to remember to carry a defibrillator and other advanced life support (ALS) equipment, but will he remember a urinal? A seated patient may suffer unexpected cardiac instability during the journey necessitating a restriction in mobility. Any equipment packs should therefore contain appropriate equipment in order to facilitate the holistic nursing care of the patient, examples of which will be described within this chapter.

When selecting appropriate equipment, it is important to consider the space limitations inherent with caring for patients within the aeromedical environment. Within a hospital, patients at high risk from pressure area breakdown may be effectively nursed on a pressure distribution mattress, but this is obviously impracticable in flight. Furthermore, AC electricity powered equipment is not suitable for use in flight, unless the aircraft is equipped with a power inverter. Even then, consideration must be given to the availability of electrical power during ground transfers. Attention should also be paid to the availability of oxygen. Different systems, connections and flow rates will be available according to the type of aircraft or its continental base. European flow meters are of no value on an American aircraft as the systems are incompatible. Similarly, nebulisers driven by oxygen are of little use on commercial aircraft. They require a flow rate in excess of 6L/min in order to nebulise liquid and most airlines only supply oxygen at a maximum flow rate of 4L/min.

Medicolegal competence

It is vital that a comprehensive hand-over is received when accepting an elective aeromedical repatriation, not least to ensure that the patient's condition falls within the practitioner's level of competence. Consideration should be paid not only to the patient's primary presenting condition, but also to any relevant past medical history and co-morbidities. An extreme example of this could be the cardiologist tasked to transfer a patient following myocardial infarction who also happens to have a significant psychiatric condition that has destabilized during the current illness.

The issue of working within a field of personal competence is especially relevant for nurses. Aeromedical transport often involves autonomous (and lone) practice. The laws of many countries do not support nurse prescribing of medication unless the nurse has undergone specific training in this 'extended' role. Yet, as an autonomous and lone worker, a nurse will often be placed in a position where prescription and supply (dispensing) of medications may be necessary. It is important, therefore, to ensure that a robust *Patient Group Directives*[1] should be in place so that the prescription and administration of medication in these circumstances adheres to relevant laws and guidelines or, alternatively, to ensure that any medication that may have to be administered is correctly prescribed by a medical practitioner.

Positioning and handling of patient

Seated versus stretcher

An important consideration in facilitating effective nursing care is the mode of transport. Some conditions necessitate a stretcher for the transfer (such as many spinal injuries, hip fractures prior to formal repair, dense hemiparesis, and so on), but moving a patient on a stretcher can cause its own problems. Self-care should always be encouraged, but the patient's ability to be self-caring on a stretcher is severely limited. For instance, once on a stretcher, an immobile patient requiring to urinate or defecate will need a bedpan or urinal, as it is usually too difficult to mobilize to a toilet in the confined environment of an aircraft cabin. This adversely affects privacy and dignity. Many airlines now provide upgraded seating that reconforms to provide a flat bed so, as long as a patient can sit upright for taxi, take-off and landing, this may be appropriate for many patients who previously would have been moved on a stretcher.

The stretcher patient – head forward versus backward

This debate has been raging for many years, and from every angle! When transferring a patient commercially, different airlines fit stretchers in different directions, even on the same types of aircraft. The aeromedical escort may have little choice in which direction to position a patient because the securing straps (which normally consist of a five-point harness) will only permit loading in one direction. Furthermore, attention should be paid to stretchers with elevating 'backrests' and appropriate positioning of patients who may need to be nursed sitting.

---

1   A Patient Group Directive is a specifically written instruction for the administration of named medicines in an identified clinical situation. It is drawn up by doctors and pharmacists, and approved by the employer, advised by professional advisory committees. It applies to groups of patients and other service users who may not be individually identified before presentation for treatment.

Use of wheelchairs

Although it is accepted that with most clinical conditions ambulation is important to prevent the complications of reduced mobility, the use of wheelchairs for semi-ambulant patients is advised. Distances needed to walk at airports can be long, queues are stressful and clinical conditions can be exacerbated by the need to climb stairs to aircraft, or even a sloping walkway. Airlines provide wheelchairs according to three different categories (Table 17.1).

During the check-in process, it is important to ensure that the correct category of wheelchair is indicated on the patient's booking, as the support that airlines will provide is dependant on this. For example, if a scheduled repatriation necessitates a change of aircraft, and each aircraft is parked off stand, that is, not attached to a terminal via an airbridge, and a patient is categorised as WCHS or WCHC (see definitions in table below), then the airline will provide (at best) a high lift and transfer between aircraft or (at worst) an 'aisle chair' to lift a patient down steps, and wheel them to the next aircraft. If the patient was categorized as WCHR, in this scenario he would be expected to walk down and up aircraft steps (which on a Boeing 747 or Airbus A340 means four floors in each direction!).

Table 17.1   Airlines' classification of wheelchair usage

WCHR	Wheelchair to aircraft steps, but can manage steps independently
WCHS	Wheelchair to aircraft door, but can walk to seat
WCHC	Requires assistance directly to seat

Respiratory system and oxygen delivery

General considerations

Oxygen, available at 21 per cent in ambient air, is the most important substance that may need to be administered during an aeromedical mission. It is also arguably the substance that causes most problems in relation to its delivery. If a patient is dependant on oxygen at sea level, he will definitely need it at a higher concentration at altitude. If a patient needs it intermittently at sea level, he will require it continuously at altitude. Other patients who do not require oxygen on the ground may well need it at altitude. Patients lying flat on stretchers often suffer a degree of hypoxia, especially in the obese, or in the presence of mechanical obstructions preventing high tidal volumes during normal respiration. The latter can be caused by stretcher straps, vacuum mattresses, and diaphragmatic splinting following abdominal surgery. Patients with weakness of the muscles of respiration (such as those with a cerebrovascular accident [CVA]) and postural pooling of secretions (such as those in heart failure) will also deteriorate if left to lie flat.

Prior to transfer, special attention should be paid to the availability and usability of the calculated required amount of oxygen at every stage of the journey. A fully equipped air ambulance with on-board piped oxygen is an excellent facility, but does the ground ambulance in the economically challenged country you are collecting the patient from have any oxygen at all? Even if flying on a Boeing 747-400,[2] in which the oxygen supply often originates from an excellent ring main, care must be taken to plan effectively. The oxygen source is a fixed outlet above the patient's head and if mobilising a patient to the toilet, for example, there is also a need for portable cylinder oxygen.

Oxygen delivery – mask versus nasal cannulae

If oxygen is required in the non-ventilated patient with no tracheostomy, there are two options readily available for its delivery – oronasal mask and nasal cannulae. Each has its own benefits. The flow rate for each will primarily be dependant on the patient's clinical requirement, and judicious use of a pulse oximetery is recommended. It is difficult to estimate the inspired oxygen fraction (FiO_2) when delivering oxygen via nasal specs, but Table 17.2 gives manufacturers' estimations, based on a nose breathing patient at sea level. Flow rates are slightly increased at altitude.

Table 17.2   Manufacturers' estimations of inspired oxygen fraction at various flow rates through nasal cannulae at sea level

Flow rate (L/min)	Approx FiO_2 at sea level
1.0	24%
2.0	28%
3.0	32%
4.0	36%

Indications and nursing care related to nasal cannulae: Nasal cannulae should be positioned with one cannula in each nostril, and therefore are contraindicated in patients with nasal trauma, obstruction of nasal passages, and those with a nasogastric tube in situ. The oxygen tubing should be placed over and around the patient's ears, and secured under the chin (like wearing a pair of glasses). Hence, they are colloquially known as nasal specs. They should not be secured too tightly, and regular checks should be made to potential pressure points (the nostrils and behind the ears) as tissue breakdown related can occur quickly at these points.

---

2   There are oxygen access nipples on the service panel overhead every second seat row on the Boeing 747-400 and on some Boeing 757s and 767s.

Oxygen delivery by this method causes the nasal mucosa to dry very quickly. The nostrils should be moistened every two hours, or when the patient complains of discomfort. Patients receiving oxygen via nasal cannula generally find the method more comfortable and less claustrophobic than an oxygen mask, and they are able to eat and drink more freely.

Indications and nursing care related to oxygen delivery by mask: Inspired oxygen can be more accurately controlled by mask delivery as both the mouth and nose are exposed to the inspired gas. Some patients who have symptoms related to hypoxia or shortness of breath feel more confident with an oxygen mask, especially if they have been using them on the ground. However, some patients find oxygen masks to be more restrictive than nasal cannulae, and sometimes the smell of the mask can precipitate nausea. Patients are often less inclined to eat and drink, and the mouth and nose quickly become dry. Humidification is not normally possible in flight, so patients should be encouraged to sip water frequently and regular mouth care should be given. Also, moisturising cream should be administered around the nares. Consideration should also be paid to potential pressure sore formation with oxygen masks. The most common points are the bridge of the nose and back of the head where elasticated straps are used to secure the mask. Straps should not be placed over or behind the ears as these areas quickly become sore.

Cardiovascular system

Thromboembolic precautions

The prevention of complications related to reduced mobility is an inherent part of nursing care for all patients. One such group of complications is the development of thromboembolic phenomena such as deep vein thrombosis (DVT) and pulmonary embolus (PE). Many patients being transferred will have already had a period of inactivity in the hospital of origin and, although the use of subcutaneous prophylactic anticoagulation is common around the world, the use of antiembolic stockings is not. Considering the dehydrating impact of the aviation environment, and the further restrictions to mobility imposed during transfer, the use of correctly sized and fitted antiembolic stockings is recommended except in the presence of peripheral vascular disease, venous ulcers or cellulitis.

However, even antiembolic stockings are not without their complications. Creases should be avoided and the tops of the stockings should not be allowed to roll down, exerting a tourniquet effect on the leg. Pressure points around the heels and ankles should be observed closely and any sign of pressure breakdown should be treated by relief of the pressure every two hours. During long distance transfers, antiembolic stockings should be removed every 12 hours, legs should be washed and dried, and stockings re-applied to maintain good skin hygiene. There is ambiguous and conflicting evidence relating to effectiveness of knee length versus thigh length antiembolic stockings and, as such, the use of knee length stockings is recommended as these feel more comfortable and less restricting, and are easier to manage in the confined aircraft environment.

Exercise tolerance and use of wheelchairs for cardiac patients

Distances at airports are often long and exhausting. In patients at risk, it is always sensible to minimize cardiac demand prior to the commencement of any journey by air. The onset of cardiac pain in the preceding minutes to a flight is a clinical contraindication to undertaking a transfer until it has resolved or has been further investigated. Most commercial airlines gate staff would also decline to carry a patient if they became aware of a recent onset of cardiac symptoms. As such, judicious use of wheelchairs is advised, bearing in mind that some cardiac patients may feel a wheelchair is not required, as they have become asymptomatic with appropriate medical care that they may have received. However, given appropriate explanations, most patients will readily agree to this strategy.

Relaxation and seating

Appropriate seating arrangements can prevent potential exacerbations of anxiety or stress in cardiac patients. Spacious, relaxed environments (such as those in business class cabins) should be used whenever possible. This would have the additional benefit of the use of First Class lounges and waiting facilities and often speedy passage through the necessary airport formalities, thus contributing to effective holistic patient care. Aeromedical escorts should sit next to their patients from where continuous assessment and immediate treatment can be provided if required. Although insurance companies may resist the extra cost, family members or friends should be kept with the patient whenever possible, to avoid undue patient separation anxiety.

Stress and anxiety are significant contributing adrenergic factors in acute cardiac events. It is important that precipitators that could potentially lead to stress are addressed early. Whilst the practitioner caring for a patient will be familiar with aeromedical transport and the associated occurrences and issues, the patient will probably not be and, as such, full explanations and reassurances should be given prior to any event occurring wherever possible. Patients should be encouraged to ask questions and articulate concerns, and the aeromedical escort should ensure that the questions are answered, wherever possible, to the satisfaction of the patient. Appropriate terminology should be used at all times – medical jargon is pointless where it will not be understood. Patients should be encouraged to articulate the onset of symptoms at an early stage. Mild transient angina is easier to treat acutely than angina that develops into an acute cardiological event.

Neurological impairment

It is important to consider that there may be a past medical history of central nervous system (CNS) impairment unrelated to the reason for transporting the patient. For example, a patient being transported for a gastrointestinal problem may have had a CVA with residual hemiplegia in the past.

Visual impairment

Visual disabilities will have an impact throughout a transfer. It is important to gain an early understanding of the patient's abilities and requirements, and to consider how the patient normally manages his visual impairment. Visually impaired patients in unfamiliar environments need constant reassurance to prevent high levels of anxiety. Simple things such as help with nutritional intake, guidance to the toilet, and explanation of the immediate environment are imperative. When undertaking any procedure or element of care, it is vital to talk to the patient before touch occurs. It can be very disconcerting for a partially sighted or blind patient to suddenly feel an intravenous drug being administered, or a blood pressure cuff being inflated without first being warned.

Auditory impairment

There are also significant impacts that the aviation environment poses on those with auditory impairment. It is important when caring for a patient with hearing disability to agree a method in which to communicate most effectively. The degree of impairment will obviously be the biggest consideration, and it is extremely important to determine how much he lip-reads. If the aeromedical escort is not sitting where a lip-reading person can easily see him, it is important to agree a way of getting the patient's attention. Being tactile before you attempt communication is often the agreed solution. Once that attention is gained, it is important not to restrict sight of the lips – this is even more important when using headsets and microphones inside the cabins of smaller air ambulances. Furthermore, If a patient uses a hearing aid, remember that the aid also amplifies ambient sound, such as aircraft engine noise. In helicopter air ambulances, this often causes such significant problems that it may be better to turn the hearing aid off.

Motor and sensory impairments

One of the more common symptoms related to CVA with residual deficit is the lack of perception of the affected side. Whilst it is accepted that during the rehabilitation phase healthcare practitioners should address this lack of perception by working with patients on the affected side, it is suggested that during aeromedical transfer, for reasons of safety and patient confidence, the aeromedical escort should approach patients from the unaffected side. This ensures that patients are always fully aware of the availability of any help or support they may require. This should include sitting next to the patient's unaffected side wherever possible, and requesting the positioning of stretchers appropriately so that anyone approaching the patient does so towards the unaffected side. This is not always possible, and patients may need assistance when people who may not be aware of these issues approach them from the affected side.

The impact of loss of sensation should also be considered. Limbs with no sensation should be positioned appropriately, thereby preventing pressure necrosis or contractures. Also, unless clinically contraindicated, they should be moved at least every two hours through a full range of movement.

Confusional states

Although the safety of the patient must be the primary concern of the aeromedical escort, the safety of other passengers and the aircraft are clearly also important. A risk benefit analysis should be made in relation to the appropriateness of moving confused patients by air. This analysis should include the competency of the aeromedical escort in dealing with acute exacerbations of the confusional state and its cause, if known.

Appropriate strategies must be planned to effectively manage all possible problems en route. Both acute and chronic psychiatric conditions should be managed by appropriately qualified and experienced psychiatrists and/or psychiatric nurses. Other pathophysiological confusional states, such as sometimes seen after CVA and head injury, should be stabilized prior to transfer with use of appropriate strategies such as the utilization of relatives. Patients often relate better to people they knew prior to the acute event causing their confusion. Alternatively, spending extra time with such patients may be of benefit, so that they may gain some form of recognition prior to undertaking the transfer.

Musculoskeletal system, mobility and patient handling

The method of moving a patient is dependant not just on his need, but also on length of transfer, type of vehicle (small fixed wing, helicopter, road ambulance, commercial airliner and so on), and the decisions made are often made remotely or by treating physicians and nurses who are not fully conversant with retrieval techniques. For example, a two-sector commercial repatriation of a semi-mobile patient with a stable L4 fracture from Sydney to London could be undertaken using a stretcher. As discussed earlier, there are considerable issues and potential complications associated with a stretcher transfer. If the patient could sit upright for take-off and landing (in terms of clinical safety and pain control), then this same transfer could easily be undertaken on a business class commercial seat, many of which can now recline to a fully flat position.

Every element of the transfer should be considered, not just the flight. As well as movement within an aircraft, the transfer may also involve ground transfers by ambulance, elevators, stairs and through other confined spaces. It is important to be aware of these implications in the planning stage. If a patient is on a stretcher, how is he going to be transferred from a ground ambulance to an aircraft? A scoop stretcher is a useful tool in these circumstances, but on some aircraft there is not enough space to turn the stretcher round the acute corner near the entrance door, and so patients must be loaded on a wheelchair. This would obviously be contraindicated in some patients, for example unstable spinal injuries, certain hip or pelvic fractures or completely immobile patients.

A vacuum mattress is helpful in managing stretcher patients. By ensuring a snug fit around the patient, it provides safe and effective immobilisation. It works by forming a cocoon around a patient as air is sucked out of a mattress containing small beads. However, during ascent, any residual air between the beads expands with the decrease in ambient air pressure, and the aeromedical escort must check the mattress frequently during ascent, aspirating more air if appropriate.

The restriction of mobility associated with many presenting complaints is often compounded when undertaking an aeromedical transfer, especially long distance. There is a common list of complications that need to be considered when caring for patients (including appropriate nursing interventions):

- pressure areas
- chest infection
- urinary tract infection
- contractures and joint stiffness
- muscle wasting.

Pressure area formation

Stretcher patients should be nursed on an appropriate pressure distribution mattress and clean, wrinkle-free sheets. A vacuum mattress can also be used where appropriate immobilization or enhanced patient support is required. A vacuum mattress should never be used as the primary method of lifting a patient. A scoop (or clam-shell) stretcher should be used under the vacuum mattress in order to prevent disruption of the formed shape. Patients should have their position changed at least every two hours. This may be difficult in the confines of an aircraft, but whatever can be done to promote relief of pressure will be of benefit, even if it is just redistributing weight away from a particular area by using pillows to roll the patient slightly. Straps and securing aids should be loosened after take-off, but kept secured in the event of unexpected turbulence.

Close attention should be paid to areas of the body which are unable to move, for instance in those with hemiplegia or fractures preventing movement. Sheets should be wrinkle-free and oxygen cylinders monitors, syringe pumps, or other machines should not be placed directly on the patient. Drainage tubes, intravenous lines and monitoring cables should not be left underneath the patient. As a guide, every time an aeromedical escort feels the need to adjust position, it is likely that the patient will also need to be moved.

Chest infection

Whenever possible, patients should be sat upright and encouraged to breathe deeply and expectorate any sputum. Many stretchers come with a backrest which can be raised; otherwise a backrest may be constructed out of pillows or rolled up bedding.

Since cabin air is derived from cold outside ambient air, its water content is much less than warmer air at lower altitudes. If dried secretions or mucosal membranes are an issue, a battery operated nebulizer can be used to humidify air intermittently as required. Continuous use is logistically difficult because of the volume of water required, and gas driven nebulizers also consume large volumes of oxygen.

Urinary tract infection

Patients should be encouraged to drink two to three liters of fluid per day unless there is a clinical contraindication such as renal failure. If catheterised, urine should be monitored for cloudiness or debris and, in the latter case, bladder washouts may be considered, especially if partial obstruction of the catheter is suspected.

Contractures, muscle wasting and joint stiffness

Patients should be encouraged to move joints and muscles actively at least every two hours. Unless clinically contraindicated, patients who are unable to comply should have passive exercises carried out on their behalf.

Elimination

The restricted environment of the aircraft cabin poses particular problems when dealing with elimination and patient assessment prior to transfer should include recent gastrointestinal and urinary history. Thought should also be made of the patients presenting symptoms and how they may affect gastrointestinal management. Wherever possible, for reasons of normality, privacy and dignity, patients should be encouraged to use toilets for all elimination needs. However, this is not always possible, especially if a patient is being transferred commercially on a stretcher, or is in a small air ambulance which does not have toilet facilities.

Elimination (stretcher patients)

The process of fecal or urinary elimination on a stretcher can be very embarrassing for patients, especially on a commercial aircraft. It is the job of the aeromedical escort to minimize this embarrassment and promote patient privacy and dignity. Wherever possible, patients should be encouraged to defecate prior to commencement of the transfer. Frequent diarrhoea or fecal incontinence is likely to be a contraindication to commercial transfer. The correct equipment should always be available to support patient elimination needs. Bedpans and urinals (both male and female) should be available. Incontinence pads should be placed underneath the patient so that any spillage can be disposed of quickly and effectively, leaving sheets clean and dry. It is a good idea to line bedpans, prior to their use, with plastic bags (with no holes!), to aid disposal of eliminated matter into an appropriate place at the earliest opportunity. There are, after all, no bedpan washers at altitude!

While there is some evidence to support an increase in the incidence of sacral pressure area development when incontinence pads (adult nappies or diapers) are kept underneath patients as an aid to patient hygiene, it could be argued that their judicious use in the aircraft cabin would be of benefit in the event of known or unexpected incontinence.

Following any elimination, patient hygiene needs should be met. The patient's skin should be left clean and dry, and hand hygiene should be offered. Understandably, patients on stretchers become anxious when needing to eliminate, and the aeromedical escort should endeavour to support the patient in dealing with these uncomfortable feelings. Because of this, patients are often disinclined to drink, but they should be encouraged to avoid exacerbating the dehydrating effects associated with cabin air.

Patients with occasional or stress incontinence should be offered bedpans or urinals with a greater frequency than their usual pattern, to prevent occurrence during transfer. This should include encouragement of any elimination during ground portions of the transfer, when management of the situation is far easier and less concerning for the patient.

Although urethral catheterisation is not a long term answer for urinary incontinence and there are risks associated with the presence (and insertion) of a urethral catheter, a risk/benefit analysis should be carried out for catheterisation prior to a long transfer. Taking into account the problems associated with incontinence (such as pressure area breakdown, lack of dignity and privacy, lack of facilities to change bedding and linen, difficulty in maintaining hygiene and so on), the sensible view may be that informed consent for urethral catheterisation may be the most appropriate action.

Elimination (ambulant and semi-ambulant patients)

Even with seated patients, thought should be given to the elimination requirements of those with special needs. If a WCHC patient is being transferred commercially, the airline should provide an aisle chair so that the patient can be transferred to the aircraft toilet. That same patient may prefer a urinal to urinate, but this can only be provided if a satisfactory degree of privacy can be guaranteed. The aeromedical escort must also be mindful of the feelings of other passengers in this situation, as a commercial aircraft is, in reality, a public place. Female urinals cannot be used with any degree of ease or privacy in a seat.

If a patient is oxygen dependant, then a mobile oxygen cylinder should be requested from the airline or air ambulance company so that the correct inspired oxygen fraction can be maintained whilst the patient is mobilizing to the toilet. Oxygen demand will increase with the effort and anxiety of the move to the toilet and also during the elimination process itself. On commercial airlines, it is also useful to enlist the help of cabin crew to ensure that the toilet is unoccupied, thus preventing a potential long wait for the patient in a queue.

Stomas

The presence of a stoma itself should pose no concern to the aeromedical escort. However, there are some obvious issues to be considered. Stoma bags should be filtered to prevent over expansion of any contained gas and potential bag rupture as the cabin altitude increases (Boyle's Law). Spare bags should also be carried. It is a good idea to empty feces prior to loading onto an aircraft. Urostomy bags, of course, do not require a filter as there should not be any gas in the bag, with the notable exception of patients with a fistula or surgical connection between bowel and urinary tract.

Nutrition and hydration

Feeding

Nutrition and hydration should always be maintained to a satisfactory level during transfer. Patients requiring supplementary nutrition as part of their treatment regime should have uninterrupted feeding where practicable. It is, however, suggested that continuation of nasogastric or gastrostomy feeding should only be continued on long distance transfers of greater than 12 hours in duration, as the difficulties associated with continuing administration of nutrition in the aircraft environment outweighs the benefits. The problems include the requirement for special feed pumps (mostly requiring AC mains electricity) and the lack of feed preparation areas.

Total parenteral nutrition (TPN) is very difficult to maintain during a long transfer, especially if administered through a centrally placed venous catheter, due to the difficulties with storage which requires precision temperature control and aseptic conditions, as well as AC electrical supply to charge or power the required infusion devices. The aeromedical escort must seriously consider the benefits of continuing TPN for the duration of transfer, against the perils of a nutritional pause. If enteral or parenteral nutrition is paused, it is important to ensure that patients remain hydrated, either by encouraging oral intake or by intravenous administration.

Whilst it is accepted that aeromedical escorts easily recognize patients with overt dexterity problems such as hemiplegia who may not be able to cut food into manageable portions or drink fluids with normal cups or glasses, there are many other patients who may have similar problems. Patients with arm fractures or even painful intravenous catheters are such examples. It is also very difficult for patients lying on stretchers to eat and drink normally and it is important for the aeromedical escort to assist.

Food should be presented appropriately, in manageable proportions and portions. Feeding aids such as beakers with spouts and straws should be used, but many patients will have to be fed. Patients should be offered hand hygiene before and after eating. There are also a large number of special diets (available for both medical and social or religious reasons) that can be ordered on commercial airlines (with 24 hours' notice for most airlines), and it is often left to the aeromedical practitioner to arrange.

Nasogastric feeding and drainage

A nasogastric tube (NGT) should pose no problems in flight. If it has been inserted for feeding purposes, and is not being utilized for feeding, it can just be connected to a drainage bag and secured. Spigoting is less satisfactory because it eradicates one way of venting trapped gastrointestinal gas should the need arise. If the NGT is there for reasons related to gastrointestinal drainage, it should be secured to a drainage bag with tap, positioned below the level of the abdomen – gravity still works at altitude! Clearly, great care must be taken with a patient with gastrointestinal obstruction, as the associated expansion of bowel gas with the increase in cabin altitude could lead to gut perforation.

Mouthcare

Mouthcare should be carried out at least every two hours in those patients unable to eat or drink. The mouth should be kept moist and clean. The best method is with a toothbrush and toothpaste, but it is important to ensure that the mouth is rinsed effectively afterwards. Alternatively, pre-packed mouthcare swabs are easy, cheap and effective. In hemiplegic patients with disorder of mastication, it is important to ensure that the affected side of the mouth is cleaned after meals as patients often neglect to do this. Naturally, a suction device should be handy for those patients with poor swallow and cough reflexes.

Emotional Support

Most individual people requiring aeromedical transfer have not been in a similar situation before. The unfamiliar environment and procedures associated with any such transfer therefore have the potential to be stressful, even more so if they are alone and without the support of family or close friends.

Given that patients are more likely to be compliant if they are informed and certain about what is coming next, it is important to offer explanations for any impending events or plans. In that way they can give informed consent and even feel part of the team undertaking the transfer.

A transfer also provides an opportunity for the aeromedical escort to ensure that the patient understands the events surrounding their health problems. Often, patients have been cared for in a country where they do not speak the native language. In these circumstances, full and thorough explanation of procedures and diagnoses may not only allay many of the fears that patients have, but is also likely to instil a degree of confidence in the aeromedical escort. In essence, the patient will develop trust in the abilities of the nurse and/or doctor or team. It is important to realize that although patients will generally welcome the arrival of aeromedical personnel, it is likely to be the first time that the two parties have met and, as such, a little time building rapport, and gaining the patient's trust is time well spent.

There may be political, economic or psychosocial factors concerning the country from which the patient was transferred. Commonly, the care received is believed to be of a lower standard than expected in the home country. This may or may not actually reflect the truth. On the other hand, this may be the reason the patient is being transferred, that is, to receive appropriate care in an appropriate place by the appropriate person or team. However, great caution should be taken when discussing the treatment a patient has received prior to being handed over to the aeromedical team. Although possibly not optimum, it is the care the patient has received, and to openly criticize is unprofessional and is likely to give the patient anxiety and cause for concern.

It is often difficult to gauge how much information to give. Too much may cause data overload followed by poor retention of important explanations given. On the other hand, too little may cause anxiety and mistrust. Each patient should be assessed individually.

Privacy and confidentiality

Privacy is of considerable concern when transferring patients on commercial aircraft, especially for those on stretchers. Other passengers, tend to take a significant interest! This can be intrusive and embarrassing for the patient. Privacy and dignity should always be maintained, curtains and blankets should be used where appropriate and both patients and relatives should be given an explanation of this occurrence before starting the transfer. If the situation should become overly intrusive, the aeromedical escort can enlist the support of cabin crew to address the issue with other passengers.

It is also important to consider issues related to confidentiality, not just with other passengers but also with the aircraft crew, airport and ambulance personnel and those working for the air ambulance and insurance organizations. On a similar theme, consent should be obtained to discuss any health issues with travelling companions, especially if they are not near relatives. It should not be implied just because the companion is travelling on the same flight.

The use of appropriate terminology is also imperative. Medical jargon is not understood by most patients, yet over-simplification may be interpreted as being condescending. 'An obstruction to the blood supply to a portion of your heart' may be understood, alongside a picture depicting the explanation whereas 'ischemic changes on your ECG' and a copy of the ECG will likely not.

Conclusion

It should be remembered that the nursing needs of patients do not disappear when there is not a nurse present, and that the harsh environment of the air ambulance or commercial aircraft compounds many of the problems that require nursing care to resolve. Patients can be transferred far more effectively, safely and comfortably by thinking about them holistically and by anticipating problems before they arise, rather than by simply addressing their primary medical conditions.

References

Topley, D.K., Schmelz J., Henkenius-Kirschbaum J. and K.J. Horvath (2003) 'Critical care nursing expertise during air transport', *Milit Med.* **168**(10):822-6.
Bader, G.B., Terhorst, M., Heilman, P., DePalma, J.A. (1995) 'Characteristics of flight nursing practice', *Air Med J.* **14**(4):214-8.
Wilson, P. (1998) 'Safe patient transport: nurses make a difference', *Nursing Times.* **94**(26):66-7.

PART V
Organization and Administration

Chapter 18

The Administration of Aeromedical Transport Organizations

Types of services

There are wide variations in the type of aeromedical transportation services operating around the world, but several major categories have emerged. One of the most common is the hospital-based helicopter system, which serves to transport patients from outlying referral centers to the base hospital or other facilities as dictated by patient needs. The majority of these services also function as advanced life support (ALS) providers and respond to calls from prehospital EMS personnel for assistance. Flight programs are often based in academic medical centers or tertiary care facilities, and may be sponsored by a consortium of institutions. While the service may be sponsored by a hospital, the hospital may not own the aircraft. Aviation equipment, pilots, and mechanics are often leased from vendors familiar with the needs of air medical services.

Private independent services also exist, and most commonly operate fixed wing aircraft. These programs are often based out of airports and feature medically configured aircraft staffed by on-call medical attendants. They may integrate with hospital flight programs to provide aircraft and pilots while using medical crew provided by the hospital. These services may have significantly higher overhead costs and may work on fee-for-service arrangements, a subscription basis, or a combination of both.

Public service agencies may also sponsor aeromedical services. Aircraft used by these programs are often multifunctional vehicles serving in medical, search and rescue, fire suppression, and law enforcement roles. As they are sponsored by local, regional, or national authorities, costs are borne by the public at large. Any of these agents may sponsor both fixed and rotor wing services. Other types of aeromedical transportation services include those operated by military forces or voluntary agencies, or those for whom aeromedical transportation is a secondary mission.

Policies and protocols

All aeromedical services must operate under a policy and protocol umbrella in order to ensure that operations are consistent and open to objective evaluation. Both of these types of documents originate from the program's mission statement, which outlines in broad terms the goals of the service. Policies represent specific statements of intent designed to meet these targets, while protocols are the actual steps to be taken in fulfillment of the policy goal. As protocols are operational documents, they should be written in a fashion that allows quick reference, and that outlines actions to be taken in a sequential fashion, allowing minimum room for error. Policies and protocols must reflect all aspects of aeromedical transportation, and should be designed for medical, aviation, communication, personnel, and financial aspects of the operation.

Protocols should be specific and detailed to eliminate ambiguity. Within clinical protocols, it must be clearly understood when on-line medical control is to be utilized. Protocols must be constructed with sufficient flexibility to allow aeromedical crew to act in a manner consistent with the patient's best interests when unanticipated situations arise or on-line medical control is not available.

The medical director

Every aeromedical transportation service must have a designated medical director. While the scope of medical direction will vary by program mission, legal and regulatory requirements, and physician commitment and time, the medical director must always serve as the ultimate authority and bear final responsibility for all patient care aspects of the transport system.

All aspects of an aeromedical program, from salary structures to work schedules and aircraft maintenance requirements, may at some point impact upon patient care. The medical director may choose to be involved in any or all of these areas of concern. Many will opt to leave the supervision of non-clinical areas to others with the requisite training, experience, and expertise. However, patient care protocols, criteria for flight, staffing patterns, on and off-line medical supervision, and flight crew education and training all remain fully within the domain of the medical director. Participation by the supervising physician in safety, communications, and quality assurance (QA) and continuous quality improvement (CQI) programs is also of key importance.

The provision of safe and efficacious aeromedical transportation requires that the medical director be appropriately qualified. Unfortunately, there is little. The US based Air Medical Physician Association (AMPA) has published a position paper outlining the optimal background for this role, and some authors suggest that the medical director be a specialist in emergency or critical care medicine, and should have a thorough knowledge of flight physiology. The US Association of Air Medical Services (AAMS) and the Commission on Accreditation of Air Medical Services (CAAMS) propose similar qualifications. The medical director must also possess a current license to practice medicine in the state, province, or country which serves as the program's headquarters. This is especially important in those settings where the operational protocols for nurses and paramedics require physician endorsement.

Flight programs are extremely variable with respect to the type of missions they undertake. The medical director must have an in-depth knowledge of the myriad of transport difficulties and inflight patient care problems anticipated within the system. An awareness of the prehospital care environment, local hospital and physician resources, and regional referral patterns is critical to the successful completion of aeromedical assignments.

One of the most complex tasks facing the medical director is personnel management. Professionals in aeromedical transportation tend to be independent, knowledgeable, and highly motivated. To deal effectively with staff, the medical director must command the respect of the crew. This is obtained not only by clinical expertise, but by possessing the ability to listen to the concerns of the individuals within the team. Emotional maturity and conflict resolution skills are crucial to the role of mentor and guide.

The medical director should practice audit and must directly review a certain proportion of transfer documents. A forum should exist to discuss deaths, complications, or difficult cases encountered by aeromedical crew. This 'morbidity and mortality' review may be incorporated into flight crew meetings and should be an educational experience. Evaluation of team members must be a continuous process. The quality of care provided by each aeromedical escort may be assessed through case presentations, skills may be assessed in animal or mannequin training sessions, and performance on flights may be evaluated through on-line observation and retrospective reviews of medical docuents. The medical director may conduct these reviews or delegate this responsibility to other qualified parties. All reviews should provide constructive feedback for individual staff and must be documented.

Many medical directors believe that they do not need documented terms of reference, but a written contract or agreement is imperative. Some have informal verbal agreements with their employers and may be unaware of the responsibilities of directorship imposed by governmental agencies, and of the liability associated with supervision of physician surrogates in the field. Those that provide medical direction for services with flight physicians may wrongly assume that the presence of the other doctor mitigates their liability for the care provided (see Chapter 19).

If one accepts that the medical director is responsible for the establishment, maintenance, and monitoring of the quality of medical care delivered within the service, it follows that any legal action concerning the medical care delivered will involve the medical director of that service. Informal agreements made with administration may disappear as personnel change, or in response to evolving perceptions or priorities within the sponsoring organization. In addition, the decisions and opinions of the medical director may not always be popular. Without a written contract, an organization may find it more convenient to change medical directors than to change operations!

The medical director of an aeromedical service who wishes to avoid conflict and confusion in fulfilling his duties must therefore have his role and terms of reference clarified in writing. Essential elements of this agreement include responsibility, authority, liability, and compensation. Defining these elements offers both the contracting organization and the medical director a clear understanding of performance expectations. As the needs of the service change, additions or deletions can be agreed by both parties, in order to accommodate the director's evolving role.

Quality assurance and continuous quality improvement

The implementation of QA and CQI programs are key to maintaining quality control, measuring efficacy, and ensuring the cost effectiveness of any aeromedical transportation system. The work of QA and CQI must involve all members of the transport team.

The clinical CQI plan should address overall program issues. Examples include appropriate utilization of the aircraft, the level of care provided prior to flight crew intervention, and the care provided by receiving hospitals for given patient populations (especially when the program assists in determining patient destination). Clinical staff should actively participate in the CQI plan developed by the communication and aviation components of the air transport system. The converse is also true, as communications and aviation staff can often make valuable contributions to patient care.

A model QA/CQI program has been described by the United States Joint Commission on Accreditation of Hospitals (JCAH). This '10 Step Plan' is outlined in Table 18.1.

Integration of EMS, hospital, and transportation services

Aeromedical services should seek to develop and maintain good professional relationships with all prehospital care agencies within their service area. In many EMS systems, paramedics are empowered with the ability to request a helicopter for scene response. Given the expense and intensity of resources used in a prehospital response, it is essential that the aeromedical program provides the field paramedic with the appropriate triage criteria, the means to access the aircraft, and possibly the tools to locate, secure, and mark landing zones. Ground providers must also know how to prepare patients for air transport, and how to safely approach the aircraft and assist the flight crew in patient loading. The aeromedical program must take the initiative in developing triage criteria and offering educational programs for local EMS providers. The cultivation of close working relationships with local EMS teams, based upon the shared goal of enhancing patient care, allows for quality improvement information and recommendations to flow in both directions. By establishing regular channels of communication and feedback, the occasional problem incident is easily addressed and maybe even prevented.

Aeromedical services may also interact with ground EMS services during interfacility transports, especially when the use of fixed wing aircraft necessitates ground ambulance transfer of the patient to and from an airport. A knowledge of the capabilities of local EMS services can assist the flight team in determining the safety of patient transport to the airport, the need for carriage of equipment, and the degree of assistance that can be expected from local personnel.

Table 18.1   Model quality assurance/continuous quality improvement program

1	Assign responsibility	Responsibility for QA and CQI activities should be specifically delineated and assigned.
2	Describe the scope of service	The mission statement should be a concise description of the services offered, structural components of the program, and types of patients the program serves. QA and CQI activities will focus on the organizational goals established in the mission statement.
3	Identify aspects of care that are high risk, frequent, or problem prone	Aspects of care considered high risk, frequent, or prone to difficulties must be identified. The individuals responsible for CQI within a program should discuss these points in detail and studies may be designed to result in the most effective improvement in quality.
4	Develop indicators and measurable components	Indicators must be identified to facilitate data collection on specific aspects of care. Indicators are utilized to establish proposed standards. An example of an indicator is the statement, All hypoxic patients receive supplemental oxygen.
5	Establish thresholds	A threshold is a predetermined optimal level of compliance with an indicator. In establishing a threshold, one must take into account a balance between the ideal world and reality. It is best to be conservative in the early stages of establishing thresholds. CQI may opt to continually increase the threshold over time.
6	Collect and organize data	Methods for data collection appropriate to the measurement of indicators and thresholds must be determined.
7	Analyze data	Review of the data collected should take place at specified intervals using appropriate descriptive and analytical statistical techniques. A uniform interval of study should be established to aid in the determination of trends.
8	Create an action plan	If trends are identified which require correction, an action plan should be developed. Methods for implementing, recording, and updating progress on the action plan must be devised.
9	Evaluate the effectiveness of action	After a problem has been identified and an action plan enacted, the problem should be restudied at a designated time to insure that the action plan has been effective.
10	Communicate relevant information	Any information generated from CQI data analysis should be communicated to aeromedical personnel and the administration of the organization. Communication may also include individuals who are the customers of the service (that is, the patients and health care providers who refer patients to the system).

Good relations between aeromedical programs and hospital staff are also essential. Both medical and nursing staff need to be made aware of aeromedical resources. They must be educated as to when flight is the most appropriate transfer medium, and the need for proper patient packaging prior to departure. In addition, they must possess an understanding of the role of the aeromedical team so they do not feel demeaned or slighted if patient management is altered in preparation for transport. For their part, aeromedical crew must be sensitive to the feelings of hospital staff, and never undermine their efforts unless a patient's wellbeing is at stake (and then only with appropriate on-line medical support). Communication is the key to conflict resolution and prevention.

Often, aeromedical teams make the mistake of underestimating the capabilities of local personnel. As a result, flight crew may be perceived as having a negative, condescending attitude towards ground EMS or hospital staff. This attitude is to be discouraged at all times. Not all medical care can be provided at the tertiary care level familiar to aeromedical crew. Given limited resources and training, many prehospital and hospital personnel provide exemplary care. Flight crew should offer praise and support when appropriate, and education, not criticism, when it is not.

Regulatory aspects

Every aeromedical transport program, whether public or private, civilian or military, will be bound by specific regulatory authorities. These authorities may exist at the national, regional, or local levels, and may concern themselves with aviation activities, medical management, communications programs, or the financial practices of the transport system. The regulatory system can be complex and replete with legal pitfalls. Each program must investigate the regulatory environment in which it exists and tailor its operations accordingly. Flight programs should participate actively in the regulatory system to ensure that high standards of patient care are mandated.

Research in aeromedical transportation

It may seem unusual to consider research as an administrative issue but, in fact, research activities give flight service managers and medical supervisors the ability to make informed decisions. The image of research as a laboratory-based entity is not applicable, nor appropriate, to the aeromedical industry. Research may be descriptive, demographic, operational, or economic in nature. All of these formats can provide vital information, given proper study design, data collection, and interpretation of results.

Research has the power to identify and solve problems, but the relative youth and continuing evolution of aeromedical services mean that research into the needs for, and efficacy of, aeromedical transportation has been lacking. The small database that currently exists lends itself to heated discussions regarding the efficacy of aeromedical transportation, and personal opinions often remain based on anecdote and intuition.

While we know that many kinds of patients with a variety of conditions can be transported safely by air, very little data exists to authoritatively state which patient groups should be transported, at what stage of their illness or recovery they should be flown, and the efficacy of such flights. At present, the research base in aeromedical transportation can be said to have proven only four hypotheses (Table 18.2).

Table 18.2   Proven hypotheses in aeromedical transport

1. There are limitations in patient care imposed by the flight environment.
2. Patients in cardiopulmonary arrest without signs of life noted by EMS providers gain no benefit from helicopter transport.
3. Aeromedical helicopters are involved in accidents.
4. Aeromedical transportation is expensive.

There is a critical need for continued research, and expansion of the industry's common database should be an important goal of every flight service. Future research efforts should be directed towards the further exploration of the limitations of patient care while aloft and the development of solutions to those obstacles. Safety, cost-benefit analyses, and patient outcomes research (particularly for the non-trauma patient) are fields ripe for investigation.

References

Air Medical Physician Association (2002) 'Medical direction and medical control of air medical services. Position statement of the Air Medical Physician Association', *Prehosp Emerg Care.* **6**(4):461-3.

Balazs, K.T. and C. B. Thompson (1996) 'Quality assurance and continuous quality improvement within air transport programs', *Air Med J.* **15**(3):104-7.

Benson, N.J., Jacobsen J.T. and J.S. Wynn (1990) 'Quality assurance models for air medical services', in Eastes L. and J. T. Jacobsen (eds.), *Quality Assurance in Air Medical Transport*, Word Perfect Publishing:Orem, Utah.

Berns, K.S., Caniglia, J.J., Hankins, D.G. and S.P. Zietlow (2003) 'Use of the autolaunch method of dispatching a helicopter', *Air Med J.* **22**(3):35-41.

Carrubba, C. (1994) 'Empowerment of the medical director: the written contract', in: Blumen, I.J. and H. Rodenberg (eds), *Air Medical Physician's Handbook*, AMPA: Salt Lake City.

Department of Transportation (DOT) (1990) 'National Highway Traffic Safety Administration and the American Medical Association Commission on Emergency Medical Services air ambulance guidelines', *Emerg Med Serv.* **19**(12):220.

Gabram, S.G.A. and N.J. Benson (1994) Quality improvement: an introductory guide for air medical physicians', in Blumen, I. J. and H. Rodenberg (eds), *Air Medical Physician's Handbook*, AMPA: Salt Lake City.

Gibbons, H.L. (1984) 'Regulations and the air ambulance', *Aviat Space Environ Med.* **55**(3):239-43.

Hotvedt, R., Kristiansen, I.S., Forde, O.H., Thoner, J., Almdahl, S.M., et al. (1996) 'Which groups of patients benefit from helicopter evacuation?', *Lancet.* **347**(9012):1362-6.

Hunt, R. (1994) 'Research in air medical transport', in Blumen' I. J. and H. Rodenberg (eds), *Air Medical Physician's Handbook*, AMPA: Salt Lake City.

Polsky, S., Krohmer, J., Maningas, P., et al. (1993) 'Guidelines for medical direction of prehospital EMS', *Ann Emerg Med.* **22**:742-4.

Poulton, T.J. and P.A. Kisicki (1987) 'Medical directors of critical care air transport services', *Critical Care Medicine.* **15**:84-5.

Thomas, F., Gibbons, H. and T.P. Clemmer (1986) 'Air ambulance regulations: a model', *Aviat Space Environ Med.* **57**(7):699-705.

Thomson, D.P. and S.H. Thomas (2003) '2002-2003 Air Medical Services Committee of the National Association of EMS Physicians: Guidelines for air medical dispatch', *Prehosp Emerg Care.* **7**(2):265-71.

Walker, R. (1994) 'Qualification and training of the air medical director', in: Blumen I. J. and H. Rodenberg (eds), *Air Medical Physician's Handbook*, AMPA: Salt Lake City.

Chapter 19

Medicolegal Aspects of Aeromedical Transport

Introduction

Any text written on the medicolegal aspects of aeromedical transport can never be complete. Although general principles are likely to be relevant throughout the world, it would be impossible in a book of this size to discuss the legal implications of every possible dilemma, situation, or incident that may arise. The discussion in this chapter is therefore an illustration based on experience in English speaking nations, especially Britain and the USA. Jurisprudence in all English speaking countries has its origins in centuries of English (not British[1]) common law. Compared with this, the history of aviation, and specifically of aeromedical transport, is short. Outside of North America, few legal cases involving air ambulance organizations or personnel have so far found their way into the legal literature. However, we live in an increasingly litigious society, and aeromedical organizations, and those that work for them, should be aware of their potential liabilities. Medical directors must take responsibility for the selection, assessment, training, and supervision of personnel, for documentation, quality assurance, and the periodic review of medical protocols and guidelines used by the service. The issues of standards of care, consent, liability, documentation, confidentiality, and clinical management guidelines, within the constraints imposed by operating in the flight environment, reflect those that are important in normal terrestrial practice. However, for flights that cross international borders, these problems are compounded by such issues as jurisdiction, importation and exportation of drugs, international health regulations, and birth and death in flight.

Aeromedical practice is separated into helicopter and fixed wing services, and the potential liability differs significantly in each group. The operation, and hence the liability, of a helicopter emergency medical service in the prehospital environment is similar to that of a ground ambulance. Although it is normally the employer who is vicariously liable (literally *'second-hand liability'*) for the acts and omissions of an employee, the medical director of the HEMS system may also be deemed responsible for the actions of emergency medical personnel under his supervision.

---

1   UK has two major legal systems: English law (actually England and the principality of Wales) and Scottish law. Great Britain and United Kingdom are not synonymous terms. The UK is the United Kingdom of Great Britain, Northern Ireland and the Channel Islands.

This is the legal concept of *respondeat superior* ('let the master answer', that is, the 'master' is liable in certain cases for the wrongful acts of his 'servant').

Fixed wing air ambulance services are principally used for interhospital transport. These organizations may be considered under the stricter standards that normally apply to airlines and charter carriers. Medical directors share responsibility for the negligent action of their medical personnel but may have their liability superseded by another doctor, such as the one who requests the transport and who gives the transfer orders.

It is a striking but hardly surprising observation by the author, that everyone in the aeromedical industry seems concerned with liability and its risks. Inflight medical personnel, flight crew, air ambulance operators, medical assistance companies, and medical directors each face the risk of liability, not only for their own actions, but also for those working under or for them. The issues are complex but, to take the most simplistic approach first, let us consider a fully qualified and registered British doctor, escorting a patient of British nationality, on board a British aircraft, belonging to a British airline, in UK airspace (or, similarly, for a flight physician of any other nation in like circumstances). In this situation, the responsibilities and obligations of that doctor are no different than they are in normal everyday practice.

Medicolegal issues general to all medical transport flights

Good Samaritan acts

A Good Samaritan act has been described as *'the provision of clinical services related to a clinical emergency, accident or disaster when you are not present in your professional capacity but as a bystander'*.

The ethical body for British doctors, the UK General Medical Council (GMC), changed its guidance on Good Samaritan acts following the 9/11 atrocities in 2001, and these changes have significant implications for doctors in the UK. All registered medical practitioners now have an enforceable ethical obligation to provide Good Samaritan assistance where appropriate. The GMC states:

> In an emergency, wherever it may arise, you must offer anyone at risk the assistance you could reasonably be expected to provide.

There have been no cases of successful litigation against a doctor in a British court arising from a Good Samaritan act and, at the time of writing, only one known case in the USA. In spite of this, fear of litigation is often quoted as a reason why American doctors appear to hesitate to volunteer assistance. At least 40 of the states in America have therefore passed legislation to protect Good Samaritan doctors.

Some medical malpractice organizations (such as the Medical Defence Union in the UK) insure their members for Good Samaritan acts worldwide. However, doctors should clarify the situation with their own medical malpractice organization because discretionary indemnity may only give them the right to ask for legal assistance, not to receive it. The prospect of giving assistance as a Good Samaritan therefore still causes anxiety among some doctors.

The doctor's ethical duty is not in doubt, but under English (and USA) civil law, a doctor has no legal duty of care to volunteer as a Good Samaritan. In other words, it is not open to a patient to sue a doctor when there is no pre-existing duty of care. In contrast, failure to offer assistance to a person in distress in France is a criminal offence under paragraph 2 of article 63 of the French penal code, and this applies to everyone, not just doctors.

The standard of care expected of health care professionals is described below, but it is worth noting that the GMC requires all doctors to recognize the limits of their competence and, where appropriate, a doctor should step back and allow someone else to take over, such as a paramedic.

Standards of care

The doctor/patient relationship is a rather special one and, to some extent, the flight nurse or paramedic acting alone during medical missions shares many of the fundamental obligations and responsibilities of this relationship. Under normal circumstances, a form of contract exists between the parties. In other words, a patient requests diagnostic and therapeutic services, and the doctor agrees to provide his or her professional advice and accepts a duty to provide the appropriate standard of medical care.

In the prehospital or emergency environment, this traditional view of the contract does not seem to apply. After all, the patient is likely to be unconscious or even moribund and will not have purposefully and intentionally sought a doctor's advice before the emergency actually occurs. However, once a doctor or other health professional offers diagnostic or therapeutic advice, in other words, he *undertakes to treat* a patient, he is, in effect, forming a contract, even in the absence of any mutual consent.

Liability only occurs when the health professional fails to meet the accepted standards of care (that is, to exercise the degree of knowledge, skill and due care expected of a reasonably competent practitioner in the same class, acting in the same or similar circumstances). This means that the ATLS trained surgeon will be expected to exercise a greater degree of knowledge, skill and due care than, perhaps, the public health doctor who never intentionally sees acute trauma patients. There is an issue here for inflight physicians. It would be expected that those doctors employed by air ambulance organizations have a greater understanding of aviation physiology and transport medicine than, say, a doctor who is traveling as a passenger and who happens to volunteer his services in an emergency. Although the volunteer may not be aware of the potential dangers of gaseous expansion at altitude, such ignorance in an employee paid for his expertise as an aeromedical escort would be considered to fall short of the expected standards of care.

Despite the doctor's own self-imposed moral code, or those ethical obligations imposed by professional organizations, in most countries there is no legal duty to rescue or resuscitate another person. Technically then, from the legal standpoint, the doctor who encounters an emergency by chance (such as our example, above), need not offer his services. Unless that is, it is his own patient who is involved (even if he were not specifically called to treat that patient).

However, once treatment is started, a legal duty exists to do all that is reasonable to complete the resuscitation successfully, although the law would not expect anyone to put his own life at risk in doing so. Many are worried about the possibility of litigation for negligence or malpractice under such circumstances. However, many governmental bodies and medical defense organizations have initiated *Good Samaritan* regulations to encourage potential rescuers to render aid in emergency situations. In point of fact, litigation in such instances is virtually unheard of.

Consent

In an emergency situation, when life is at risk, the law will infer consent, even if it is not formally or informally obtained. The law presumes that any reasonable person would want his life saved under such circumstances. Having said that, adult individuals of sound mind do have the right to refuse treatment, as do courts acting on behalf of those who are minors or those incapable of making such decisions. The rider is, of course, that the patient must be fully aware of the consequences of such refusal.

An 'Advance Statement' (*Living Will*) allows a person, when healthy and of sound mind, to state how he would wish to be treated if unable to express an opinion. These documents are becoming increasingly common among those who do not wish to be resuscitated, kept artificially alive, or who have no wish to have life prolonged after suffering serious damage with no prospect of normal recovery. An Advance Statement is legally binding upon doctors but, clearly, only when its existence is known.

Technically, a *battery* (an *assault* in some countries) is committed whenever there is an intentional and unpermitted *touching* of another person. The provision of medical care in the absence of consent may therefore be considered as an act of assault. Nevertheless, as already mentioned, the law will normally presume consent in life threatening circumstances.

Liability

No doctor or other medical professional need fear litigation if diligence and due care is exercised during the management of the patient. To reiterate, the standard of care is the degree of knowledge, skill and due care expected of a reasonably competent practitioner in the same class, acting in the same or similar circumstances. A successful law suit would be required to prove that the health professional had performed in a grossly negligent manner, for instance in failing to recognize unsuccessful intubation, or forgetting to stabilize the cervical spine during resuscitation. Furthermore, negligence requires the plaintiff to prove four elements which are set out in Table 19.1.

Table 19.1   Elements of proof required in cases of negligence

- To establish the standard of care by expert medical testimony.
- To establish a breach of that standard.
- To demonstrate an injury.
- To establish that the breach of duty was the logical and legal cause of the claimed injury.

Careless conduct may constitute grounds for legal liability, even though the fault upon which it is predicated is attributable to a lack of care or skill, rather than to a conscious design to do wrong. A patient who suffers an injury through the act of another person, in which the requisite elements of negligence and cause are present, is entitled to invoke the process of law to obtain compensation. Injury in itself, though, confers no legal rights. When the misfortune of the plaintiff is not attributable to any person, the law has no redress. Many argue that compensation should be paid to those who suffer disability or distress, despite no fault being attributable. Some countries have adopted such *No Fault Liability* laws, and compensation is paid from government or other central funds.

Negligence, in itself, is not liability. The basic determinant of liability for negligence is fault, a breach of a duty imposed by law or contract. In theory, any person (for example, flight nurses and paramedics, as well as doctors) can be held liable for negligence, but only where there is failure to observe the standard of care which the law requires him to observe in the performance of a duty owed by him to the injured person. Clearly, these standards differ between the professions and, in a team situation, the most senior person may carry responsibility for his juniors. When a doctor is present, final responsibility for the wellbeing of the patient will be his, although liability may be shared by medical directors and supervising physicians, especially if consulted in flight, by radio or telemetry.

Air ambulance management may also face liabilities and should attempt to minimize risk appropriately. Screening of applicants for flight and medical crew employment, maintaining an active QA/CQI program, and budgeting for adequate malpractice and other insurance premiums are essential to the air ambulance administration. Medical managers must take an active interest in documentation, quality assurance, assessment and supervision of aeromedical personnel, and the currency and accuracy of the medical care protocols used by the transport service. Relationships between members of the team must be carefully delineated. Since the medical staff, operators, and flight crew are all mutually dependant upon one another, a rapport is crucial to minimize potential liabilities. Furthermore, doctors employed by aeromedical organizations should ensure that they have personal medical malpractice insurance for work overseas, and that it offers sufficient cover.

Documentation

A common problem in cases of malpractice liability is the poor standard of documentation. Good notes are essential; memory cannot be relied upon and, even if it could be, amounts to nothing more than unsubstantiated evidence in a court of law. An aeromedical transfer is in continuum with the pre and post-transport phases of patient management, and cannot be viewed in isolation. As a result, there is a requirement for aeromedical personnel to maintain accurate, legible, clear, and concise documentation, annotating all treatments, incidents, interventions and other significant interactions with the patient, relatives or other third parties which may have a bearing on the patient's clinical condition or management. Every entry must be preceded with the current date and time (local, and also UTC/GMT on international flights), and signed when completed. Alterations to records must be signed and similarly annotated with the date, time and reason for the correction clearly stated, at the time the alteration was made. Lawyers are normally highly suspicious of changes made retrospectively to medical notes and charts. On the other hand, if a notable event has not been documented then, in the eyes of the law it has not happened. Proof may not necessarily be the same as truth!

Many air ambulance organizations maintain their own transfer records (Figure 19.1). When these are not provided, it is permissible to continue documentation in the hospital notes. The first entry in interhospital transfer cases, and when collecting patients for repatriation, must be a preflight assessment to identify or exclude problems which may be important to the safe and efficient conduct of the transfer. Included at this stage should be the results of any investigations or special examinations necessary before decisions on fitness to fly, or on the conditions of the transfer, are made. During the journey, itself, clear details of the transfer process should be entered, along with an aeromedical summary at the safe conclusion of the transfer. Although dictaphone tapes are not considered legal documents, they may be used for contemporaneous note taking, as long as they are transcribed into written form at the earliest opportunity.

At the destination, hand-over of the patient to the receiving medical team should include transfer of all notes, radiographs and investigations received from the referring hospital, along with the aeromedical summary which should outline the logistic details of the journey, stopovers, delays, and time zones crossed, as well as the clinical details described above.

Notes taken during primary missions will inevitably be shorter and specifically relevant to the prehospital emergency situation (Figure 19.2). Despite the need for brevity, the same considerations must apply, that is, that they are written in a clear, concise, accurate, and legible manner, appropriately dated and signed, with the timings of the incident, arrival on scene, and arrival at hospital duly noted. If necessary, fuller notes can be sent by fax or e-mail once the emergency transfer has been completed.

In many countries patients have open access to their medical documents. In the European Community these powers have been extended to include all written

europ assistance

Europ Assistance Holdings Limited, 252, High Street, Croydon, Surrey CR0 1NF
Tel No: 0181-680 1234   Fax No: 0181-680 8992

SURNAME:	FILE REF:
FIRST NAMES:	DATE OF TRANSPORT:
ADDRESS:	AGE: D. OF B:
	MALE ☐ FEMALE ☐
	TELEPHONE:
G.P.:	TELEPHONE:
RELATIVE IN ATTENDANCE: NAME:	
RELATIONSHIP:	TELEPHONE:

	OVERSEAS	DESTINATION
HOSPITAL		
WARD / ROOM		
TOWN		
COUNTRY		
DOCTOR		
TELEPHONE		

TIME (UK)	DEPART HOSPITAL / HOTEL	ARRIVE HOSPITAL / HOME

AIR AMBULANCE ☐	JET ☐	TURBO ☐	TYPE:		
AIRLINE ☐	SEATED [1] [3]	STRETCHER ☐	COMPANY:		
HELICOPTER ☐	FERRY ☐	OTHER ☐			
ROUTE:		CHARTER ☐	SCHEDULED ☐		

ORIGINAL FLIGHT: [Y] [N]

CLASS:	FIRST ☐	CLUB ☐	ECONOMY ☐
LEVEL OF ASSISTANCE:	WCHR ☐	WCHS ☐	WCHC ☐
OXYGEN:	SUPPLIED [Y] [N]		USED [Y] [N]
	L / MINUTE		CONTINUOUS [Y] [N]
CABIN ALTITUDE:	THOUSAND FEET		
UK TRANSPORT:	AMBULANCE ☐	TAXI ☐	COMPANY:

PATIENT TRANSPORT TIME:	HOURS
PATIENT FLIGHT TIME:	HOURS

WHITE TOP COPY TO HOSPITAL / GP   WHITE CARD COPY TO EA

Figure 19.1   Typical air ambulance transfer documentation

documents as well as computer records. It would be unwise, therefore, to write anything which would later prove embarrassing if read out in a court of law, or which one would not wish the patient or his relatives to see.

Confidentiality

Patients are entitled to expect that information learned by members of the medical team during the course of the transfer will remain confidential. Doctors carry the prime responsibility for the protection of this information, whether it is verbal, written, on tape, or computerized, but clearly this responsibility will be delegated when flight nurses or paramedics escort patients alone.

Patients (or those acting legally on their behalf) must consent to the disclosure of information and specific refusal for permission to disclose must normally be respected. However, if in the opinion of the medical escort, disclosure is considered essential and in the best interests of the patient, he must be prepared to justify that decision later. For instance, the captain of a dedicated air ambulance is usually informed of the general nature of the patient's condition because of any constraints or limitations that it may impose on the operation of the aircraft. The flight physician or other medical escort must use his judgment to ensure that disclosure does not exceed the level of information that the third party really needs to know. It is also wise for the medical escort to inform the patient that a disclosure has been made and, if the patient raises objections, full details should be documented in the transfer notes.

Clinical management guidelines

Until comparatively recently the medical profession has been free to exercise the science of medicine according to its traditions, standards and knowledge, without interference or regulation. Clinical practice is now increasingly being governed by practice policies, protocols, guidelines and codes of practice. Although some argue that these changes are designed to modify or control the clinical behavior of individual practitioners, most are comforted by the knowledge that adherence to such policies offers some protection against liability. However, while the evidential basis for many clinical guidelines remains to be confirmed, their legal status may also be questioned.

In America, steps are underway to produce legally validated clinical guidelines to ensure that doctors who comply with them are shielded against liability in malpractice cases. However, in English courts, since guidelines and policies are written documents (and therefore cannot be cross-examined) they are considered only hearsay evidence. They may be accepted as customary standards of care, but are no substitute for expert testimony. An expert witness can be questioned on such issues as how the guidelines were developed, how effectively they have been adopted, and whether there is a significant body that rejects them in favor of a different approach.

Helicopter Emergency Medical Service

Forename: **Surname:** **M/F** **Age:**

Date: **Incident time:** **HEMS Dr:**

Mechanism: RTA Sport Domestic Assault Industrial Fall<2m >2m

Type: Blunt Penetrating Burn Inhalation

Vehicle: Car M/C Bicycle Commercial PSV Other

Person: Pedestrian Driver Front Pass. Rear Pass.

Involved with: Bicycle Other Veh. Street Furniture Loss of Control

Detail: Ejection Entrapment Assoc Fatality

Protection: Seat Belt Helmet Other: | **RTA Data** |

Map Ref/Postcode:

Apparent Injuries:

Interventions: DC Shock x
Oxygen Surgical Airway NETT OETT
Chest Drain Collar Splint RED MAST
IV Lines x Cutdown CVC
Hartmanns: Haemaccel:

Drugs:

Time	Pulse	B.P.	Resps	Eyes/4	Verbal/5	Motor/6	G.C.S.	Sat%

Reason for Triage Decision: Signed:

Figure 19.2 Typical HEMS documentation

DNR orders

Perhaps one of the more contentious issues is when to stop resuscitation efforts or, indeed, whether they should be started at all. Although brain death criteria are useful in the intensive care unit scenario, during the prehospital phase, especially in the transport environment, such a diagnosis cannot be made. DNR (*Do Not Resuscitate*) policies are popularly used by HEMS operators in the USA, but there remains a reluctance in many parts of the world to legislate on an issue which is seen to carry so much emotional impact and potential for litigation. Under these circumstances the best measure of failure to resuscitate is cardiac unresponsiveness. The law simply requires that reasonable medical judgment has been used in making the decision to stop resuscitation attempts. In other words, that the medical facts have been considered, and that a logical conclusion has been drawn after exercising diligence and due care during the diagnostic process. Naturally, when medical judgment is reasonable, it can easily be confirmed and substantiated by colleagues.

Medicolegal issues specific to international missions

Jurisdiction

Earlier in this chapter, an example of the most simple medicolegal scenario was described as a British Doctor with a British patient in a British registered aircraft in British airspace. The situation is easily clouded when different national interests are at stake, not least because some legal systems vary significantly from the English law model. Islamic law is a prime example.

The unfortunate destruction of Pan Am Flight 109 over Lockerbie, Scotland, in 1988 clearly demonstrated the many legal complexities that can occur with incidents on international flights. The question of jurisdiction depends on a number of factors, and potential for dispute is high. Jurisdiction is defined as the power or the right to administer justice and to apply laws. When an aircraft is in international airspace, the country with jurisdiction may well be disputed, depending on the nature of the incident or situation in question. Jurisdiction may belong to the country of origin of the aircraft, or the airline or carrier, the country in which the aircraft is registered (sometimes different from the above), or where the crew are based, the country most recently overflown, or the one most recently departed. In addition, the national interests of the passengers may be paramount (and they may come from a multitude of countries), as well as those of the flight, cabin or medical crew.

In some countries, in particular in the USA, the patient population is much more litigious than in others. If an incident occurs on an American registered aircraft, or involves an American patient on a foreign aircraft, an action might be brought in an American court. In Great Britain, the level of damages awarded after a successful action is usually determined by the judge. In the USA, the award is set by a civil jury and the amounts involved are usually staggeringly in excess of those awarded in

Britain. Because of this, British malpractice insurers specifically exclude cover for litigation expenses in the United States resulting from the policy holder's activities, wherever they may have taken place. For this reason, all medical personnel working in international repatriation must be sure of adequate supplemental insurance cover for liability in the American courts.

Another unique concern in air ambulance operations is the issue of licensing and professional practice across national borders (and State boundaries in the USA). There is potential for liability, or even criminal action, if medical care is carried by an aeromedical escort, or under the authority of a medical director, not licensed to practice medicine at the site of patient pickup or delivery. International transfers also raise concerns about visas, border controls, and the carriage of controlled substances.

Importation and exportation of drugs

Most countries prohibit the importation and export of medicines unless they are required for an individual's personal treatment or unless import/export permission has previously been authorized. Some drugs appear on controlled lists in some countries but not in others, and it would be wise to maintain an inventory of all drugs carried and also a record of those actually used during the transfer.

In the United States, controlled drugs are supplied only if the DEA (Drugs Enforcement Agency) registration number of the prescribing physician is known. This is not so in the UK, where any registered practitioner can write a prescription for controlled drugs, as long as that prescription is correctly completed with the dose prescribed written in both words and numbers. In both countries, though, it is incumbent upon the doctor to ensure absolute security of the drugs. This means that a close watch must be kept on all equipment bags (especially when they are opened), and accurate records of drug use must be kept.

Annual export licenses are available through air ambulance and medical assistance companies so that named individuals can take drugs out of the country but, equally as important, can also bring them back again if unused. A letter from the medical director (preferably written in the language spoken at the destination or pickup point overseas) explaining the medical nature of the mission may ease problems at immigration and customs. In any case, an inventory should be available for presentation, and the equipment bag available for inspection. Even then, problems may still arise, for instance, diamorphine (*heroin*), a commonly used analgesic drug in the UK, is prohibited in the USA, even in controlled medical use.

International Health Regulations

The problems of global spread of disease, in an age of rapid long distance travel made easily available to millions have been known for many years. Most countries are signatories to the World Health Organization's (WHO) International Health Regulations (IHRs), or have adopted their own (usually more stringent) regulations based on IHRs. An example of the latter is the United Kingdom's Public Health (Aircraft) Regulations of 1979. The original IHR code of practice was established in 1969 with the stated aim 'to ensure the maximum security against the international spread of disease with minimum interference to world traffic'. The current IHRs which were revised in 2005 go beyond the 1983 revision (designed to tackle the worldwide eradication of smallpox). The regulations cover immunization procedures, quarantine methods, and the prevention of transmission of disease and of disease vectors.

In the 1983 IHRs, there were only three diseases which were 'subject to the regulations' and for which special provisions are made. These were cholera, yellow fever, and plague. A further five diseases (poliomyelitis, influenza, malaria, louse-borne relapsing fever, and louse-borne typhus) were added as 'diseases under surveillance', and countries were free to add other diseases of local concern. In the UK, the list included Lassa fever, Marburg disease, viral hemorrhagic fever and rabies, but the regulations were loose enough to cover 'any other infection or infestation in a person or aircraft arriving or departing'.

The WHO felt that the 1983 revision of IHR(1969) did not address the multiple and varied public health risks that the world faces today. In addition, some unwarranted and damaging travel and trade restrictions led to reluctance by some countries to promptly report disease outbreaks. The 2005 IHRs, which are firmly grounded in practical experience, broaden the scope of the 1969 regulations to cover existing, new and re-emerging diseases, including emergencies caused by non-infectious disease agents.

It is impossible in this text to describe the provisions of the IHRs and other local regulations in any great detail and medical directors are advised to keep current copies of all regulations for reference as and when required. Within the IHRs, health measures en route and at airports are described in Articles 23 to 49. These cover the actions required to prevent the departure of persons with any of the diseases subject to the regulations or under surveillance. They also cover the medical inspection of passengers and aircraft, and the circumstances under which a passenger may be isolated. Articles 50 to 75 describe the provisions to be undertaken if a patient carrying one of the subject diseases is discovered on board an arriving aircraft.

It is the captain's responsibility to complete the *Aircraft General Declaration* on landing. Included in this report is a *Health* section in which must be recorded details of any passenger who has shown signs of illness in flight, other than air sickness or accidental injury. The medical escort might be asked to assist with the completion of this report. Arrival formalities can be expedited if destination authorities can be notified in advance that ill patients are on board, especially when the captain is able to confirm that there is no risk of infection to others.

In general, requests for the transportation of patients with active and dangerous infectious diseases should be refused. In any case, airlines will likely refuse to carry such patients, and most air ambulance and charter organizations will require daunting and probably extremely expensive isolation facilities and procedures. Such a flight places innumerable people at risk and should only take place in exceptional circumstances. The Royal Air Force undertook just such a flight in 1985, when a patient with Lassa fever was transferred from Sierra Leone back to the UK for specialist treatment. The patient was transferred in a mobile patient isolation facility housed in a dedicated VC-10 aircraft which was stripped of all but the bare essentials for the flight. A full medical and nursing team practiced barrier techniques for the complete journey, and the aircraft was thoroughly disinfected before refitting. One has to consider the risks and benefits very carefully in patients such as these who often have an extremely poor prognosis.

Birth and death in flight

Most airlines will refuse to carry terminally ill patients. For those who feel the need to travel in their final days, or who wish to return home to die, the only answer is usually by private air ambulance. Few medical insurers are sympathetic to this expenditure, and some patients may charter their own aircraft. Nevertheless, death may occur unexpectedly during planned aeromedical missions, and may even happen to passengers not being carried as patients (British Airways reported 14 inflight deaths between April 1991 and March 1992; only two of these were patients known to the medical department before departure). The medicolegal problems again center around the question of jurisdiction. When a death occurs en route, five options present themselves to the aeromedical and flight crews (Table 19.2).

Table 19.2   Options when death occurs in flight

- Notify the nearest air traffic control service and land at the designated diversionary airfield.
- Record the exact navigational position at the time of death and return to the point of origin to notify the authorities.
- Record the exact navigational position at the time of death and continue on to the planned destination before notifying the authorities.
- Continue resuscitation attempts until able to divert to a 'friendly' country with the same or similar laws as those which are familiar to the medical and flight crew, and then notify the authorities.
- Continue resuscitation attempts until entering airspace of the planned destination, and then notify the authorities.

There are no clear rules or guidelines on how to manage death in flight and each case must be dealt with on its merits. A decision may be made based on which particular jurisdiction has interest in the death, and knowledge of the difficulties that may be encountered. It may be that some countries have laws with regard to the payment of death taxes, or over the distribution of the estate of the deceased. The medical escort must also consider the bereaved relatives. Not only will they have the major problem of arranging for the return of the body from overseas, but they may also become entangled in complex and expensive legislation.

Under such circumstances, there may be a case for continuing resuscitation attempts until the aircraft enters 'friendly airspace', be it at the planned destination or a more suitable diversion en route. Decision making in these situations may be complicated by the fact that the medical escort is not a qualified doctor. In many countries, only medically trained personnel may certify death. In this case the patient cannot be legally dead until certified by a doctor at the next available landing. All circumstances should be fully discussed with the captain of the aircraft who inevitably takes responsibility for such decisions. In the case of a doctor not wishing to certify death (or, more correctly, pronounce life extinct), until the aircraft is in friendly airspace, few would argue that brain death criteria are impossible to decide in the confines and restrictions of an aircraft, and patients can be kept 'alive' by minimal resuscitation attempts. Whatever decision is taken, it is incumbent on the medical escort to keep the captain, his cabin crew and, above all else, any accompanying relatives, fully informed of the actions to be taken, and the justification for these actions.

Births en route are less of a problem. Although most airlines will refuse carriage to any woman over 35 weeks pregnant, labor may be premature and some passengers in the late stages of pregnancy may travel unannounced and only be brought to the attention of the medical team by chance. Clearly, there are many problems associated with delivery on board an aircraft but, from a legal point of view, the only issue is of nationality and place of registration of birth of the newborn. This, once again, is a problem of jurisdiction.

Personal protection and accident insurance

In terms of self-protection during an emergency, in 1995 the GMC stated:

> 'You must not refuse or delay treatment because you believe that the patient's actions have contributed to their condition, or because you may be putting yourself at risk.'

However, since one of the basic rules of first aid is to ensure one's own safety, the GMC clarified the position in 1998:

> If a patient poses a risk to your health or safety you may take reasonable steps to protect yourself before investigating their condition or providing treatment.

The decision to act may have to be made instantly and the word 'reasonable' is not defined, so each doctor will have to decide at the time what they consider to be reasonable. However, as a general rule, if the doctor feels comfortable with his justification and the possible prospect of being asked to defend his actions (or inactions) at a professional conduct meeting, it is very probably defensible.

Nevertheless, patient transport, by whatever means, is not without its risks and health care professionals working in transfer and retrieval sytems are strongly advised to acquire appropriate insurance cover. This may be possible through professional organizations. Two such examples are the Association of Anaesthetists of Great Britain and Ireland (AAGBI) and the UK Intensive Care Society (ICS) which both provide worldwide insurance for members who escort patients in ambulances, helicopters, aircraft and boats, for both the escorted and staging (or returning) sectors. Accidents while driving personal cars to an emergency are also covered. The key features of the cover are detailed in Table 19.3.

Table 19.3   Details of AAGBI/UK ICS personal accident cover

- Up to £1 million GBP per member
- £5 million GBP limit per vehicle
- The cover is worldwide
- Protection for patient escort duties when undertaking usual occupation
- There is a scale of payouts for injuries that are not fatal

References

Chapman, P.J.C. (1993) 'Legal aspects of inflight emergencies', in Harding R.M. and F.J. Mills (eds) *Aviation Medicine*, (3rd Ed.), BMJ: London.
Faux, G.A. and M. M. MacPherson (1988) 'International Health Regulations', in: Ernsting, J. and King, P.F. (eds) *Aviation Medicine* (2nd Ed.), Butterworth: London.
General Medical Council (1995) *Confidentiality*, GMC: London.
General Medical Council (2001) *Good Medical Practice*, GMC: London.
General Medical Council (2005) *The Duties of a Doctor*, GMC: London.
Glendenning, J.A. (1998) 'A patient requests DNR and then arrests: agonizing decisions, haunting questions', *J Emerg Nurs*. 24(4):335-6.
Hopson, L.R. Hirsh, E., Delgado, J. et al. (2003) 'Guidelines for withholding or termination of resuscitation in prehospital traumatic cardiopulmonary arrest: joint position statement of the National Association of EMS Physicians and the American College of Surgeons Committee on Trauma', *J Am Coll Surg*. 196(1):106-12.
Hurwitz, B. (1995) 'Clinical guidelines and the law', *Brit Med J*. 311: 1517-8.
Macnab, A.J., Noble,R., Smart, P., Green, G. (1998) 'Narcotics and controlled drugs: a secure system for access by transport teams', *Air Med J*. 17(2):73-5.
McNeil, E.L. (1983) *Airborne Care of the Ill and Injured,* Springer-Verlag: New York.
Mitchell, M. (1993). Legal ramifications in air medical transport, in Rodenberg, H. and I. J. Blumen (eds) *Air Medical Physician's Handbook*, AMPA: Salt Lake City.
Mookini, R. K. (1990) 'Medical-legal aspects of aeromedical transport of emergency patients', *Legal Medicine*, 1-30.

Robinson, K. J., Murphy, D.M., Jacobs, L.M. (2003) 'Presumption of death by air medical transport teams', *Air Med J.* **22**(3):30-4.

Strong, C. and C.B. Thompson (2000) 'Documentation of decision-making during air transport', *Air Med J.* **19**(3):77-82.

Williams, A. (2001) 'Diversion: air medical liability issue?', *Air Med J.* **20**(6):11-2.

Williams, A.R. (2001) 'More than poor care can lead to legal liability', *Air Med J.* **20**(4):8-9.

Williams, A.R. (2001) 'Who pays when air medical personnel are injured?' *Air Med J.* **20**(3):6-7.

World Health Organization (1983) *International Health Regulations* (3rd Ed.), WHO: Geneva.

World Health Organization (2005) *International Health Regulations* http://www.who.int/csr/ihr/en.

Chapter 20

Planning the Successful International Repatriation

Travel insurance, medical assistance and repatriation

It takes about the same length of time to fly from Heathrow airport near London to JFK airport in New York as it does to drive from London to York. A century ago, the road journey to York would have taken two days. In that time, a traveler can now circumnavigate the globe, and almost every part of it is accessible. There is hardly a recess or corner that has not been exploited in some way by the travel and tourism industry. Even the remaining communist countries are now fair game for the dedicated tourist and for the business traveler seeking opportunities in new territories. Swathes have been cut through jungle, often in the name of eco-tourism, and tourists can now be found in deserts and on mountains alike. Even the Antarctic continent has a tourist trade!

Since international travel is such an unexceptional experience, and well within the pocket of most people (at least in the western world), a certain amount of illness among travelers is only to be expected. There is a normal incidence of illness in any population. Some, perhaps, should never have traveled in the first place, especially those with known chronic illness. Despite the traveling public's fears, very few fall ill as a result of exotic or tropical diseases.

In addition, for some reason, many travelers overseas seem to leave common sense at home. The normally careful American or European driver might habitually click into his seatbelt for even the shortest journey at home, but will think nothing of driving on unfamiliar badly-repaired roads without restraint, and at the mercy of local road users. Similarly, accidents often occur with motorcyclists declining to wear crash helmets, and after over-exuberance with alcohol (a major cause of swimming, diving and other accidents). Lastly, there are those injuries common to specific holiday adventure activities such as skiing, SCUBA diving and parasailing.

The repatriation of these unfortunate patients is usually a matter for travel insurers, since few individuals can afford the expense of their own return flights when complicated by the addition of inflight medical care. However, insurance companies rarely have the expertise (or, quite frankly, the interest) in medical matters. The actual work of repatriation is therefore usually subcontracted to a medical assistance organization.

Those taken ill or injured overseas will telephone their 'emergency number' (actually the medical assistance company) for any one of a number of reasons. Quite possibly, all that is required will be the payment of local bills, for instance, after a visit to a family doctor, a clinic, or for prescription items overseas. At the other end of the scale, a seriously ill or injured traveler may be in urgent need of treatment that cannot be offered locally. This patient requires full air ambulance facilities with an aeromedical escort or team, and monitoring and therapeutic facilities en route back to his home country.

Many cases fall somewhere in between, for instance, patients who have fallen ill or who have required a surgical operation, but have almost fully recovered, at least, enough for the flight home. In this group, some will still need an aeromedical escort. This may be a nurse or doctor, depending on the severity of the condition and the likelihood of inflight complications. A proportion will be fit enough to return without a medical escort, although some (especially the frail elderly) may require some other traveling companion and special arrangements at airports (for example, wheelchairs).

A medical assistance organization is the interface between the insurers and the patients. Doctors and nurses working for these organizations may find themselves working in the office ('on the desk') or actually flying as aeromedical personnel. Most combine both, with periods on assignment interspersed by days on the desk, acting as the medical adviser for new cases seeking assistance.

This type of employment is unusual for doctors, who find themselves with loyalties, not just to the patient, but also to the insurers. This rather tenuous relationship is often an uneasy one, and doctors are advised to keep the best interests of the patient in mind at all times, albeit tempered by the need to comply with the policies of the insurers.

To facilitate a successful repatriation, medical personnel must work closely with operations staff (who provide linguistic expertise and act as contacts with local agents, and so on) and travel experts (who find the most appropriate and available travel options, arrange ticketing, and obtain medical clearance from the airline, if needed).

Between the three groups of staff, a team approach helps the decision-making process, not least on the urgency of repatriation, the destination hospital or facility, the mode of transport (dedicated air ambulance, air taxi, charter or scheduled airliner, or military flight). This chapter identifies the roles and responsibilities of both the office medical staff and inflight repatriation personnel, and discusses the problems that may be encountered in the planning and execution of an assignment.

The medical assistance desk doctor

The role of the desk doctor is difficult, yet it carries a lot of responsibility. He must collate medical information received from overseas, the medical regulations of the major airlines, the guidelines and procedures established by national regulatory bodies and the organization for which he works. Furthermore, he may seek advice from the medical director, medical (hospital) specialists and other agencies. He must have a good working knowledge of the physical, physiological and psychological stresses of flight, and must confidently be able to assess and decide upon each patient's fitness to fly. Finally, he must coordinate arrangements for a safe, acceptable and comfortable repatriation. These duties are summarized in Table 20.1.

Table 20.1   The duties of the medical assistance desk doctor

- To obtain medical reports on patients who require assistance
- To complete repatriation request documentation
- To complete airline medical information forms (MEDIF)
- To liaise with accepting medical team and family practitioner
- To assist operations personnel on medical matters
- To assign and brief the inflight medical escort or team

Medical reports

Obviously it is essential to have good, clear clinical information about the subject patient. There are a number of ways of achieving this, and the most immediate is by telephone. Some referring doctors give excellent medical reports of their own volition, but it is a mistake to rely too heavily on information given solely by the overseas doctor. He does, however, have the distinct advantage of being on the spot, having seen and (hopefully) examined the patient before starting treatment. Unfortunately, it is often necessary to question medical decisions, especially those related to length of hospital stay. In some countries the treatment of tourists is a lucrative trade, and unnecessary treatments or admissions and delayed discharges are not uncommon. Remembering cultural differences and professional pride, it is best to avoid antagonizing the overseas doctors, since they supply the 'fitness to fly' certificates demanded by the airlines. If they refuse, the patient is grounded. The provision of these certificates is often a moot point, since most referring doctors have no expertise in transport medicine. In any case, the 'fitness to fly' certificate is only really meaningful at the time it was signed. Therefore, although an essential piece of bureaucracy for many airlines and aircraft operators, the certificate usually has no real clinical value.

Language is often a problem, and it is always worth asking the initial contact (sometimes the patient, but usually a relative, friend, or tour operator) if the local doctor speaks English or has access to an interpreter. Most medical assistance organizations employ linguists in the operations department, specifically for this purpose. Even in the most difficult of situations, there is usually a common language that can be found. It may mean, for example, asking questions through an English speaking French interpreter to a French speaking Romanian doctor, and so on.

It is essential to remember that medical reports are legal documents. As such, they must be written in legible, clear, accurate and concise language, and should be signed and dated. The name of the correspondent and the times of all telephone calls should also be documented, as should all intentions and actions which result from the report. All medical reports, whether they are received by fax, telegraph, electronic mail or post, must be seen and signed by a doctor before filing in the case notes. It is crucial that any questions arising from the report are referred back to the overseas doctor by the most suitable means as soon as possible.

If it becomes clear that the case is serious, details should be entered into a serious case file and brought to the attention of the medical director. A case may be considered serious for medical, logistical or financial reasons (Table 20.2).

Table 20.2   Patients considered to be 'serious'

Medical	• Any patient who is intubated and/or ventilated.
	• Any patient who would be admitted to an ICU, CCU or SCBU, with the exception of those with uncomplicated myocardial infarcts.
	• Patients who have suffered spinal cord transection.
	• Patients who have suffered subarachnoid hemorrhage.
	• Moribund patients.
Logistic	• When the medical facilities are substandard and the patient needs transportation to another country for adequate treatment.
Financial	• Any case where the medical fees are rising excessively.

The serious case file is a way of summarizing the important issues faced by the medical desk and is the easiest way for the medical director to keep in touch with significant events. Although HIV infection does not, in itself, merit inclusion in the file, many feel that these patients should be included. To avoid potential problems with medical confidentiality, some advocate that the case notes of known or suspected HIV infected patients should themselves remain unannotated, apart from a referral to the serious case file, where such details can be recorded in relative confidentiality.

Urgent repatriation

There are at least four criteria for moving patients urgently (Table 20.3), but all assume that there is an immediate requirement for a treatment or procedure that is not available locally, and which cannot be brought expeditiously to the patient. All other patients are transported at the earliest opportunity. Actual travel details will depend on many variables, including the availability of flights, aircraft seating, medical clearance from the airline, positioning flights for medical escorts, and so on.

Table 20.3   Key essentials for urgent and immediate repatriation

- The condition must be life or limb threatening.
- The patient must be fit enough to survive the physical, physiological and psychological stresses of flight
- A suitably qualified, skilled, equipped and insured doctor or team is available to escort the patient.
- Arrangements have been made for the patient to be collected by ambulance from the destination airport and transferred immediately to the receiving hospital.

Repatriation documentation

A correctly completed repatriation document is needed by the travel organizers before final transportation details can be arranged. The earlier that this form is received, the greater the chances of a successful and early repatriation. This can only be achieved by close cooperation and liaison between the operations, travel and medical departments. Great care is needed in the completion of these forms, especially when indicating the need for stretcher, wheelchair or upgraded seating. Patients with limb injuries, and others who need to stretch out, may require a row of three seats booked. This decision may well be influenced by the age and general condition of the patient, and by the estimated flight duration (Table 20.4). Stretchers take up nine seat positions (plus seats for the aeromedical team and accompanying relative). Availability at short notice can be a great problem.

Stretcher patients should never travel without a medical or nurse escort, but, because of the expense and the difficulty that may be encountered in trying to reserve such a large number of seats at short notice, advice about the absolute need for stretcher travel should be sought from the referring doctor. Only rarely is it acceptable that a relative or doctor from the referring team may act as an escort, and then only with the permission of the medical director. It should be remembered that these people will have no equipment with them and are unlikely to be trained in the aeromedical considerations of transportation of the ill and injured. They may not have the necessary language skills, and their ability to deal with an onboard emergency will be unknown.

There may be other decisions which must be made with respect to the flight arrangements, for instance it may be necessary to organize a 'turnaround'. This is useful if a rapid departure is necessary, when the patient is escorted by the referring team to meet the arriving aircraft at the airport of origin.

Table 20.4   Indications for upgrading of seats

To Business Class	• Within 3 weeks of major illness (for example, myocardial infarction [MI]).
	• Within 3 weeks of major operation (for example, laparotomy).
	• Within 3 weeks of multiple trauma (for example, motor vehicle accident [MVA]).
(More than one indication must apply)	• There is an extremely urgent need for repatriation (for example, in serious cases when local facilities are poor).
	• Duration of flight over 5 hours.
	• Duration of total journey over 9 hours.
	• Space needed for escort's attention.
	• Justified opinion of the overseas doctor.
To First Class	• If the patient would otherwise be on a stretcher and needs to lie down for much of the journey.
	• Patient must be continent and able to walk to the toilet.
	• There must be no requirement for screening or special privacy.

MEDIF forms

The medical information form (MEDIF) is the interface between the assistance company and the airline. Obtaining medical clearance can be expedited if the form is fully and correctly completed. In particular, it is important to ensure that the date of onset of illness is correct, and not confused with the dates of admission to hospital, or date of travel (a common error). It is vital to give as much clinical information as possible, taking great care to accurately describe the patient's current condition. If the patient is not fully recovered and stable, it is pointless to try and mislead the airline medical staff. They will inevitably discover the truth and any good reputation and trust between the organizations will be lost. The key is to put yourself in the airline doctor's position when reading back the MEDIF. Does it contain the answers to all the questions that you would ask? The airline doctors will inevitably carry the responsibility in the event of any inflight emergency causing a diversion or unnecessary delay. It is not surprising that they are cautious.

Considerable care must be taken over the decision to request oxygen. At least 50 per cent reserves must be added to the calculated requirements for the journey. Most airlines will not yet accept liquid oxygen (LOX), which is considered 'dangerous air cargo'. On the other hand, if oxygen is not necessary, it should not be requested. There is no doubt that medical clearance is easier to obtain without the complications of oxygen.

The information that is written on the MEDIF will inevitably be read by non-medical staff. Here lies an important issue. The profession teeters on the edge of the medical confidentiality guidelines. We assume that the patient would give permission to divulge clinical information to effect his safe and speedy repatriation. However, this is rarely explicit. Although every effort should be made to elicit consent before disclosure, this is rarely possible. Care must be taken to ensure that non-medical staff are aware of their responsibilities (just as clerical staff in a hospital or clinic).

Information is produced by all major airlines, listing their regulations with regards to medical clearance for flight. These rules are advisory, not absolute, but any deviations must be discussed with the medical personnel of the airline concerned.

Assistance with repatriation arrangements

When planning the repatriation, early consideration must be given to the need for special items of equipment, such as monitoring devices, vacuum mattress, suction apparatus, oxygen, ventilator, and so on. The office medical and nursing staff are also tasked with finding a suitable and available aeromedical team or escort who are able to accept the assignment. When the transportation arrangements are finalized, the escort or team must be informed and updated of any changes, and fully briefed about the mission when they arrive to collect the equipment. It may also be necessary to brief the ambulance company tasked with collecting the patient from the destination airport, in order to give them the opportunity to send the most appropriate crew and any extra equipment that they think may be necessary.

If the repatriated patient is to be admitted to a hospital, the desk doctor must contact the nearest suitable hospital to the patient's home address, and ensure that he can be accepted. He must also pass relevant clinical information to the admitting doctor. In addition, it is advisable to inform the patient's family doctor of the repatriation date, and request a home visit for those returning directly home.

Assistance to operations personnel

Operations personnel may ask the opinion of office medical personnel on the suitability of certain travel arrangements. These might seem totally inappropriate with middle of the night departures, long road journeys, or flights of many sectors, but each case must be assessed on its own merits. It is not simply a case of fitness to travel; it may be that the patient needs to move quickly in order to receive more appropriate care, or that the next available direct flight may be many days later, for instance. In some cases it may be preferable to move a patient to the nearest suitable medical facility overseas, rather than undergo a multi-sector flight home which is complicated by stopovers and long delays.

When to refer to the medical director

The medical director should be trained in aviation medicine and will be able to advise on problems specifically related to the flight environment. He must also be able to advise on specialist medical problems, although often after referral to an external expert specialist. In addition to these strictly medical areas, some operational decisions are usually referred to the medical director for authorization.

Air ambulance flights: Air ambulances are defined as dedicated aircraft used only for the transport of serious cases. They inevitably involve the transfer of very ill patients between hospitals, usually between intensive care units. They are, in effect, flying intensive care units, staffed by a mixed nurse/doctor (usually an anesthesiologist) team.

Air taxi flights: An air taxi may be defined as a light aircraft or business jet used for the non-urgent transfer of patients when, for operational or logistic reasons, such means of transport is considered more appropriate than a scheduled flight.

Whenever an air taxi or air ambulance is arranged, it may be possible to fill empty aircraft seats or stretcher space with other patients who may be located nearby. There is, of course, no necessity for these patients, themselves, to be serious cases, but the inclusion of any 'extra' patients must not in any way detract from the care given to the primary patient. The indications for both modes of transport are given in Table 20.5.

Table 20.5   Indications for air ambulances and air taxis

Air ambulance	• If the patient requires ventilation or invasive monitoring.
	• If the patient is suffering from a condition which may be a danger, disruptive or offensive to other passengers (that is, he has been refused carriage by an airline).
	• Any other reason for failure of medical clearance by the airline (for example, oxygen requirements).
	• When there is an extremely urgent need for repatriation (for example, in serious cases when local facilities are poor).
Air taxis	• If a scheduled or charter flight is not available (for example, because of infrequent services).
	• When scheduled aircraft facilities are inadequate (for example, no stretcher capability).
	• When there is no major airport in the vicinity, since air taxi aircraft can operate into/out of very small airfields that larger scheduled aircraft could not use.
	• Occasionally it is cheaper and easier to use an air taxi than to organize road transportation and/or a sea crossing.

Upgraded seating It is worth remembering that the standard and quality of airline seats, and other factors such as seat pitch (leg room), vary considerably between aircraft and between airlines. In some cases economy seats may vary little from business class seats on the same airline, or may actually be better than business class seats on an alternative carrier. A further concern is the use of 'double decker' aircraft (such as the new Airbus 380, Boeing 747, and military Lockheed C5 Galaxy). Patients should always be accommodated on the lower deck.

General points

There may be specific times of day when doctors in some countries can be contacted in their clinics. If they are missed, contact may be impossible until the next day, and 24 hours can be unnecessarily wasted.

By the nature of the work, close daily contact will be made with distressed patients and relatives who may feel stranded and helpless overseas. These people are often frightened, anxious and depressed, and may be frustrated by what they perceive to be inactivity on the part of insurers and medical assistance organizations. They are often quick to become angry and may even resort to complaint or litigation. Things said by aeromedical personnel (and some which are not) will be remembered and may be repeated at a later date. It is important to be cautious and careful in what is said, but to be accurate and polite at all times. It is most unwise to enter into conjecture about past treatment or prognosis, or to offer a service which you are unable or not authorized to provide.

Dealing with difficult clients

Each case should be treated on its merits and with the compassion that it deserves, but most people are quite reasonable when they are given clear, concise and calm explanations about policies with regard to repatriation. It is, perhaps, best to explain that the organization is working in the best interests of the patient and should be regarded as an interface between the patient and insurers. Under these circumstances, part of the doctor's role is to advise the patient, or his representative, what the insurers will pay for. One of the aims is to protect them against unclaimable expenses. An example is the relative who demands immediate repatriation in a dedicated air ambulance for a patient who is not seriously ill. An illustration of the costs of an air ambulance will often suffice, especially if it is made clear that these costs would not be borne by the insurer.

Release of confidential medical information

Whenever a medical condition or description of signs and symptoms is associated with a name (or any descriptor which can be easily linked with an individual), there is potential for a breach of confidentiality. Confidentiality is an implied condition of the contract between patient and doctor, and unauthorized disclosure gives grounds for civil proceedings in many countries. Occasionally, repatriation organizations may have to release information in order to act in the best interests of the patient (for instance, to ascertain the level of insurance cover) and this, although verging on the unprofessional, should be seen as essential for the best management or transportation of the patient. Every endeavor should be made to ensure that patients are made aware that information may be disclosed, so that any objections can be raised at an early stage. Finally – a word of warning. Aeromedical cases are often newsworthy, and journalists have been known to impersonate medical and nursing personnel in an effort to find a story. It is foolhardy to accept the word of a telephone caller who requests medical information. The caller must always be referred to the medical director so that identity can be verified before deciding on the release of information.

Inflight aeromedical escorts

The role of the inflight team is not limited to the medical and nursing care of patients while airborne. During international assignments (much more so than for flights within national borders and for primary missions), there are many stages that have to be considered (Table 20.6).

Preflight

The successful assignment starts with good communication and planning. Teamwork between the office staff and inflight personnel is crucial to the success of the transfer, and no mission should start until the inflight escort or team is fully briefed on both the clinical and logistic aspects of the transfer. Preflight briefing should therefore include, not only the patient's clinical details and the latest medical report, but also the travel details, such as the airports of departure and arrival (and these may differ for the outbound and inbound sectors of the assignment), check-in and departure times, airline and flight details, type of aircraft, requirements for passports, visas and other special documents, information on the ground ambulance connections at either end of the transfer and, clearly, details of the destination hospital and receiving team.

If the transfer is to be undertaken in a dedicated air ambulance, it is likely that a regional airport will be used, at least for the outbound departure. When a conventional passenger aircraft is used, tickets must be collected usually direct from the airport. Sufficient time must therefore be allowed for travel to the airport and for parking and check-in formalities. An assignment is put at risk if the time taken for this stage is underestimated.

Table 20.6   Logistic stages in repatriation assignments

• Preflight	• Medical briefing
	• Visas, passports and medical documentation
	• Suitable equipment, checked and prepared
	• Journey to airport, tickets, check-in formalities
	• Equipment to be kept as hand baggage
• Outbound	• Telephone base office
	• Adequate rest
• Patient collection	• Hand-over, notes, reports, radiographs
	• Translations
	• Patient's baggage and personal documentation
	• Arrangements for accompanying relatives
	• Transfer to ambulance
	• Compatibility of equipment
• Airport	• Loading, lifting
	• Stretchers, wheelchairs, and seats in aircraft
	• Confined space
	• All equipment in cabin
• En route	• Airborne sectors and sector times
	• Time zone changes
	• Stopovers and facilities
	• Potential for diversions
	• Time and temperature at destination
	• Emergency funds (suitable currencies)
• Arrival	• Airport arrival formalities
	• Transfer to ambulance
	• Length of road journey
	• Total out-of-hospital time
• Destination hospital or home	• Hand-over to receiving medical team or family practitioner

At this point, it is worth considering the wide variety of assignments that may be undertaken. To illustrate the extremes, a flight nurse might utilize a simple light aircraft (air taxi) for a flight across the English channel to collect and immediately return with a reasonably fit and ambulant patient. On the other hand, an air ambulance assignment might require a full inflight team who, for instance, might fly from Houston to collect a critically injured patient from an intensive care unit in Cairo and return him to a similar facility in Chicago. In transfers (as opposed to retrievals) the outbound sector is the medical team's staging flight, and the inbound sector is the flight during which the patient is carried. However, the principles remain the same, whether the patient is being 'delivered' (outbound) or 'retrieved' (inbound). The length of the flight will determine if the patient is collected immediately or whether the escort or team need to rest and transfer the patient the next day. There may be other logistic considerations, such as the time of arrival at the destination (some airports close early in the evening, others may stay open specially for an aeromedical flight), and the receiving hospital (it is usually unacceptable to arrive late at night or in the early hours of the morning).

When satisfied that logistic arrangements are the best that can be made (and there must often be a compromise when so many agencies are involved), the medical escort must ensure that all necessary equipment is carried, and that it is thoroughly checked and prepared prior to leaving the base office. This includes portable oxygen supplies, medications, fluids, special dietary requirements, and other consumables that will be needed for the entire transfer. A good principle is to carry at least 50 per cent reserves to cater for possible delays or diversions.

Another sensible precaution is to telephone back to the base office before embarkation, in case of any last-minute information that may influence the assignment (although, of course, the desk staff will have the travel details and should be able to contact inflight personnel through the airline or airport concerned). Most medical staff now carry triple or quad band mobile telephones with worldwide coverage.

Outbound

Depending on the length of the outbound leg and the time of arrival, the inflight team may wish to travel directly to see the patient, even if the return flight is not until the following day. This is advisable to ensure that all necessary preparations have been made by the referring hospital, and that there is no bar to departure. This is the time to sort out any problems, not when the ambulance is waiting to take the patient to the airport.

Patient collection

The adequacy of the hand-over from the referring team can be extremely variable. It may be very thorough with medical reports already translated and typed, and copies of the investigations and radiographs included. On the other hand, there may be no investigations, a referral letter handwritten in the local language, and only the briefest of verbal hand-overs, mediated through an interpreter. In either case, it is recommended that the medical escort fully examines the patient. Often, the referring team will have little knowledge of the limitations and dangers of the flight environment, and it will remain the escort's duty to ensure that the patient is, indeed, fit to travel. Even when relative contraindications exist, if they are identified prior to departure, steps can be taken to prevent or ameliorate problems occurring later. As an example, the multiply injured victim of a road accident might require a blood transfusion to elevate the hemoglobin above 7 g/dl, the placement of a nasogastric tube to decompress the stomach, chest radiography to exclude pneumothorax, and for freshly applied orthopedic casts to be bivalved. Finally, if required by the air carrier, a certificate of fitness to fly must be completed and included in the medical notes.

As the time for departure approaches, patients must be adequately prepared and 'packaged' for movement between hospital bed and both ground and air vehicles. This entails ensuring that all lines, tubes, and other medical paraphernalia are secure, will not become displaced, and are correctly working, before departure. At this stage, the patient will be transferred to the inflight monitoring devices and equipment, although advantage should be taken of any offer from the referring team or ambulance, to supply oxygen or other consumables for the journey to the airport. Similarly, it is always advantageous when the referring hospital can supply any essential medications, although proper planning should ensure that the inflight team carry all essential items overseas. Reliance should not be placed on the referring team.

Stretchers come in a variety of forms and are supplied by most of the major airlines. There is continuing debate about whether the patient should lie with the head or foot towards the front of the aircraft and, although there is no good evidence for any physiological advantage of one over the other, most agree that the 'head

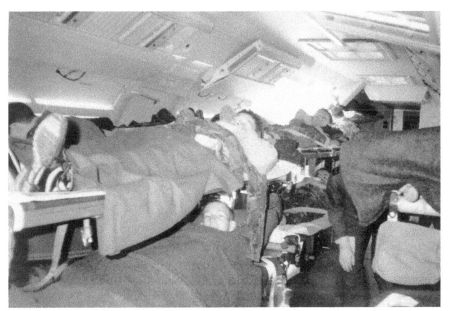

Figure 20.1 Stretchers stacked on special mountings

first' position is safer from a crash restraint point of view. Most stretchers are fixed to existing seats which are folded down, but some aircraft can be fitted with special frames secured to conventional seat mountings on the cabin floor. These frames can accommodate up to three stretchers stacked from floor to ceiling (Figure 20.1). Medical teams should be aware that stretcher patients are usually sited at the rear of the cabin. Although most international flights are non-smoking, and cabin conditioning in modern aircraft is very efficient, the build-up of stale air around the stretcher can be problematic. On those flights that still allow smoking, medical personnel may have to ask neighboring passengers for their indulgence. Curtains or screens are often provided, but are usually badly designed, allowing little privacy or quiet to the patient, and causing difficulty in access to equipment and maneuvering for the team. Backrests are only available on the most modern stretchers, otherwise extra pillows may be required for those who need, or wish, to sit up.

In addition to strictly medical matters, the patient (and any accompanying relative) must have baggage (up to any weight limitation set by the airline or imposed by the center of gravity limitations of a smaller aircraft), passports, visas and any other essential documents easily at hand. If baggage is to be placed in the aircraft hold,

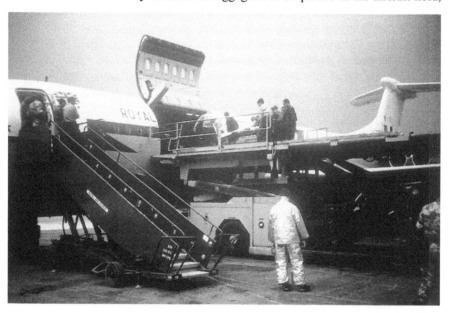

Figure 20.2 Embarkation may best be achieved by means of an elevator

documents, medications and any other items needed in flight must be kept separate and taken as hand baggage. Medical flight crew may need to remind patients and relatives of the types of items that are banned in hand luggage.

A small selection of local currency may also be necessary to pay for telephone calls, reading materials, snacks and so on, especially if delays are encountered. Stopovers in endemic areas may require special immunization or prophylaxis arrangements and, finally, the patient must be dressed or wrapped for the coldest environment, whether it be at the point of origin, destination, or in the aircraft (especially so in some tactical military types where cabin heating is a luxury!).

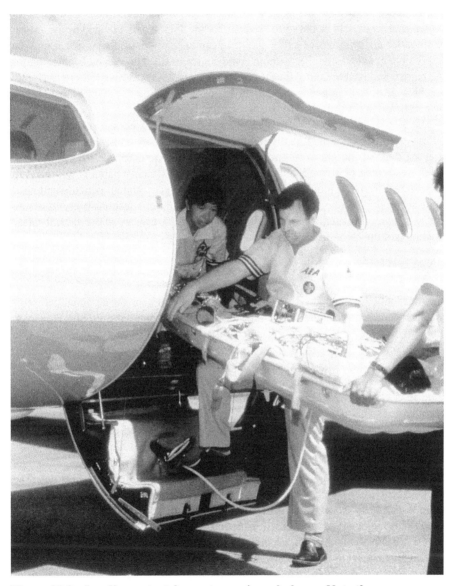

Figure 20.3   Loading a stretcher onto an air ambulance. Note the difficulty with access and lifting

Airport

Although most international airports now load passengers via enclosed walkways or piers, many smaller airfields still rely on external stairs. Loading may therefore need some careful thought. An otherwise ambulant patient may not be able to climb stairs, and embarkation may best be achieved by means of an elevator (Figure 20.2). This will certainly be required for loading stretchers and wheelchairs which, in the case of passenger aircraft, will be designed specially for the aircraft and provided by the airline.

Smaller air ambulances suffer the disadvantages of small doors, and it may be impossible to load a stretcher without some degree of tilt. This can be frightening for the patient and backbreaking for the loaders (Figure 20.3). Although there is usually no shortage of willing hands to help, the lifting and loading of patients must always be controlled and supervised by the aeromedical escort.

As a rule, patients are usually enplaned before able bodied passengers and, unless disembarkation is urgently required, will be offloaded last. Prior to take-off, it is the duty of inflight personnel to ensure that all equipment is readily at hand, safely restrained or stowed, and working correctly. Stretcher patients will need to be screened from the inquisitive eyes of other passengers, and all patients will need to be securely restrained. It is also the aeromedical escort's responsibility to ensure that accompanying relatives (and patients, when able) are aware of the aircraft safety briefing and the location of emergency exits.

En route

Having planned and prepared meticulously for the assignment, the aeromedical escort may feel confident enough to relax once the patient is on board the aircraft. However, although much of the hard work has been done, there is still every possibility of an inflight incident, and attention must not waiver from the supervision of the patient. Without doubt, the main concerns during a long transfer are most likely to be of a nursing nature. Good care of the patient must not stop once the aircraft doors are shut. Every effort must be made to continue (or improve on) care that has already been started. This may take more planning. For instance, equipment and supplies that will be required throughout the journey must be placed close at hand in the cabin, and simple needs such as fresh water and waste disposal must be nearby.

Medical emergencies that occur en route may fall into two categories, those that are caused or exacerbated by the flight environment and those that are not. The management of these incidents may include descending the aircraft to a lower altitude or, in an extreme, diverting to a nearby airfield. Aeromedical personnel should not make these decisions in isolation. Clearly, the flight crew will want to do the very best for the patient, but they will be reluctant to divert (especially a scheduled airliner) unless it is absolutely essential. In coming to the decision, one must consider the options available – to carry on, return to the departure airport, or divert to the nearest or most appropriate destination. There is no single and universal answer. The inflight escort must ask himself where the patient's needs can best be met. If the aircraft's medical team is more skilled and better equipped than the nearest hospital, then clearly there is no advantage to a diversion. When flying over oceans or vast stretches of wilderness, the luxury of a diversion may not even be an option, and it may be more appropriate to turn back, rather than to fly on. There may be other considerations, such as inhospitable regimes or outright warfare in the nearest country, or there may be legal or political implications if the aircraft is diverted. On these matters, the aircraft captain must be the best judge, but although the best interests of the patient should be paramount to the medical crew at all times, the captain of the aircraft also has to consider the safety and welfare of all the other passengers on board.

It is impossible to closely supervise a patient when the aeromedical escort is seated some distance away. Late flight bookings may dictate unfavorable seating positions and, when airlines are unable to rearrange seating, or are uncooperative, efforts must be made to ensure co-location, even if it means asking neighboring passengers to exchange seats. If separate seating is absolutely inevitable (which is most unlikely), then the purser or cabin flight director must be informed that the escort is traveling with the patient and should be called if needed. In any case, there can be no excuse for failing to visit the patient frequently during the flight. It is always good practice for aeromedical personnel to inform cabin crew of their presence onboard, and that their services may be called upon, if required for any inflight emergency. This will foster harmonious links with the airline staff, and may help with additional favors, free upgrades, and so on.

At all costs and wherever seated, aeromedical personnel must avoid falling asleep. The patient and relatives consider that the escort is on duty, and they are absolutely correct. If personnel are unfit for the mission, or the schedule is likely to be too tiring, the assignment must be declined. During long haul missions, when the patient needs constant attention or supervision, a minimum team of two will always be required. This allows each to rest at alternate times. Some organizations have issued guidelines about duty times and rest periods (see Chapter 6). A general rule of thumb is illustrated in Table 20.7.

Arrival

When safely arrived at the destination airfield, patients will appreciate being taken smoothly through the arrival formalities. For the severely ill, disembarkation directly on to an ambulance is the usual rule.

Base office personnel will notify the receiving team of the patient's impending arrival, and a bed will have been booked. This speeds the admission procedure and allows the transfer escort to effect a timely hand-over. As well as the medical notes and investigations collected from the referring hospital, a transfer document should be completed, annotating the travel details and information on any treatments or untoward incidents that occurred in flight. When the receiving team members are happy to accept the patient, the handover is complete, and the inflight escort may return to the base office, being sure to take all items of equipment and unused consumables. Medical waste and used sharps should be correctly disposed of at the receiving hospital. On return to the base office, a copy of the transfer document should be placed on file and all equipment returned and replenishment arranged, ready for the next assignment.

Table 20.7   Suggested medical escort flight time limitations

Definitions	• Duty time	• Period between arrival at base office for briefing and collection of equipment, and arrival at destination hotel for first rest (that is, after seeing patient, if applicable).
	• Minimum rest time	• Minimum time between arrival and departure from the patient's location. This period should not include time spent traveling to or attending the patient, nor the transfer of the patient to the airport.
Optimum minimum rest time		• 1.5 x the previous *duty time* plus one hour for every time zone crossed.
Flexibility		• In the interests of economy, if the next available flight departs more than 12 hours after the end of the minimum rest time, or involves an extra overnight stop, the minimum rest time can be reduced at the discretion of the medical director and with the escort's agreement.

References

Air Medical Physician Association (2003) 'Medical condition list and appropriate use of air medical transport', *Air Med J.* **22**(3):14-9.

Dewhurst, A.T., Farrar, D., Walker, C., Mason, P., Beven, P. and J. C. Goldstone (2001) 'Medical repatriation via fixed-wing air ambulance: a review of patient characteristics and adverse events', *Anaesthesia.* **56**(9):882-7.

Fairhurst, R.J. (1992) 'Health insurance for international travel', in: Dawood R. (ed.) *Travellers' Health* (3rd Ed.), Oxford University Press: Oxford.

Macnab, A.J., Noble, R., Smart, P. and G. Green (1998) 'Narcotics and controlled drugs: a secure system for access by transport teams', *Air Med J.* **17**(2):73-5.

Martin, T.E. (1993) 'Transportation of Patients by Air', in Harding and Mills, *Aviation Medicine* (3rd Ed). BMJ: London.

Neri, M. and R. De Jongh (2004) 'Medical and trauma evacuations', *Clinics in Occupational & Environmental Medicine.* 4(1):85-110.

Parsons, C.J. and W.P. Bobechko (1982) 'Aeromedical transport: its hidden problems', *Can Med Assoc J.* 126(3):237-43.

Preston, F.S. (2003) 'Commercial aviation and health – general aspects', in Ernsting J., Nicholson, A.N., and D.J. Rainford (eds) *Aviation Medicine* (3rd Ed.), Arnold: London.

Wilde, H., Roselieb, M., Hanvesakul, R., Phaosavasdi, S. and C. Pruksapong, (2003) 'Expatriate clinics and medical evacuation companies are a growth industry worldwide', *J Travel Med.* 10(6):315-7.

Chapter 21

Primary Transfers: The Casualty Evacuation Conflict

Of the many controversial issues surrounding the prehospital management of the victims of trauma, the decision to evacuate or stabilize on site is probably the one most often criticized. In a mass casualty situation this decision takes on a much greater significance. In brief, a multi-casualty incident can be defined as an incident where more than one patient requires transportation and treatment, but where the local facilities are able to cope. On the other hand, a mass casualty situation occurs when the local emergency services are initially overwhelmed and are only later able to respond with reinforcements. A disaster, however, is a poorly defined term which implies that the emergency services are totally overwhelmed or are themselves impaired by the incident. It can be qualified by information on the circumstances surrounding the incident, such as the cause, location, environmental conditions and so on.

Since the very first ambulance units were formed (originally by the military), speedy evacuation from the scene of wounding has been a major objective in the management of the injured. During the Vietnam War, this 'scoop and run' concept may have been partly responsible for the saving of many lives, thanks mainly to the rapid transportation system afforded by helicopters, and the proximity of excellently equipped, multi-speciality medical facilities. Had these patients to face the 'treatment vacuum' of a long and arduous journey, many of those who survived initial wounding might have perished during what has been called the 'golden hour'.

Since the 1960s there has been growing concern over the management of civilian victims of trauma, not least in the standard of prehospital care which they receive. Following the lead taken by the USA, Advanced Trauma Life Support (ATLS) training was introduced into the UK in 1988 and was rolled out worldwide in the subsequent decade. Although it is a hospital-based training package it provides an excellent gold standard by which to measure all levels of trauma management. The newer Prehospital Trauma Life Support (PHTLS) course was designed specifically for those who work at the coalface of emergency medicine, and this has been followed by the Prehospital Paediatric Life Support (PHPLS) course in the UK.

Most ambulance authorities now aim to provide all frontline emergency vehicles with equipment and personnel able to provide basic trauma life support. Paramedic training has been introduced in many western countries and is constantly under review. In addition, the training of doctors in immediate medical care skills is increasing in popularity, thanks largely to the British Association of Immediate Care

Schemes (BASICS) and the establishment of the Faculty of Immediate Care at the Royal College of Surgeons in Edinburgh, as well as similar programs in Europe, North America and Australasia.

Globally, there is an increasing awareness of the need to correctly treat the seriously injured before evacuation to hospital and we are gradually acquiring the skills, expertise, equipment and personnel to do so. There is little doubt that the best treatment occurs in countries with abundant well equipped hospitals, good road communications, reasonable coverage by emergency vehicles, and a network of EMS helicopters which can cater for large urban expanses (where there is a high density of trauma) and for large rural gaps (where there is a low density of ambulance cover). How, then do we decide whether to 'scoop and run' or to 'stay and play' with the trauma casualty? Clearly, there is no single answer for all situations, and a few examples will highlight the difficulties:

1. In some geographic locations and under some circumstances, the environment and availability of assets dictate the answer. For instance, when search and rescue helicopters are utilized to retrieve casualties from mountains, moors or the sea. In most cases the survivor is rescued from a hostile environment and, although limited medical care may be possible onboard the helicopter, little or nothing can be done at the scene.

2. At the roadside, in the single casualty situation, if a road ambulance is on scene within a few minutes and the nearest emergency room is nearby, although much could be done for the patient, with appropriate facilities so close, speedy evacuation is warranted and only the essentials should be attempted.

3. If entrapment delays evacuation, one must ask how serious are the injuries, and will the patient survive the extrication process without the provision of advanced resuscitation skills? Resuscitation and stabilization on scene may be essential in these cases, but it should not unnecessarily delay extraction. The caveat is, of course, that the extrication process, itself, must not prevent urgent medical actions.

4. In a multicasualty situation, other ambulances will be required and the surrounding roads may be congested as a result of the accident. The nearest hospital may not have the required specialist facilities, such as burns, neurosurgery and cardiothoracic surgery. The questions then to ask are: who needs to be evacuated immediately, and to where? Who can be retained, and why? Care must be taken to avoid a bottleneck at the nearest emergency room, thereby delaying definitive care for those in most need.

Who should provide immediate medical care? Ambulance technicians are familiar with roadside scenarios and, although trained and equipped paramedics quite clearly influence the survival and outcome of many casualties, they are still limited by the extent of their skills. At the other end of the scale, most hospital doctors, without proper training in prehospital management, work best in a familiar environment, with familiar equipment, and with the teamwork and support services that are normally provided in a hospital.

Immediate care trained doctors, whether community or hospital-based, are likely to be able to cope with most incidents, even more so if they have anesthetic and surgical skills. Many family practitioners are now vastly experienced in the roadside management of serious injuries. They work closely alongside their paramedic colleagues, supporting, supplementing and supervising their medical capabilities in complicated and multiple trauma situations. Some hospitals are now able to provide mobile medical teams (previously known as 'accident flying squads') for complicated incidents. In general, these teams will have been trained and equipped for the prehospital environment and will have suitable transport and communications to act independently, yet under the control of the medical incident officer at the scene.

When evacuation of many casualties is needed, decisions must also be made about the most suitable mode or methods of transport. Perhaps by using road ambulances, buses or trucks, by rail or underground, by sea or by air. However, the old adage that 'evacuation is important but resuscitation is a priority' is still true. Every medical student knows that shocked patients travel poorly. In fact, any patient who has an unstable airway, breathing or circulation undertakes a perilous journey when he is scooped away from the scene of injury. Although speed is important in transferring critically injured patients from the incident to hospital, it is secondary to safety and ongoing management of life threatening conditions. When faced with a delay in evacuation or a journey lasting more than a few minutes, each patient should preferably be stabilized and 'packaged' appropriately for a safe transfer. Monitoring and continual reappraisal during transportation is essential.

It is now common to see military and civilian helicopters at the sites of major accidents and disasters. At incidents on or near airports, it should be remembered that fixed wing aircraft can be used to transfer patients over long distances, although this mode of transfer is usually utilized for secondary or tertiary referrals, and for repatriation from overseas after life-saving treatment has been completed.

Often a mixture of ground and air ambulances is required, and it should be remembered that helicopters can be used to bring skills and equipment to the accident scene in addition to taking patients away from it. For small contained incidents, though, the helicopter can usefully be utilized as a mobile intensive care unit, thereby extending the therapeutic arm of the hospital into the community.

So, having started with a grand aim – to resolve the casualty evacuation conflict – the situation is perhaps now more confused by the illustration of the many pitfalls that may be encountered. Ideally, the aim is to provide the best possible care for those patients with greatest need. However, to ensure the maximum benefit to the largest number, triage must be used, and it must be performed by the most experienced resuscitation trained person on site (not always a doctor). Triage will not only decide the priorities of treatment, but also the priority for evacuation, since the patient with an unresolved airway problem (A) is likely to die before the patient with a breathing problem (B) who, in turn, is likely to die before the patient with a circulatory problem (C), and so on. Triage is essentially a dynamic process. Casualties must be continually reassessed and priorities must be changed in the light of clinical deterioration or improvement.

And so to the decision-making process. The essential point is that there is no single, simple, universal answer. Decisions must be made by the person in control at the scene. If that person is not aware of the extent of the incident (and that may not be easy in the early minutes or hours of a significant catastrophe), or if he is not in communication with those at the workface, any decisions made will be based on an inappropriate model of events. There is no authoritative advice, but the aim must always be to treat those who are salvageable, and in most urgent need, first. Delay in definitive care will cost lives. If nearby hospitals are blocked by an early wave of minor injuries and these hospitals are unaware of the extent of the backlog still to come, those in most need will die waiting for attention.

Table 21.1 lists the information which is therefore essential before making decisions on which casualties should be held, which should be stabilized, which should be evacuated first, and of course, by which means. Although there are no easy answers, it is essential, at least, to be aware of the potential problems. If all else fails, ask yourself 'where is the potential medical bottleneck going to be and what can I do to prevent it?'.

Table 21.1   Considerations in casualty evacuation

- Number of casualties.
- Numbers in each triage group.
- Will there be delays in extrication?
- Are further casualties expected?
- Quality and quantity of medical assets on site.
- Quality and quantity of medical personnel on site.
- Access to incident site and transport available.
- Distance and time to nearest medical facilities.
- Appropriateness of local hospitals (for example, neurosurgery, burns).
- Capabilities of local hospitals (for example, beds, operating rooms).
- Capabilities of nearest specialist hospitals.
- Ability to hold and treat casualties on site.
- Possibility of on-site medical reinforcement/supplies.
- Condition of roads and communications.
- Availability of helicopter landing sites.
- Flight times to medical facilities.
- Local weather and environmental conditions.

References

Berns, K.S., Caniglia, J.J., Hankins, D.G. and S.P. Zietlow (2003) 'Use of the autolaunch method of dispatching a helicopter', *Air Med J.* **22**(3):35-41.

Cameron, P.A., Flett, K., Kaan, E., Atkin, C. and L. Dziukas (1993) 'Helicopter retrieval of primary trauma patients by a paramedic helicopter service', *Aust N Z J Surg.* **63**(10):790-7.

Falcone, R.E., Herron, H., Werman, H. and M. Bonta (1998) 'Air medical transport of the injured patient: scene versus referring hospital', *Air Med J.* 17(4):161-5.

Garner, A., Rashford, S., Lee, A. and R. Bartolacci (1999) 'Addition of physicians to paramedic helicopter services decreases blunt trauma mortality', *Aust N Z J Surg.* 69(10):697-701.

Hotvedt, R., Kristiansen, I.S., Forde, O.H., Thoner, J. et al. (1996) 'Which groups of patients benefit from helicopter evacuation?' *Lancet.* 347(9012):1362-6.

Law, D.K., Law, J.K., Brennan, R. and H.C. Cleveland (1982) 'Trauma operating room in conjunction with an air ambulance system: indications, interventions, and outcomes', *J Trauma.* 22(9):759-65.

Martin, T.E. (1993) 'Resolving the casualty evacuation conflict', *Injury*, 24(8)514-6.

McCann, J.P., Burnett, J.R. and F.M. Holmstrom (1970) 'Potentials of the Aeromedical Evacuation System in the overall treatment process for the seriously ill patient', *Aerosp Med.* 41(3):323-8.

Royal College of Surgeons of England (1988) 'The management of patients with major injuries', RCS: London.

Skogvoll, E., Rygnestad, T. (1997) 'Helicopter emergency medical service', *Lancet.* 348(9026):543-4.

Thomson, D. P. and S.H. Thomas (2003) 'Guidelines for air medical dispatch', *Prehospital Emergency Care.* 7(2):265-71.

Tomazin, I. and T. Kovacs (2003) 'Medical considerations in the use of helicopters in mountain rescue', *High Alt Med Biol.* 4(4):479-83.

Travis, D.T. and M. Lozano (2004) 'No-fly zones: Hillsborough County defines urban grids where ground transport of trauma patients makes the most sense', *J Emerg Med Serv.* 29(5):116-8.

Trunkey, D. D. (1983) 'Trauma', *Scientific American,* Vol 249, pp. 20-27.

Trunkey, D. D. (1985), 'Towards optimal trauma care', *Arch Emerg Med,* Vol 2, pp. 181-195.

Index

Milton Keynes UK
Ingram Content Group UK Ltd.
UKHW031144141024
449569UK00024B/1084